Frontiers in Myocardia

(*Volume 2*)

(Clinical Nuclear Cardiology: Practical Applications and Future Directions)

Edited by

Shinro Matsuo
Department of Nuclear Medicine, Kanazawa University, Dunkerque, Graduate School of Advanced Preventive Medical Sciences, Kanazawa, Japan

Frontiers in Myocardia

Volume # 2

Clinical Nuclear Cardiology: Practical Applications and Future Directions

Editor: Shinro Matsuo

ISSN (Online): 2451-8352

ISSN (Print): 2451-8344

ISBN (Online): 978-1-68108-760-3

ISBN (Print): 978-1-68108-761-0

Bentham Science Publishers Ltd.
Executive Suite Y - 2
PO Box 7917, Saif Zone
Sharjah, U.A.E.
Email: subscriptions@benthamscience.org

BENTHAM
SCIENCE

CONTENTS

FOREWORD i

PREFACE ii

LIST OF CONTRIBUTORS iii

CHAPTER 1 DIAGNOSIS OF CORONARY ARTERY DISEASE WITH MYOCARDIAL PERFUSION IMAGING 1

Shinro Matsuo

INTRODUCTION 1

Diagnosing Ischemia or Infarction 2

Cardiac Function 2

SPECT/CT 2

Risk Stratification 2

Normal Myocardial Perfusion Imaging 3

Evaluation of Ischemia 4

IQ-SPECT (SMARTZOOM Collimator) 5

Quantitative Myocardial Flow Measurement with CZT Camera 7

Mitochondrial Function Imaging 7

CONSENT FOR PUBLICATION 9

CONFLICT OF INTEREST 9

ACKNOWLEDGEMENTS 9

REFERENCES 9

CHAPTER 2 GATED MYOCARDIAL PERFUSION IMAGING AND RISK-STRATIFICATION IN CORONARY ARTERY DISEASE AND HEART FAILURE 15

Tomoaki Nakata, Kenji Sato and *Kei Nakata*

GATED MYOCARDIAL PERFUSION IMAGING TECHNOLOGY 15

Clinical Implications of Gated MPI 17

Risk-Stratification in Coronary Artery Disease 18

Risk-Stratification in Heart Failure 20

CONSENT FOR PUBLICATION 23

CONFLICT OF INTEREST 23

ACKNOWLEDGEMENTS 23

REFERENCES 23

CHAPTER 3 MYOCARDIAL VIABILITY ASSESSMENT IN PREDICTING PROGNOSIS AND PROVIDING OPTIMAL MANAGEMENT FOR ISCHEMIC LEFT VENTRICULAR DYSFUNCTION 29

Tokuo Kasai

INTRODUCTION 30

Impact of Myocardial Viability on Patient Management 30

Pathophysiology of Reversible Ischemic Dysfunction 33

Structural Alteration of Hibernating Myocardium 34

Metabolic Alteration in Reversible Ischemic Dysfunction 35

Role of Imaging in Assessing Reversible Ischemic Dysfunction 35

Amount of Residual Ischemic Myocardium 45

LV Remodeling 46

Viability and Cardiac Resynchronization Therapy 47

CONCLUSION 48

CONSENT FOR PUBLICATION 48

CONFLICT OF INTEREST 49

ACKNOWLEDGEMENTS 49
REFERENCES 49

CHAPTER 4 CARDIAC HYBRID OR FUSION IMAGING AND FUTURE PROSPECTIVE 57
Shinro Matsuo
INTRODUCTION 57
Anatomic and Physiological Stenosis 58
Quantitative Evaluation of Myocardial Ischemia 58
Fusion Imaging of CT Angiography and SPECT 59
The Benefits of Fusion Imaging 61
The Coronary Artery Calcification Evaluation by SPECT / CT 61
Fusion Diagnosis of Functional Information and Blood Flow 62
CONCLUSION 63
CONSENT FOR PUBLICATION 63
CONFLICT OF INTEREST 63
ACKNOWLEDGEMENTS 63
REFERENCES 63

CHAPTER 5 POSITRON EMISSION TOMOGRAPHY MYOCARDIAL PERFUSION IMAGING 67
Keiichiro Yoshinaga and *Osamu Manabe*
TRACERS FOR PET MYOCARDIAL PERFUSION IMAGING 67
Rubidium-82 68
^{15}O-labeled Water 70
^{18}Fluorine-labeled Myocardial Perfusion Agents 70
C-11-labeled PET Agents 71
^{11}C-acetate 71
^{11}C-HED 72
CLINICAL INDICATION AND IMAGING PROTOCOLS 72
Clinical Indication 72
Imaging Protocol 72
Patient Preparation 72
Stress Protocol 73
Pharmacological Vasodilator Stress 73
Dobutamine Stress 73
Image Acquisition and Processing 74
^{82}Rubidium 74
^{15}O-labeled Water 74
Assessment of Absolute Myocardial Blood Flow 74
CLINICAL APPLICATIONS 75
Diagnosis in Coronary Artery Disease 75
Visual Assessment 75
MBF Assessment 77
Prognosis in Coronary Artery Disease 78
Visual Analysis 78
Quantitative Analysis 79
CONSENT FOR PUBLICATION 80
CONFLICT OF INTEREST 80
ACKNOWLEDGEMENTS 80
REFERENCES 80

CHAPTER 6 **MYOCARDIAL PERFUSION IMAGING AND OTHER MODALITIES** 87
Yasuyo Taniguchi
CARDIAC MAGNETIC RESONANCE IMAGING (CMR) IMAGING 87
Assessment of Myocardial Perfusion 88
Assessment of Area at Risk in AMI 89
Assessment of Myocardial Viability 90
Tissue Characterization 91
CARDIAC COMPUTER TOMOGRAPHY (CCT) 92
Standardized Reporting of CCTA 93
Anatomical CCT Imaging and Other Functional Imaging 95
Functional Imaging with Coronary CTA 96
CT Myocardial Perfusion Imaging 96
Triple Rule Out with CT 97
APPROPRIATE CRITERIA 98
CONSENT FOR PUBLICATION 100
CONFLICT OF INTEREST 100
ACKNOWLEDGEMENTS 100
REFERENCES 100

CHAPTER 7 **FATTY ACID IMAGING FROM BASIC TO CLINICAL** 104
Iichiro Osawa, Takashi Ushimi, Nanami Okano, Eito Kozawa and *Ichiro Matsunari*
INTRODUCTION 104
BASIC PRINCIPLES 105
Myocardial Fatty Acid Metabolism 105
Radiopharmaceuticals for PET and SPECT 107
PET Tracer 109
SPECT Tracer 109
BMIPP 111
Kinetics 111
Imaging Protocols 112
Serial Changes of BMIPP Imaging 114
CLINICAL APPLICATIONS 115
Ischemic Heart Disease 115
Myocardial Infarction 115
Angina Pectoris and Acute Coronary Syndrome 123
Chronic Coronary Aartery Disease 128
Nonischemic Cardiomyopathy 132
Dilated Cardiomyopathy 134
Takotsubo Cardiomyopathy 136
CONSENT FOR PUBLICATION 137
CONFLICT OF INTEREST 137
ACKNOWLEDGEMENTS 137
REFERENCES 137

CHAPTER 8 **RECENT ADVANCES IN BMIPP IMAGING** 147
Takashi Kudo, Altay Myssayev and *Reiko Ideguchi*
BMIPP: MECHANISM OF UPTAKE AND THEORY FOR DIAGNOSIS 147
Recent Findings on the Uptake/Metabolism Mechanism CD36 148
Single Ischemic Insult 149
ISCHEMIC HEART DISEASE 149
Acute Conditions: Unstable Angina and ACS 150
Subacute Conditions and After Interventions 150
Chronic Ischemia 152

Vasospasm ... 153
SPECIFIC DISEASE GROUPS ... 154
CKD/HD ... 154
Hypertrophic Cardiomyopathy ... 157
Dilated Cardiomyopathy ... 157
Takotsubo Cardiomyopathy ... 158
Heart Failure ... 160
NEW CLINICAL APPLICATIONS ... 161
Radiation Injuries in the Myocardium ... 161
Cardiac Sarcoidosis ... 162
Chronic Thromboembolism Pulmonary Hypertension ... 163
Triglyceride Deposit Cardiomyovasculopathy ... 163
Mitochondrial Cardiomyopathy ... 163
METHODOLOGICAL ASPECTS ... 164
How to Quantify BMIPP ... 164
Technical Advances in Imaging Equipment ... 165
GUIDELINES ... 165
RADIATION DOSE ... 166
SUMMARY ... 166
CONSENT FOR PUBLICATION ... 167
CONFLICT OF INTEREST ... 167
ACKNOWLEDGEMENTS ... 167
REFERENCES ... 167

CHAPTER 9 POTENTIAL USES OF ^{123}*m*IBG AND ANALOGOUS PET TRACERS TO GUIDE USE OF CARDIAC IMPLANTABLE ELECTRONIC DEVICES IN HEART FAILURE AND ASSOCIATED ARRHYTHMIAS ... 177
Mark I. Travin
INTRODUCTION ... 178
NEUROHORMONAL REGULATION OF CARDIOVASCULAR FUNCTION ... 178
RADIONUCLIDE IMAGING OF CARDIAC SYMPATHETIC INNERVATION ... 179
CLINICAL APPLICATIONS OF ADRENERGIC IMAGING IN HEART FAILURE ... 180
Risk Stratification Power in Patients with Heart Failure ... 180
Risk Stratification for Risk of Ventricular Arrhythmias and Sudden Cardiac Death ... 181
USE OF CARDIAC ADRENERGIC IMAGING TO GUIDE THERAPY ... 184
^{123}I-*m*IBG Imaging to Guide Use of Cardiac Resynchronization Therapy (CRT) ... 185
^{123}I-*m*IBG Imaging to Guide Use of a Left Ventricular Assist Device (LVAD) ... 187
^{123}I-*m*IBG Imaging to Guide Use of an Implantable Cardioverter Defibrillator (ICD) ... 189
^{123}I-*m*IBG Imaging as a Potential Tool for Guiding Electrophysiological Procedures ... 193
CONCLUDING REMARKS ... 194
CONSENT FOR PUBLICATION ... 195
CONFLICT OF INTEREST ... 195
ACKNOWLEDGEMENTS ... 195
REFERENCES ... 195

CHAPTER 10 NEUROTRANSMITTER IMAGING FOR CARDIOMYOPATHY AND TAKOTSUBO SYNDROME ... 204
Takayuki Warisawa and *Yoshihiro J. Akashi*
INTRODUCTION ... 204
HYPERTROPHIC CARDIOMYOPATHY ... 205
Relationship Between Cardiac Sympathetic Activity and Clinical Features in HCM ... 205
Usefulness of ^{123}I-MIBG Scintigraphy for Prognosis in HCM ... 206

Role as a Monitor for Medical Therapy in HCM 206
TAKOTSUBO SYNDROME 206
Evidences and Roles of ^{123}I-MIBG Scintigraphy in TTS 207
Future Prospects of ^{123}I-MIBG Scintigraphy in TTS 208
CONCLUSION 208
CONSENT FOR PUBLICATION 209
CONFLICT OF INTEREST 209
ACKNOWLEDGEMENTS 209
REFERENCES 209

CHAPTER 11 EVALUATION OF CARDIAC SYMPATHETIC NERVE FUNCTION USING IODINE-123 METAIODOBENZYLGUANIDINE SCINTIGRAPHY 213
Hiroshi Mori and *Shinro Matsuo*
RADIONUCLIDE AND UPTAKE MECHANISM 213
PATIENT PREPARATION 214
EXAMINATION METHODS 215
NORMAL FINDINGS 215
CORONARY ARTERY DISEASES 216
TRANSPLANTED HEART 217
DIABETES MELLITUS 218
CONCLUSION 218
CONSENT FOR PUBLICATION 218
CONFLICT OF INTEREST 219
ACKNOWLEDGEMENTS 219
REFERENCES 219

CHAPTER 12 STANDARDIZATION OF ^{123}I-*meta*-IODOBENZYLGUANIDINE HEART-TO-MEDIASTINUM RATIO: TECHNICAL ASPECTS 222
Koichi Okuda, Kenichi Nakajima, Chiemi Kitamura and *Yumiko Kirihara*
INTRODUCTION 222
A Software Program for Semi-Automated ROI Setting 223
HMR Calibration Methods for Characteristics of Gamma Cameras 223
SUMMARY 225
CONSENT FOR PUBLICATION 225
CONFLICT OF INTEREST 225
ACKNOWLEDGEMENTS 225
REFERENCES 225

CHAPTER 13 IMAGE DIAGNOSIS OF ARTERIOSCLEROSIS AND POSSIBILITY OF EARLY INTERVENTION 227
Shinro Matsuo
INTRODUCTION 227
A Hybrid SPECT/CT System 228
CAC in Patients with Normal Coronary Flow Reserve 229
Inflammation and Calcification 229
Evaluation of Atherosclerosis by SPECT/CT 230
Inflammation and FDG 230
LIMITATION 232
CONSENT FOR PUBLICATION 232
CONFLICT OF INTEREST 232
ACKNOWLEDGEMENTS 232
REFERENCES 232

CHAPTER 14 **NUCLEAR CARDIOLOGY FOR THE DIAGNOSIS OF TAKOTSUBO SYNDROME** 235
Shinro Matsuo
INTRODUCTION 235
Fatty Acid Metabolism Myocardial Scintigraphy (^{123}I-BMIPP) 237
^{18}F Fluorodeoxyglucose PET 238
Neurotransmitter Imaging for Cardiomyopathy and Takotsubo Syndrome 238
Fusion Image of Takotsubo Syndrome 240
Various Nuclear Medicine Tests used for Takotsubo Syndrome 241
CONCLUSION 242
CONSENT FOR PUBLICATION 242
CONFLICT OF INTEREST 242
ACKNOWLEDGEMENTS 242
REFERENCES 242

CHAPTER 15 **SMALL RODENT ANIMAL POSITRON EMISSION TOMOGRAPHY/SINGLE PHOTON EMISSION TOMOGRAPHY** 245
Hiroshi Wakabayashi
INTRODUCTION 245
Radionuclides Used for SPECT and PET 246
Myocardial Perfusion Image 246
Cardiac Function 247
Glucose Metabolism 247
Cardiac Sympathetic Nerve Imaging 248
Angiogenesis Monitoring 248
Apoptosis Imaging 249
Artifact of SPECT and PET 249
CONCLUSION 249
CONSENT FOR PUBLICATION 250
CONFLICT OF INTEREST 250
ACKNOWLEDGEMENTS 250
REFERENCES 250

SUBJECT INDEX 253

FOREWORD

How can we best practice the clinical nuclear medicine? This eBook is designed to explain some methods regarding nuclear cardiology, which would be instructive for physicians and scientists. This book would tell what is nuclear cardiology, or how non-invasive imaging is used, from clinical evidences. The Nuclear cardiology has demonstrated continuous dramatic growth over 40 years. This book is composed of recent progress of the nuclear cardiology by leading physicians and scientists in this field. I am sure that this eBook would be useful for daily practice of all the physicians and scientists interested in this field.

Seigo Kinuya
Professor of Department of Nuclear Medicine
Graduate School of Medical Sciences
Kanazawa University
Kanazawa, Japan

PREFACE

Nuclear cardiology has demonstrated continuous growth for over 35 years, and now become important tool for evaluation of patients with heart disease. A nuclear cardiology test is one of the most commonly performed non-invasive cardiac imaging tests in hospitals for the patients with heart disease as well as echocardiography.

This book is composed of four parts by leading physicians and scientists in the field. The first part describes the perfusion scintigraphy. Myocardial perfusion imaging is an established method for the primary detection of coronary artery disease. Gated myocardial perfusion single-photon computed tomography (SPECT) is essential for the diagnosis of cardiac function. The addition of ECG-gating has allowed nuclear cardiology to expand from myocardial perfusion alone to the assessment of systolic and diastolic function.

The second part provides metabolic aspects of heart disease, including fatty acid metabolism. The heart is an active organ that requires high oxygen to maintain mechanical function. The major aim of oxygen uptake in the heart is to provide sufficient energy in the mitochondria in the myocardium. Glucose and free fatty acids are major energy sources in the myocardium. Recent advances in nuclear cardiology include fatty acid metabolic tracer of iodine-12--labeled BMIPP. I-123 BMIPP provides useful information in patients with heart disease.

The third part covers cardiac sympathetic function, including sympathetic nerve imaging. ^{123}I-MIBG scintigraphy is now used as an important technique for studying cardiac neuronal function. ^{123}I-MIBG shares the same uptake and storage mechanisms as norepinephrine. It is reported that the uptake-1 system is mediated by the norepinephrine transporter, and the uptake-2 system is an extra-neuronal system. ^{123}I-MIBG imaging has an important prognostic value in patients with heart failure.

The fourth and the final part describes small animal molecular imaging, preventive medicine and Takotsubo syndrome.

Nuclear cardiology tests, including neurotransmitter imaging and metabolic imaging, are now easily preformed with new tracers to refine the diagnosis of heart disease. Nuclear cardiology studies contribute significantly to guiding management decisions for identifying cardiac risk in patients with heart disease.

Shinro Matsuo
Department of Nuclear Medicine,
Kanazawa University
Graduate School of Advanced Preventive Medical Sciences
Kanazawa, Japan

List of Contributors

Altay Myssayev	Department of Radioisotope Medicine, Atomic Bomb Disease Institute, Nagasaki University, Nagasaki, Japan
Chiemi Kitamura	FUJIFILM RI Pharma Co., Ltd., 14-1, kyobashi 2-Chome, Chuo-Ku, Tokyo 104-0031, Japan
Eito Kozawa	Department of Radiology, Saitama Medical University Hospital, Saitama, Japan
Hiroshi Mori	Department of Nuclear Medicine, Kanazawa University Hospital, Kanazawa, Japan
Hiroshi Wakabayashi	Department of Nuclear Medicine, Kanazawa University Hospital, 13-1 Takara-machi, Kanazawa, Ishikawa 920-8641, Japan
Iichiro Osawa	Division of Nuclear Medicine, Department of Radiology, Saitama Medical University Hospital, Saitama, Japan
Ichiro Matsunari	Division of Nuclear Medicine, Department of Radiology, Saitama Medical University Hospital, Saitama, Japan
Kenji Sato	Department of Cardiology, Hakodate Goryoukaku Hospital, Hakodate, 38-3 Goryoukaku-cho, Japan
Kei Nakata	School of Medicine, Sapporo Medical University, Sapporo, Hokkaidō, Japan
Keiichiro Yoshinaga	Diagnostic and Therapeutic Nuclear Medicine, National Institutes for Quantum and Radiological Science and Technology, Chiba, Japan
Koichi Okuda	Department of Physics, Kanazawa Medical University, 1-1 Daigaku, Uchinada, Kahoku, Ishikawa 920-0293, Japan
Kenichi Nakajima	Department of Nuclear Medicine, Kanazawa University Hospital, Kanazawa, Japan
Mark I. Travin	Department of Radiology, Division of Nuclear Medicine, Montefiore Medical Center, Albert Einstein College of Medicine, Bronx, New York, USA
Nanami Okano	Department of Radiology, Saitama Medical University Hospital, Saitama, Japan
Osamu Manabe	Department of Nuclear Medicine, Hokkaido University Graduate School of Medicine, Sapporo, Japan
Reiko Ideguchi	Department of Radioisotope Medicine, Atomic Bomb Disease Institute, Nagasaki University, Nagasaki, Japan
Shinro Matsuo	Department of Nuclear Medicine, Kanazawa University Hospital, Kanazawa, Japan Graduate School of Advanced Preventive Medical Sciences, Kanazawa, Japan
Tomoaki Nakata	Department of Cardiology, Hakodate Goryoukaku Hospital, 38-3 Goryoukaku-cho, Hakodate, Japan
Tokuo Kasai	Department of Cardiology, Uonuma Kikan Hospital, Niigata University, Niigata, Japan
Takashi Kudo	Department of Radioisotope Medicine, Atomic Bomb Disease Institute, Nagasaki University, Nagasaki, Japan
Takashi Ushimi	Department of Radiology, Saitama Medical University Hospital, Saitama, Japan

Takayuki Warisawa Imperial College London, Hammersmith Hospital, International Center for Circulatory Health, National Heart and Lung Institute, London, United Kingdom
Division of Cardiology, Department of Internal Medicine, St. Marianna University School of Medicine, Kawasaki, Japan

Yasuyo Taniguchi Hyogo Brain and Heart Center, Himeji, Hyogo, Japan

Yoshihiro J. Akashi Division of Cardiology, Department of Internal Medicine, St. Marianna University School of Medicine, Kawasaki, Japan

Yumiko Kirihara FUJIFILM RI Pharma Co., Ltd., kyobashi 2-Chome, Chuo-Ku, Tokyo 104-0031, Japan

CHAPTER 1

Diagnosis of Coronary Artery Disease with Myocardial Perfusion Imaging

Shinro Matsuo*

Department of Nuclear Medicine, Kanazawa University Hospital, Kanazawa, Japan

Graduate School of Advanced Preventive Medical Sciences, Kanazawa, Japan

Abstract: Myocardial perfusion imaging can be used to diagnose and make a risk stratification of the patients with coronary artery disease. Recognizing normal subjects as definitely normal is one of the critical factors in daily practice. This article describes myocardial perfusion imaging, including technical points especially in IQ-SPECT system and a new technology, semiconductor camera.

Keywords: Attenuation Correction, IQ-SPECT, Normal Perfusion, SPECT.

INTRODUCTION

Myocardial perfusion imaging (MPI) is one of the major examinations of nuclear medicine. Nine million MPI have been performed in the United States and 250 thousand in Japan for diagnosing and risk stratification of coronary artery disease [1 - 5]. Following injection of radioisotopes such as thallium or ^{99m}Tc-perfusion agents, the tracer is extracted from the blood by viable myocytes and retained within the myocyte. With single-photon emission computed tomography (SPECT) perfusion imaging, the distribution of perfusion throughout the myocardium could be represented. To differentiate between myocardial ischemia and necrosis, an exercise or pharmacologic stress test is useful. The treadmill protocol should be compatible with patient's physical capacity. The radiopharmaceutical agent is injected at the peak of exercise [6]. The pharmacological stress test is performed by administering a vasodilator, adenosine. The pharmacological stress is increasingly employed as an alternative to exercise testing.

* **Corresponding author Shinro Matsuo:** Department of Nuclear Medicine, Kanazawa University Hospital, 13-1 Takara-machi, Kanazawa 920-8641, Japan; Advanced Preventive Medical Sciences, Kanazawa University Graduate School, 13-1 Takara-machi, Kanazawa 920-8641, Japan; Tel: 81-76-265-2333; Fax: 81-76-234-4257; E-mail: smatsuo@med.kanazawa-u.ac.jp

The coronary perfusion can be expressed as coronary blood flow reserve and diagnosis of angina pectoris can be performed by exercise load or pharmacological stress. In the resting state, there is no difference within the left ventricle in the myocardial perfusion, even in presence of a stenosis of the coronary artery. The stress test can make a relative blood flow difference between normal and abnormal when there is a stenosis. Using the relative difference of myocardial perfusion, we can make a diagnosis of ischemia and myocardial infarction.

Diagnosing Ischemia or Infarction

Observing stress and rest imaging and comparing the two images give us information on ischemia and infarction [7]. When the stress image has a defect and it is normalized in the rest image, this finding is called complete redistribution, indicating ischemia, and therefore reduced coronary blood flow reserve. When stress image and rest image are similar, this points to myocardial infarction. Thus, myocardial SPECT examination can differentiate between ischemic but viable myocardium and myocardial infarction, which has therapeutic consequences.

Cardiac Function

The quantitative analysis of ventricular function could be achieved with high reproducibility by ECG-gated SPECT [6]. There are many clinical situations in which serial changes in left or right ventricular function are clinically relevant [7]. Ischemia induces a decrease of myocardial contractility and hence of its function. Cardiac function measurement is useful in patients with heart failure, valvular heart disease, or in those who have received cardio-toxic chemotherapy. Numerous quantitative variables, including ejection fraction, volumes, diastolic parameters, dyssynchrony can be derived from QGS [8 - 12].

SPECT/CT

The device called SPECT / CT can use CT information because a CT scanner is attached to SPECT [13]. A hybrid SPECT/CT system has been introduced recently in clinical settings and has been available in many countries [14]. Combined SPECT/CT acquisition in one step examination is acceptable in many clinical situations and physicians can obtain perfusion and atherosclerotic information without any extra-cost and without contrast-media.

Risk Stratification

Risk stratification is essential in the management of patients with coronary artery disease. Risk stratification of coronary artery disease can be achieved by myocardial perfusion study [1, 2]. The evaluation for known or suspected CAD using electrocardiogram (ECG)-gated myocardial perfusion single-photon emission computed tomography (SPECT) imaging had been established in the diagnosis and risk assessment by many precedent studies [2]. A number of clinical research studies have shown that the extent and severity of stress myocardial perfusion defects are the predominant predictors of major cardiac events.

A multicenter study of Japanese assessment of cardiac events and survival studies by quantitative gated SPECT (J-ACCESS) was the first large-scale prognostic study conducted in an Asian population using myocardial perfusion imaging [1]. J-ACCESS1 has been conducted since 2001 to evaluate the prognostic value of myocardial perfusion imaging. The results of this study demonstrated that an increase in summed stress score (SSS) was associated with an increase in the risk of cardiac events [1 - 3]. As a gatekeeper, precise determination of normal images is critically important for the risk stratification of the patients with coronary artery disease. Normal stress myocardial perfusion imaging (MPI) was associated with an average annual cardiovascular event rate of 0.6-0.9% [2, 15, 16]. Japanese subjects with normal perfusion imaging had an excellent prognosis if their end-systolic volume and left ventricular ejection fraction (LVEF) were also normal [2, 3]. The previous study showed that inclusion of perfusion/function measurements by stress/rest gated SPECT, in combination with pre-scan clinical risk assessment, improves significantly the risk stratification and secondary prevention strategy in patients with known coronary artery disease [3]. Regarding subjects with chronic kidney disease, it is reported that the SSS value of 9 or more is a reliable predictor of cardiac events and myocardial perfusion imaging has incremental value for predicting cardiac events and survival in chronic kidney disease [4]. The subjects included in the J-ACCESS were patients with suspected or confirmed CAD. The database of J-ACCESS did not sufficiently enrol high-risk population having concurrent diabetes mellitus (DM) or chronic kidney disease (CKD) or invasive treatment. Therefore, J-ACCESS II [17], J-ACCESS III [18], and J-ACCESS IV [19] were conducted in diabetes mellitus and chronic kidney disease patients, and post-percutaneous coronary intervention patients respectively, who had no history of coronary artery disease, to supplement the lacking data on this high-risk population.

Normal Myocardial Perfusion Imaging

A watchful waiting approach in the management of patients with normal SPECT is very important. This approach results in cost efficiency and substantial cost savings, compared with a more aggressive, invasive diagnostic workup strategy that includes diagnostic cardiac catheterization [2]. For patients with normal stress myocardial perfusion images, no additional testing is needed to be done because benign course can be expected [2]. This does not guarantee a long-term cardiac-event-free period in chronic kidney disease patients, because studies of long-term outcome after a normal stress radionuclide study in terms of various categories of estimate glomerular filtration rate (eGFR) in chronic kidney disease are scarce. The patients with lower eGFR might have higher cardiovascular event rate. Because patients may complain of an atypical symptom in greater frequency, physicians should rely heavily on imaging results to make a precise diagnosis and guide management decisions [16 - 23]. This study suggested that the use of stress myocardial SPECT images could be a key component for the evaluation of chronic kidney disease patients for better management and clinical outcome [16, 24 - 28]. By using myocardial perfusion imaging, overall hospital costs might be reduced.

Evaluation of Ischemia

Evaluating the amount of myocardial ischemia is indispensable for the cardiologist to decide for invasive therapy in patients with coronary artery disease [29 - 35]. The higher amount of ischemia is known to be related with the higher future cardiac event of the patient. Previous reports demonstrated that a prognosis after revascularization was related to the amount of ischemia (% of total myocardium ischemic) estimated with myocardial perfusion imaging [36], Among the subjects with more than 10% ischemic myocardium estimated with myocardial perfusion imaging, cardiac death was less after early revascularization than medical therapy alone. On the other hand, as for the patients with 10% or less than 10% ischemic myocardium, optimal medical therapy for the patients with ischemic heart disease alone experienced a better prognosis than an invasive revascularization treatment. The propensity scores obtained from J-ACCESS study showed a close relationship between major cardiovascular event rates and the amount of ischemia evaluated by SPECT. The study reported that early revascularization possibly resulted in a good prognosis in Japanese patients with more than 5% ischemic myocardium estimated with myocardial perfusion imaging [37]. This study showed that evaluating the amount of ischemia before invasive treatment is necessary in order to predict and improve the prognosis of patients with coronary artery disease. A good prognosis may depend on a therapeutic strategy determined on the basis of the severity of ischemic myocardium estimated with myocardial perfusion imaging. The COURAGE Trial Nuclear Sub-study reported that the reduction of ischemia resulted in improving prognosis in ischemic heart disease [32]. When myocardial perfusion imaging showed 10% or more than 10% ischemic myocardium in patients, more than 5% reduction of that ischemia would be linked to the improvement of the prognosis. In addition, ischemic reduction observed on SPECT images was greater with combined coronary intervention and optimal medical therapy than with optimal medical therapy alone. In Japan, the J-ACCESS IV trial [19], which is similar to the design of the COURAGE Trial Nuclear Sub-study, has been conducted to prove similar results. A sub-study of J-ACCESS 1 had shown the relationship between the ischemic reduction and the onset of cardiac events after treatment in Japanese patients with CAD. A good prognosis could be observed in patients who achieved ≥5% ischemic reduction, or the patients with no remaining ischemia [19]. J-ACCESS IV showed the cut-off value of 5% as ischemic reduction [32]. Both COURAGE Nuclear Sub-study and J-ACCESS IV proved a reliable target value for reduction of ischemia before percutaneous coronary intervention indispensable for revascularization is performed to improve prognosis among any racial patient with coronary artery disease [38 - 40].

The artificial neuronal network system using software can diagnose the amount of ischemia. The diagnostic ability of artificial neuronal network, which is a type of artificial intelligence, increased the usefulness of nuclear cardiology. Computer-assisted quantification and evaluation play important roles in supporting visual diagnosis of physicians. Whether the diagnostic accuracy meets the need in the clinical situation has to be validated.

IQ-SPECT (SMARTZOOM Collimator)

Recently, several types of gamma cameras, semiconductor collimator, have been introduced to clinical medicine, instead of the conventional collimators made from sodium iodine crystals [41, 42]. This big change is achieved by using a multifocal collimator that rotates around the patient in a cardio-centric orbit resulting in a four-fold magnification of the heart [42]. The IQ-SPECT system with SMARTZOOM collimator (Siemens AG, Munichi, German) was manufactured by Siemens in 2010. The IQ-SPECT made it possible to perform MPI scans in one-fourth the time or using one-fourth the administered dose as compared to a standard protocol by means of parallel-hole collimators. This article describes how to read normal imaging obtained by IQ-SPECT system [43].

The meaningful thing for interpreting normal myocardial blood flow obtained with IQ-SPECT is to understand the findings of the apex and infero-lateral wall of the myocardium. In the computed tomography (CT) attenuation corrected image, even in the case of normal myocardial perfusion, the decrease in the apex of the myocardium is sometimes observed [43]. Therefore, it is necessary to carefully read images with this point in diagnosing the patients. Fig. (**1**) depicts the characteristics of the myocardial perfusion distribution obtained by IQ-SPECT system.

The cause of decreased apical accumulation of the left ventricle is related to a thinner wall of that region. Even in the findings of magnetic resonance imaging (MRI), the apical wall thickness of left ventricle is small. Therefore, it is considered that the apparent decrease in blood flow of attenuated scattering corrected image accurately reflects this.

In the thallium-201 conventional examination using low energy high-resolution collimator (LEHR), attenuation artifact of the inferior wall is a challenging matter. In the conventional LEHR collimator, the lower wall uptake of thallium-201 in the inferior wall is often observed. The reason for inferior wall decrease in conventional SPECT is well-known especially in thallium-201 perfusion study and less marked in Tc-99m study. Attenuation artifact of the soft tissue is considered to be one of the main causes for this decrease [43].

IQ-SPECT images without CT attenuation correction resembled those of the conventional LEHR. Therefore, the attenuation and scattering of the photons in the patient's tissue must be taken into consideration as well. The location of the attenuation artifact is decided by the position of the soft tissue near the heart. A CT scan can be taken of the patients immediately after a SPECT scan. Usually, a quick scout acquisition is taken. The information of soft tissues, including a liver and a breast, can be used to correct myocardial perfusion. The IQ-SPECT with CT attenuation correction improves this decreased attenuation effect, especially in the inferior wall. Actually, our study showed that the IQ-SPECT/CT images with CT attenuation correction, improved statistically the inferior wall artifacts compared to the anterior wall, when proper attenuation correction was performed by using IQ-SPECT/CT. Furthermore, it is preferable to employ the normal clinical database completed this time, and to use the distribution as a criterion for judgment [44 - 47].

After the CT correction, the representation of the inferior wall was improved as shown in Fig. (**1**), but a tendency to decrease blood flow in the apex of the apex and the apical anterior wall was observed. IQ-SPECT by using proper CT attenuation correction improves the false positive artifact of the inferior wall even in thallium-201 study, which is susceptible to attenuation and scattering. The image quality of thallium-201 is inferior to that of technetium-99m, but it is considered advantageous for IQ-SPECT/CT in the measurement of myocardial perfusion in the inferior wall with attenuation artifact. Needless to say, a physician can diagnose normal perfusion by using gated SPECT cardiac function information. When a normal wall motion and a normal wall thickness were seen on the gated images, a normal perfusion could be confirmed. Evaluation of regional wall motion, including normal dyssynchrony, is helpful in differentiating attenuation artifacts from myocardial perfusion defects.

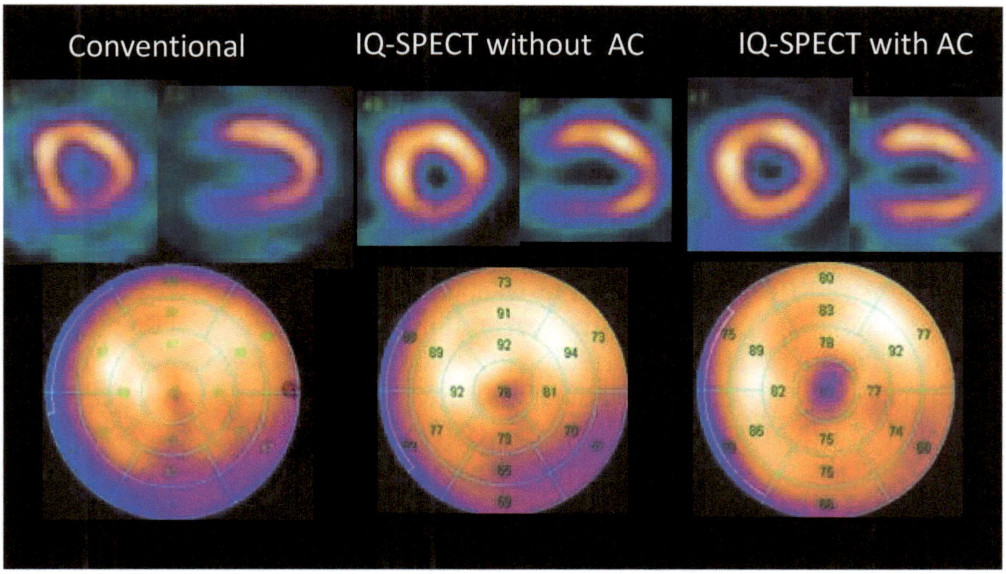

Fig. (1). A representative normal perfusion case of a 59-year-old man. Conventional SPECT has a decrease in the inferior wall of the left ventricle as an artifact. The image of IQ-SPECT without attenuation correction (AC) is similar to that of conventional SPECT. After IQ-SPECT attenuation scattering correction, the decreased uptake is significantly improved with IQ-SPECT/CT. The apex was slightly decreased after IQ-SPECT attenuation correction.

With IQ-SPECT using CT attenuation correction, it is possible to obtain high diagnostic ability, and it is a clinically useful imaging in a short time acquisition. The clinician should keep in mind these normal perfusion characteristics using IQ-SPECT.

Quantitative Myocardial Flow Measurement with CZT Camera

High resolution gamma camera with cadmium zinc telluride (CZT) semiconductors have several advantages compared to conventional Angar camera. CZT is dedicated to cardiac scan. Previous studies using this camera showed that significant differences in myocardial flow reserve between normal healthy subjects and those with coronary artery disease [48 - 50]. Quantitative assessment of myocardial perfusion and myocardial flow reserve could be achieved by using D-SPECT in patients with coronary artery disease. These new hard-wares would enlighten the way to quantitative measurement in the field of cardiology.

Mitochondrial Function Imaging

^{99m}Tc-sestamibi (MIBI) is a perfusion tracer with lipophilic cation. Myocardial uptake and retention of ^{99m}Tc-MIBI involve passive diffusion across the plasma and mitochondrial membranes [51]. ^{99m}Tc is produced from molybdenum-99m generator and emits monoenergetic gamma rays. ^{99m}Tc-MIBI behaves physiologically as a monovalent cation. ^{99m}Tc-MIBI is driven by the inside negative plasma membrane and mitochondrial inner membrane potentials, which concentrates the tracer within the cytosol and mitochondria [51]. ^{99m}Tc-MIBI is bound by mitochondria so that the retention of ^{99m}Tc-MIBI in the mitochondria is related to mitochondrial function. By analysis, the ^{99m}Tc-MIBI images on planar images to quantify cardiac ^{99m}Tc-MIBI uptake and calculate the heart-to-mediastinum (HMR) count ratio, the washout rate of ^{99m}Tc-MIBI is calculated from the segmental counts in the early and delayed images. Ischemia and mitochondrial dysfunction reportedly induce increased washout of ^{99m}Tc-MIBI [52]. In patients with congestive heart failure, including cardiomyopathies, the myocardial washout rate of ^{99m}Tc-MIBI is considered to be a novel clinical indicator for diagnosing myocardial damage or dysfunction, which provides prognostic information in patients with reduced left ventricular function [51]. ^{99m}Tc-MIBI washout is also known to be enhanced in patients with dilated cardiomyopathy or hypertrophic cardiomyopathy and anthracycline-induced cardiomyopathy. ^{99m}Tc-MIBI washout can be a sign of mitochondrial dysfunction [51].

Restrictive cardiomyopathy is a disease of idiopathic or secondary to heart muscle disease that manifests itself as a restrictive disorder, leading to heart failure [55]. The most common hemodynamic disturbance in restrictive cardiomyopathy is impaired ventricular filling due to the increased thickening and increased rigidity of the endocardium and myocardium secondary to infiltration by amyloid tissue or fibrosis. Amyloid cardiomyopathy is one of the causes of restrictive cardiomyopathy. The case of restrictive cardiomyopathy in which sympathetic and metabolic abnormalities and normal perfusion imaging were demonstrated in a report [53]. These findings of scintigraphic studies have shown us that restrictive diastole seems to cause metabolic and sympathetic abnormality as well as normal perfusion. On the other hand, alcoholic cardiomyopathy is known to be induced by chronic alcohol abuse, resulting in left ventricular dysfunction and heart failure. Up to 45% of all dilated cardiomyopathy appears to be due to alcohol abuse [54]. The first sign of myocardial function may be a decreased diastolic function in this disease. Left ventricular systolic dysfunction can be recognized later in these patients. Thereafter, cardiac enlargement is observed as a part of a compensatory Frank-Starling mechanism. Cardiac fatty acid-metabolic abnormalities of the left ventricle were imaged in a patient with alcoholic cardiomyopathy [54]. ^{123}I-MIBG, which is a sympathetic nerve tracer, identified myocardial damage in the inferior wall of the left ventricle, and mild heterogeneity of ^{123}I-MIBG uptake was observed in the myocardium. Fatty acid tracer, such as ^{123}I-BMIPP demonstrated decreased uptake in the left ventricular inferior myocardium, concordant with blood flow. These nuclear cardiology findings indicate that chronic alcoholism can cause myocardial damage, which results in metabolic and neuronal abnormalities [54]. Mitochondrial disorders manifest as heterogeneous abnormalities that were induced by abnormalities in mitochondrial DNA and function. In mitochondrial myopathy, encephalopathy, lactic acidosis and stroke-like episodes (MELAS), the cardiac involvement of the disease is manifested as hypertrophic (symmetrical or asymmetrical) or dilated cardiomyopathy [53]. In the left ventricle of the MELAS patients, decreased ^{99m}Tc-MIBI uptake is seen in the damaged myocardium and increased ^{99m}Tc-MIBI washout is also observed in the site of mitochondria dysfunction, which manifest together with reduced LVEF. Additionally, higher ^{123}I-BMIPP uptake is found at the site of reduced ^{99m}Tc-MIBI uptake [54 - 56]. ^{123}I-BMIPP is a nuclear tracer of free fatty acid, which was commercially available in Japan. ^{123}I-BMIPP after venous injection enters the intracellular triglyceride pool. Mitochondrial respiratory chain failure, and energy production shifts from aerobic to the anaerobic pathway (glycolytic pathway) result in the increased lactic acid formation and increased ^{123}I-BMIPP uptake as often seen in the patients with heart failure [54].

CONSENT FOR PUBLICATION

Not applicable.

CONFLICT OF INTEREST

The authors declare no conflict of interest, financial or otherwise.

ACKNOWLEDGEMENTS

Declared none.

REFERENCES

[1] Nishimura T, Nakajima K, Kusuoka H, Yamashina A, Nishimura S. Prognostic study of risk stratification among Japanese patients with ischemic heart disease using gated myocardial perfusion SPECT: J-ACCESS study. Eur J Nucl Med Mol Imaging 2008; 35(2): 319-28. [http://dx.doi.org/10.1007/s00259-007-0608-x] [PMID: 17926033]

[2] Matsuo S, Nakajima K, Horie M, Nakae I, Nishimura T. J-ACCESS Investigators. Prognostic value of normal stress myocardial perfusion imaging in Japanese population. Circ J 2008; 72(4): 611-7. [http://dx.doi.org/10.1253/circj.72.611] [PMID: 18362434]

[3] Hashimoto A, Nakata T, Wakabayashi T, Kusuoka H, Nishimura T. Incremental prognostic value of stress/rest gated perfusion SPECT in patients with coronary artery disease--subanalysis of the J-ACCESS study. Circ J 2009; 73(12): 2288-93. [http://dx.doi.org/10.1253/circj.CJ-09-0212] [PMID: 19797824]

[4] Hatta T, Nishimura S, Nishimura T. Prognostic risk stratification of myocardial ischaemia evaluated by gated myocardial perfusion SPECT in patients with chronic kidney disease. Eur J Nucl Med Mol

Imaging 2009; 36(11): 1835-41.
[http://dx.doi.org/10.1007/s00259-009-1165-2] [PMID: 19471925]

[5] Joki N, Hase H, Kawano Y, *et al.* Myocardial perfusion imaging for predicting cardiac events in Japanese patients with advanced chronic kidney disease: 1-year interim report of the J-ACCESS 3 investigation. Eur J Nucl Med Mol Imaging 2014; 41(9): 1701-9.
[http://dx.doi.org/10.1007/s00259-014-2781-z] [PMID: 24827603]

[6] Matsuo S, Nakamura Y, Kinoshita M. Post-stress left ventricular function in patients with coronary artery disease measured by Tl-201 ECG-gated single-photon emission tomography. Exp Clin Cardiol 2002; 7(1): 30-4.
[PMID: 19644576]

[7] Matsuo S, Matsumoto T, Nakae I, *et al.* Prognostic value of ECG-gated thallium-201 single-photon emission tomography in patients with coronary artery disease. Ann Nucl Med 2004; 18(7): 617-22.
[http://dx.doi.org/10.1007/BF02984584] [PMID: 15586636]

[8] Matsuo S, Nakae I, Matsumoto T, Horie M. Impact of endothelial dysfunction on left ventricular remodeling after successful primary coronary angioplasty for acute myocardial infarction--analysis by quantitative ECG-gated SPECT--. Ann Nucl Med 2006; 20(1): 57-62.
[http://dx.doi.org/10.1007/BF02985592] [PMID: 16485576]

[9] Matsuo S. Assessment of diastolic function using 16-frame ^{201}Tl-gated myocardial perfusion SPECT. Ann Nucl Med 2010; 24(8): 625-6.
[http://dx.doi.org/10.1007/s12149-010-0385-7] [PMID: 20425489]

[10] Matsuo S, Matsumoto T, Nakae I, *et al.* Evaluation of cardiac resynchronization therapy in drug-resistant idiopathic dilated cardiomyopathy by means of Tc-99m tetrofosmin ECG-gated SPECT. Exp Clin Cardiol 2004; 9(4): 248-50.
[PMID: 19641716]

[11] Matsuo S, Sato Y, Nakae I, Masuda D, Matsumoto N, Horie M. Evaluation of cardiac resynchronization therapy in drug-resistant dilated-phase hypertrophic cardiomyopathy by means of Tc-99m sestamibi ECG-gated SPECT. Ann Nucl Med 2006; 20(9): 643-7.
[http://dx.doi.org/10.1007/BF02984664] [PMID: 17294677]

[12] Matsuo S. Phase analysis using gated myocardial perfusion single-photon emission computed tomography imaging for evaluating cardiac dyssynchrony. Circ J 2012; 76(8): 1832-3.
[http://dx.doi.org/10.1253/circj.CJ-12-0636] [PMID: 22664418]

[13] Matsuo S, Nakajima K, Okuda K, Kinuya S. The relationship between stress-induced myocardial ischemia and coronary artery atherosclerosis measured by hybrid SPECT/CT camera. Ann Nucl Med 2011; 25(9): 650-6.
[http://dx.doi.org/10.1007/s12149-011-0517-8] [PMID: 21779962]

[14] Matsuo S, Nakajima K, Akhter N, *et al.* Clinical usefulness of novel cardiac MDCT/SPECT fusion image. Ann Nucl Med 2009; 23(6): 579-86.
[http://dx.doi.org/10.1007/s12149-009-0279-8] [PMID: 19572098]

[15] Matsuo S, Nakajima K, Yamasaki Y, Kashiwagi A, Nishimura T. Prognostic value of normal stress myocardial perfusion imaging and ventricular function in Japanese asymptomatic patients with type 2 diabetes--a study based on the J-ACCESS-2 database. Circ J 2010; 74(9): 1916-21.
[http://dx.doi.org/10.1253/circj.CJ-10-0098] [PMID: 20631452]

[16] Matsuo S, Nakajima K, Takeishi Y, Nishimura T. Prognostic value of normal stress myocardial perfusion imaging and ventricular function in Japanese patients with chronic kidney disease: a study based on the J-ACCESS-3 database. Eur J Nucl Med Mol Imaging 2018; 45(7): 1101-7.
[http://dx.doi.org/10.1007/s00259-018-3956-9] [PMID: 29502312]

[17] Yamasaki Y, Nakajima K, Kusuoka H, *et al.* Prognostic value of gated myocardial perfusion imaging for asymptomatic patients with type 2 diabetes: the J-ACCESS 2 investigation. Diabetes Care 2010; 33(11): 2320-6.

[http://dx.doi.org/10.2337/dc09-2370] [PMID: 20724653]

[18] Nakamura S, Kawano Y, Nakajima K, *et al.* Prognostic study of cardiac events in Japanese patients with chronic kidney disease using ECG-gated myocardial Perfusion imaging: Final 3-year report of the J-ACCESS 3 study. J Nucl Cardiol 2017. [http://dx.doi.org/10.1007/s12350-017-0880-5] [PMID: 28439760]

[19] Nanasato M, Matsumoto N, Nakajima K, *et al.* Prognostic impact of reducing myocardial ischemia identified using ECG-gated myocardial perfusion SPECT in Japanese patients with coronary artery disease: J-ACCESS 4 study. Int J Cardiol 2018; 267(267): 202-7. [http://dx.doi.org/10.1016/j.ijcard.2018.05.090] [PMID: 29859707]

[20] Keith DS, Nichols GA, Gullion CM, Brown JB, Smith DH. Longitudinal follow-up and outcomes among a population with chronic kidney disease in a large managed care organization. Arch Intern Med 2004; 164(6): 659-63. [http://dx.doi.org/10.1001/archinte.164.6.659] [PMID: 15037495]

[21] Go AS, Chertow GM, Fan D, McCulloch CE, Hsu CY. Chronic kidney disease and the risks of death, cardiovascular events, and hospitalization. N Engl J Med 2004; 351(13): 1296-305. [http://dx.doi.org/10.1056/NEJMoa041031] [PMID: 15385656]

[22] Herzog CA, Asinger RW, Berger AK, *et al.* Cardiovascular disease in chronic kidney disease. A clinical update from Kidney Disease: Improving Global Outcomes (KDIGO). Kidney Int 2011; 80(6): 572-86. [http://dx.doi.org/10.1038/ki.2011.223] [PMID: 21750584]

[23] De Vriese AS, Vandecasteele SJ, Van den Bergh B, De Geeter FW. Should we screen for coronary artery disease in asymptomatic chronic dialysis patients? Kidney Int 2012; 81(2): 143-51. [http://dx.doi.org/10.1038/ki.2011.340] [PMID: 21956188]

[24] Sosnov J, Lessard D, Goldberg RJ, Yarzebski J, Gore JM. Differential symptoms of acute myocardial infarction in patients with kidney disease: a community-wide perspective. Am J Kidney Dis 2006; 47(3): 378-84. [http://dx.doi.org/10.1053/j.ajkd.2005.11.017] [PMID: 16490615]

[25] Herzog CA, Littrell K, Arko C, Frederick PD, Blaney M. Clinical characteristics of dialysis patients with acute myocardial infarction in the United States: a collaborative project of the United States Renal Data System and the National Registry of Myocardial Infarction. Circulation 2007; 116(13): 1465-72. [http://dx.doi.org/10.1161/CIRCULATIONAHA.107.696765] [PMID: 17785621]

[26] Lameire N, Adam A, Becker CR, *et al.* CIN Consensus Working Panel. Baseline renal function screening. Am J Cardiol 2006; 98(6A) (Suppl.): 21K-6K. [http://dx.doi.org/10.1016/j.amjcard.2006.01.021] [PMID: 16949377]

[27] Davidson CJ, Hlatky M, Morris KG, *et al.* Cardiovascular and renal toxicity of a nonionic radiographic contrast agent after cardiac catheterization. A prospective trial. Ann Intern Med 1989; 110(2): 119-24. [http://dx.doi.org/10.7326/0003-4819-110-2-119] [PMID: 2909204]

[28] Yoda S, Nakanishi K, Tano A, *et al.* Risk stratification of cardiovascular events in patients at all stages of chronic kidney disease using myocardial perfusion SPECT. J Cardiol 2012; 60(5): 377-82. [http://dx.doi.org/10.1016/j.jjcc.2012.06.011] [PMID: 22890072]

[29] Yoda S, Nakanishi K, Tano A, *et al.* Significance of worsening renal function and nuclear cardiology for predicting cardiac death in patients with known or suspected coronary artery disease. J Cardiol 2015; 66(5): 423-9. [http://dx.doi.org/10.1016/j.jjcc.2015.01.003] [PMID: 25703693]

[30] Slomka PJ, Nishina H, Berman DS, *et al.* Automated quantification of myocardial perfusion SPECT using simplified normal limits. J Nucl Cardiol 2005; 12(1): 66-77. [http://dx.doi.org/10.1016/j.nuclcard.2004.10.006] [PMID: 15682367]

[31] Berman DS, Kang X, Gransar H, *et al.* Quantitative assessment of myocardial perfusion abnormality on SPECT myocardial perfusion imaging is more reproducible than expert visual analysis. J Nucl Cardiol 2009; 16(1): 45-53.
[http://dx.doi.org/10.1007/s12350-008-9018-0] [PMID: 19152128]

[32] Shaw LJ, Berman DS, Maron DJ, *et al.* COURAGE Investigators. Optimal medical therapy with or without percutaneous coronary intervention to reduce ischemic burden: results from the Clinical Outcomes Utilizing Revascularization and Aggressive Drug Evaluation (COURAGE) trial nuclear substudy. Circulation 2008; 117(10): 1283-91.
[http://dx.doi.org/10.1161/CIRCULATIONAHA.107.743963] [PMID: 18268144]

[33] Holly TA, Abbott BG, Al-Mallah M, *et al.* American Society of Nuclear Cardiology. Single photon-emission computed tomography. J Nucl Cardiol 2010; 17(5): 941-73.
[http://dx.doi.org/10.1007/s12350-010-9246-y] [PMID: 20552312]

[34] Yoda S, Nakanishi K, Tano A, *et al.* Diagnostic value of automated quantification of nuclear cardiology in Japanese patients with single vessel coronary artery disease: comparison between Japanese and American normal databases. J Cardiol 2013; 62(4): 224-9.
[http://dx.doi.org/10.1016/j.jjcc.2013.04.001] [PMID: 23731920]

[35] Yoda S, Nakanishi K, Tano A, *et al.* Usefulness of automated assessment of nuclear cardiology for prediction of major cardiac events in Japanese patients with known or suspected coronary artery disease: comparison with conventional visual assessment in a large-scale prognostic study. J Cardiol 2014; 64(5): 395-400.
[http://dx.doi.org/10.1016/j.jjcc.2014.02.025] [PMID: 24725761]

[36] Hachamovitch R, Hayes SW, Friedman JD, Cohen I, Berman DS. Comparison of the short-term survival benefit associated with revascularization compared with medical therapy in patients with no prior coronary artery disease undergoing stress myocardial perfusion single photon emission computed tomography. Circulation 2003; 107(23): 2900-7.
[http://dx.doi.org/10.1161/01.CIR.0000072790.23090.41] [PMID: 12771008]

[37] Moroi M, Yamashina A, Tsukamoto K, Nishimura T. J-ACCESS Investigators. Coronary revascularization does not decrease cardiac events in patients with stable ischemic heart disease but might do in those who showed moderate to severe ischemia. Int J Cardiol 2012; 158(2): 246-52.
[http://dx.doi.org/10.1016/j.ijcard.2011.01.040] [PMID: 21342709]

[38] Hori Y, Yoda S, Nakanishi K, *et al.* Myocardial ischemic reduction evidenced by gated myocardial perfusion imaging after treatment results in good prognosis in patients with coronary artery disease. J Cardiol 2015; 65(4): 278-84.
[http://dx.doi.org/10.1016/j.jjcc.2014.06.015] [PMID: 25082293]

[39] Yoda S, Nakanishi K, Tano A, *et al.* Major cardiac event risk scores estimated with gated myocardial perfusion imaging in Japanese patients with coronary artery disease. J Cardiol 2016; 67(1): 64-70.
[http://dx.doi.org/10.1016/j.jjcc.2015.04.008] [PMID: 25982667]

[40] Slomka PJ, Patton JA, Berman DS, Germano G. Advances in technical aspects of myocardial perfusion SPECT imaging. J Nucl Cardiol 2009; 16(2): 255-76.
[http://dx.doi.org/10.1007/s12350-009-9052-6] [PMID: 19242769]

[41] Du Y, Bhattacharya M, Frey EC. Simultaneous Tc-99m/I-123 dual-radionuclide myocardial perfusion/innervation imaging using Siemens IQ-SPECT with SMARTZOOM collimator. Phys Med Biol 2014; 59(11): 2813-28.
[http://dx.doi.org/10.1088/0031-9155/59/11/2813] [PMID: 24819280]

[42] Caobelli F, Ren Kaiser S, Thackeray JT, *et al.* The importance of a correct positioning of the heart using IQ-SPECT system with multifocal collimators in myocardial perfusion imaging: a phantom study. J Nucl Cardiol 2015; 22(1): 57-65.
[http://dx.doi.org/10.1007/s12350-014-9994-1] [PMID: 25273670]

[43] Matsuo S, Nakajima K, Onoguchi M, Wakabayash H, Okuda K, Kinuya S. Nuclear myocardial

perfusion imaging using thallium-201 with a novel multifocal collimator SPECT/CT: IQ-SPECT *versus* conventional protocols in normal subjects. Ann Nucl Med 2015; 29(5): 452-9. [http://dx.doi.org/10.1007/s12149-015-0965-7] [PMID: 25821018]

[44] Takahashi T, Tanaka H, Kozono N, *et al.* Characteristics of images of angiographically proven normal coronary arteries acquired by adenosine-stress thallium-201 myocardial perfusion SPECT/CT-IQ[Symbol: see text]SPECT with CT attenuation correction changed stepwise. Ann Nucl Med 2015; 29(3): 256-67. [http://dx.doi.org/10.1007/s12149-014-0935-5] [PMID: 25472779]

[45] Horiguchi Y, Ueda T, Shiomori T, *et al.* Validation of a short-scan-time imaging protocol for thallium-201 myocardial SPECT with a multifocal collimator. Ann Nucl Med 2014; 28(8): 707-15. [http://dx.doi.org/10.1007/s12149-014-0880-3] [PMID: 25038906]

[46] Ogino Y, Horiguchi Y, Ueda T, *et al.* A myocardial perfusion imaging system using a multifocal collimator for detecting coronary artery disease: validation with invasive coronary angiography. Ann Nucl Med 2015; 29(4): 366-70. [http://dx.doi.org/10.1007/s12149-015-0955-9] [PMID: 25663393]

[47] Takamura T, Horiguchi Y, Kanna M, *et al.* Validation of prone myocardial perfusion SPECT with a variable-focus collimator *versus* supine myocardial perfusion SPECT with or without computed tomography-derived attenuation correction. Ann Nucl Med 2015; 29(10): 890-6. [http://dx.doi.org/10.1007/s12149-015-1019-x] [PMID: 26307758]

[48] Shiraishi S, Sakamoto F, Tsuda N, *et al.* Prediction of left main or 3-vessel disease using myocardial perfusion reserve on dynamic thallium-201 single-photon emission computed tomography with a semiconductor gamma camera. Circ J 2015; 79(3): 623-31. [http://dx.doi.org/10.1253/circj.CJ-14-0932] [PMID: 25746547]

[49] Chikamori T. A novel Cadmium-Zinc-Telluride SPECT system: a challenge for nuclear cardiology in Japan. Ann Nucl Cardiol 2016; 2(1): 122-4. [http://dx.doi.org/10.17996/ANC.02.01.122]

[50] Miyagawa M, Nishiyama Y, Tashiro R, *et al.* Novel cardiac SPECT technology with semiconductor detectors: emerging trends and future perspective. Ann Nucl Cardiol 2015; 1(1): 18-26. [http://dx.doi.org/10.17996/ANC.01.01.18]

[51] Matsuo S, Nakae I, Tsutamoto T, Okamoto N, Horie M. A novel clinical indicator using Tc-99m sestamibi for evaluating cardiac mitochondrial function in patients with cardiomyopathies. J Nucl Cardiol 2007; 14(2): 215-20. [http://dx.doi.org/10.1016/j.nuclcard.2006.10.022] [PMID: 17386384]

[52] Matsuo S, Nakae I, Masuda D, *et al.* Noninvasive identification of myocardial sympathetic and metabolic abnormalities in a patient with restrictive cardiomyopathy - in comparison with perfusion imaging - *Ann Nucl Med* 2002; 16: 569-572. oto T, Horie M. Scintigraphic evaluation of cardiac metabolism and sympathetic nerve function in alcoholic cardiomyopathy. Intern Med 2006; 45: 57-62. [PMID: 16484740]

[53] Matsuo S, Nakae I, Masuda D, Matsumoto T, Horie M. Scintigraphic evaluation of cardiac metabolism and sympathetic nerve function in alcoholic cardiomyopathy. Intern Med 2006; 45(7): 465-7. [http://dx.doi.org/10.2169/internalmedicine.45.1696] [PMID: 16679703]

[54] Bruder O, Wagner A, Jensen CJ, *et al.* Myocardial scar visualized by cardiovascular magnetic resonance imaging predicts major adverse events in patients with hypertrophic cardiomyopathy. J Am Coll Cardiol 2010; 56(11): 875-87. Epub [http://dx.doi.org/10.1016/j.jacc.2010.05.007] [PMID: 20667520]

[55] Matsuo S, Nakajima K, Kinuya S, Sato Y, Matsumoto N, Horie M. Cardiac scintigraphic findings of mitochondrial myopathy, encephalopathy, lactic acidosis and stroke-like episodes: A case report. Exp Clin Cardiol 2008; 13(2): 93-5.

[PMID: 19343124]

[56] JCS Joint Working Group. Guidelines for clinical use of cardiac nuclear medicine (JCS 2010) – digest version –. Circ J 2012; 76(3): 761-7.
[http://dx.doi.org/10.1253/circj.CJ-88-0019] [PMID: 22293456]

CHAPTER 2

Gated Myocardial Perfusion Imaging and Risk-Stratification in Coronary Artery Disease and Heart Failure

Tomoaki Nakata[1,*], **Kenji Sato**[1] and **Kei Nakata**[1,2]

[1] *Department of Cardiology, Hakodate Goryoukaku Hospital, Hakodate, 38-3 Goryoukaku-cho, Hakodate, Japan*

[2] *School of Medicine, Sapporo Medical University, Sapporo, Hokkaidō, Japan*

Abstract: Recent advances in gated stress myocardial perfusion imaging (MPI) have facilitated the clinical use for assessment of inducible ischemia, viability and cardiac event risks in patients with known or suspected coronary artery disease (CAD). This is because gated MPI enables simultaneous quantitative analysis of regional and global myocardial perfusion and function and because cardiac functional information improves diagnostic efficacies of conventional clinical and myocardial perfusion data in the risk-stratification of CAD patients, more definitively clarifying into a low- or high-risk category. Gated stress MPI can be also applied for early identification of patients with suspected or known CAD at a high-risk for future manifestation of heart failure (HF), for differentiation of HF etiology and for improvement in risk-stratification of HF patients. In addition to clinical risks, left ventricular mechanical dyssynchrony assessed by gated MPI can be a novel powerful prognostic marker in HF patients. Thus, ECG-gating approach in stress and/or resting MPI study can contribute to better risk-stratification and to appropriate selection of prophylactic or therapeutic strategy, including optimal drugs or electrical device treatment, in a cost-effective manner in suspected or known cardiac patients.

Keywords: Coronary Artery Disease, Heart Failure, Ischemia, Mechanical Dyssynchrony, Myocardial Perfusion Imaging, Risk-Stratification.

GATED MYOCARDIAL PERFUSION IMAGING TECHNOLOGY

MPI technique using single photon emission computed tomography (SPECT) is widely used in routine clinical practice [1 - 4]. Because of a greater photo-peak (140 KeV), a shorter half-life (6 hours) and easy preparation for urgent use, ^{99m}Technetium (Tc)-labeled myocardial perfusion traces such as sestamibi and

* **Corresponding author Tomoaki Nakata**, Department of Cardiology, Hakodate Goryoukaku Hospital, Hakodate. 38-3 Goryoukaku-cho, Hakodate 040-8611, Japan; Tel: +81-138-51-2295; Fax: +81-138-56-2695; E-mail: tnakata@sapmed.ac.jp

tetrofosmin overcomes disadvantages of ^{201}Thallium chloride (^{201}Tl). This contributes to an improvement in image quality and diagnostic accuracy and to less radiation exposure and allows electrocardiogram (ECG)-gating approach. In particular, a high-count image enables ECG-gating approach in MPI which evaluates myocardial perfusion and left ventricular function with a single study. ECG-gated MPI can simultaneously evaluate myocardial perfusion and cardiac function using three-dimensional data, contributing to time-saving and precise assessment and to improvement in cost-effectiveness of this technique by reducing necessity of two-dimensional echography, conventional radionuclide or contrast left ventricular angiography for cardiac function assessment.

Technological advances in computerized analysis and displays of 3- and 4-dimesional SPECT data have remarkably facilitated clinical application of this technique to nuclear cardiology practice in patients with coronary artery disease (CAD) or heart failure. There are several established softwares available which are reproducible, practical and easily operated; *Cedars-Sinai QGS (Quantitative Gated SPECT), Sapporo P-FAST (Perfusion and Function Assessment for gated-SPECT) program, Emory Cardiac Toolbox, Michigan 4D-MSPECT*, *Heart function view/Heart risk view* and *CardioREPO* softwares. Regional perfusion abnormality is conventionally evaluated visually using a semi-quantitative analysis with a 5-point, 17-segment model then global perfusion abnormality is calculated as summed stress sore (SSS), summed rest score (SRS) and summed difference score (SDS) when stress imaging is performed (Fig. **1**). Food and Drug Administration guidelines recommend independent semi-quantitative visual interpretation of MPI by multiple experts in clinical investigations for minimizing inter- and intra-observer errors. Multiple-expert assessment, however, is not necessarily available for routine clinical practice at a community hospital. In addition to quantitative analysis of cardiac function, recent softwares for gated MPI can provide automated quantitative perfusion data which are well compatible with expert visual semi-quantitative results [5 - 7]. These automated scoring systems are more reproducible and objective than a visual scoring. ECG-gated MPI provides global and regional functional information, such as left ventricular end-diastolic volume (EDV), end-systolic volume (ESV), left ventricular ejection fraction (LVEF), regional wall motion and wall thickening (Fig. **2**). Regional wall motion is visually assessed using a cine-mode display as performed conventionally by two-dimensional echocardiography. In addition, gated MPI can evaluate regional wall thickening by comparing differences in myocardial counts between at end-diastole and at end-systole.

Thus, computerized analysis of gated MPI can provide regional and global quantitative data on myocardial perfusion and function in a highly objective, reproducible and cost-effective manner.

Clinical Implications of Gated MPI

A mismatched appearance between myocardial perfusion and function is often observed in injured but viable myocardium in patients with CAD and/or heart failure. As its typical example, myocardial stunning and hibernation are well known. The pathological conditions can be identified by simultaneous comparison of regional myocardial perfusion and functional using gated stress/rest MPI. During a recovery process from acute coronary syndrome, more reduced wall motion relative to better perfusion (^{99m}Tc-labled) tracer uptake indicates post-ischemic myocardial stunning which is often observed in patients undergoing urgent coronary reperfusion/ revascularization procedures. Even if myocardial ischemia is successfully treated, regional wall motion abnormality persists during a several-day-to-week but gradually recovers depending on the grade and duration of acute ischemic event and residual myocardial viability [8]. This dis-concordant phenomenon between depressed regional wall motion and preserved perfusion tracer uptake without significant residual myocardial ischemia is identified as post-ischemic myocardial stunning by gated MPI. When severer myocardial ischemia persists for a relatively long time in patients with chronic CAD, regional wall motion is impaired and LVEF reduces, sometimes being responsible for ischemia-induced heart failure. Impairment of cardiac function improves regionally and globally during a several-week-to-month following appropriate revascularization treatment [9]. The dys-functioning but viable myocardium with persistent ischemia is identified as hibernating myocardium by gated stress/rest MPI. Identification of stunned or hibernating myocardium, both of which are ischemia-related myocardial injury but have residual myocardial viability, is crucial clinically to predict functional recovery after therapeutic intervention using drugs and/or revascularization procedures.

Another important clinical application of gated MPI is for the improvement in differentiation of artefactual appearance of perfusion abnormality particularly when perfusion findings are equivocal [10, 11]. Myocardial perfusion-wall motion correlation is evaluated using a cine-mode display or by comparing myocardial perfusion polar maps at end-diastole and end-systole. Reduced tracer uptake with normal or near normal wall motion is considered as an artefactual or no significant (negligible) perfusion abnormality, increasing specificity in myocardial perfusion study. In contrast, near normal-to-mild or equivocal perfusion abnormality is more clearly diagnosed as pathologic rather than artefactual when definitive wall motion abnormality is present, improving sensitivity in myocardial perfusion study. Overalls, the addition of a gating approach to traditional MPI improves the diagnostic accuracy by 5 to 10%. Stress-induced reversibility of both regional perfusion and wall motion abnormalities indicates ischemic and viable myocardium, but myocardium is necrotic and less viable (*i.e.*, nearly infarcted) when both regional perfusion and wall motion abnormalities are fixed (non-reversible) at stress and resting studies. For viability assessment, quantification of resting regional tracer uptake is also useful. When myocardial uptake of perfusion tracer relative to that of a normal area (*i.e.*, a percent tracer uptake) is 50% or more, myocardial viability is significantly present, whereas a percent tracer uptake of 40% or less indicates no or little myocardial viability [12]. It is also worth addressing here that when resting regional and/or global cardiac dysfunction is present in viable but non-ischemic myocardium without reversible perfusion abnormality, non-ischemic etiology should be considered if stunned myocardium in a recovery process following acute ischemic event is ruled out.

Thus, simultaneous assessment of regional wall motion and myocardial perfusion by gated stress/rest MPI enables better differentiation of pathologic *versus* non-pathologic, ischemic *versus* non-ischemic or stunning *versus* hibernating myocardium. These evaluations are clinically crucial for selecting therapeutic approaches and predicting efficacies of therapeutic interventions.

Risk-Stratification in Coronary Artery Disease

Assessment of myocardial ischemia and viability is indispensable and central to the issue for appropriate management based on risk-stratification in patients with suspected or known CAD. This includes evidence-based selection of therapeutic interventions using optimal drugs and/or coronary revascularization and precise prediction of improvement in cardiac function and clinical outcomes. This also implies that when neither myocardial ischemia nor viability is present, no coronary intervention is effective for functional or prognostic improvement. The prognostic values of the following functional derangement in combination with myocardial perfusion abnormality have been identified in stress myocardial perfusion study without an ECG-gating approach in the past [13]; stress-induced manifestation of left ventricular enlargement, reduction in LVEF and an increase in lung uptake of perfusion tracer (^{201}Tl). There are robust data on the ability of stress/rest MPI using a semi-quantitative scoring system for risk-stratification in patients with suspected or known CAD; particularly SSS and %ischemia have been shown to be powerful prognostic biomarkers [14 - 23] (Fig. **1**). A moderate-to-severe ischemic burden assessed by SSS (9 or more) or a percent ischemia (10% or more) is closely related to fatal and non-fatal myocardial infarction, cardiac death, heart failure and coronary revascularization treatment as shown by the Clinical Outcomes Utilizing Revascularization and Aggressive Drug Evaluation (COURAGE) trial [19, 23] and the Japanese Assessment of Cardiac Events and Survival Study by Quantitative Gated SPECT (J-ACCESS) [17]. The high risk category identified by SSS and % ischemia, therefore, is an appropriate target for invasive strategy such as coronary revascularization together with optimal medical treatment, contributing to significantly reducing an ischemic burden of 5% or more, to prevention of future cardiac events and to better clinical outcomes. In contrast, no-to-mild ischemic burden (SSS of 0-8 or %ischemia less than 10%) indicates a low-risk category which needs second prevention and heart failure control by modifying coronary risks together with optimal drug treatment rather than invasive strategy.

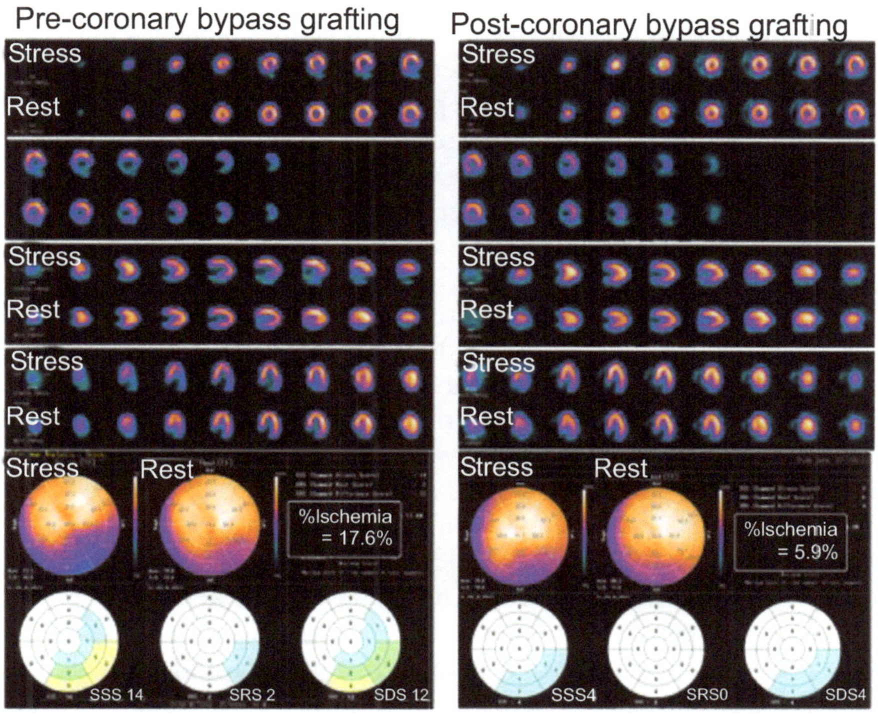

Fig. (1). A 68-year old male patient presenting with exercise-induced chest discomfort who underwent coronary artery bypass grafting because of the high-risk category identified by adenosine-stress gated myocardial perfusion imaging; the severe reversible ischemia with summed stress score (SSS) of 14 and % ischemia of 17.6% together with transient ischemic dilatation of left ventricle (as shown by visual assessment). After a 3-vessel coronary grafting, the high-risk ischemia improved together with reduction in SSS (4) and % ischemia (5.9%).

The addition of functional information to semi-quantitative data on myocardial perfusion abnormality derived from gated stress/rest MPI improves risk-stratification by conventional stress myocardial perfusion data alone. Post-stress LVEF and ESV, of which cutoff values are 45% and 70mL, respectively, can be incremental prognostic biomarkers to stress perfusion score (SSS) for more precisely discriminating high-risk or low-risk CAD patients from others [21, 22]. Patients at intermediate risk shown by mild-to-moderate perfusion abnormality such as SSS of 4-13 are more definitively clarified into higher or lower risk by identifying whether LVEF is less than 45% or not, or whether ESV is greater than 70mL or not, respectively [21]. Furthermore, severe perfusion abnormality with SSS more than 13 does not necessarily indicate high-risk when LVEF is 45% or more or ESV is 70mL or less in these studies. Stress induced-reduction in LVEF by 5% or more is related to reversible ischemia and cardiac events, contributing to improvement in risk stratification in both diabetic and non-diabetic patients [24 - 27]. Cutoff values f LVEF, ESV or ESVI at rest or at stress, however, could be affected by clinical variables such as outcomes (lethal or non-lethal, cardiac or non-cardiac, and ischemic or non-ischemic end points), age, gender, coronary risks, disease severity and imaging procedures in each facility [28, 29]. Nevertheless, a 2-year risk assessment on lethal ischemic event is demonstrated by creating risk-based nomograms using %ischemia, rest and/or post-stress LVEF based on robust stress myocardial perfusion data [30]. Post-stress transient ischemic dilatation (TID) can be an important marker of severe myocardial ischemia and adverse outcomes due to multi-vessel or left main disease complementary to standard perfusion assessment in patients with known or suspected CAD [13, 31] (Figs. **1** and **2**). Although the mechanism is still controversial, TID is due to extensive sub-endocardial ischemia [32] and/or cavity enlargement induced by global left ventricular dysfunction. Besides conventional visual assessment, TID is quantitatively defined by a 1.2 or more increase in a stress-to-rest ratio of left ventricular volume assessed by gated myocardial perfusion study and has incremental prognostic values together with clinical risks and stress myocardial perfusion data [33, 34]. Likewise, post-stress transient reduction in regional wall motion or global wall thickening is likely to be predictive of adverse cardiac outcomes independently of LVEF and SSS [35 - 37]. It is also worth noting that normal gated stress myocardial perfusion findings defined by SSS, LVEF and/or ESV indicates a low risk category with a high probability of excellent prognosis [38] even in asymptomatic diabetic patients, in whom a major cardiac event rate of 0.8%/year was reported in the J-ACCESS study [39], and in patients at a clinically high risk [40].

Thus, gated stress/rest MPI with quantitative analysis of cardiac function and perfusion contributes to facilitation of risk-based (high-risk or low-risk) management not only by maximizing efficacies of therapeutic interventions but also by minimizing unnecessity procedures and medical costs in patients with suspected or known CAD.

Risk-Stratification in Heart Failure

Heart failure (HF) is another central issue for healthcare policies and appropriate use of limited medical resources at the era of aging population in developed countries. Gated stress perfusion imaging is useful for the determination of types and etiologies of heart failure as follows; HF with reduced LVEF (HFrEF) *versus* HF with preserved LVEF (HFpEF) and ischemic *versus* non-ischemic HF, respectively. The clinical process is indispensable not only for precise diagnosis but also for selecting optimal management strategy and predicting clinical outcomes. HFrEF is defined as heart failure with LVEF less than 40% and HFpEF is defined as heart failure with LVEF of 50% or more. The definition, however, is still equivocal and controversial when LVEF is between 40-50%. Some investigators names as HF with moderately reduced EF (HFmEF). Technical problems especially using tow-dimensional assessment of LVEF with a low reproducibility make the precise definition of LVEF difficult. Left ventricular volume data (EDV/ESV) can identify left ventricular remodeling or enlargement. When patients have HFrEF, it is of great importance to evaluate the presence and grade of myocardial ischemia, viability and infarcted myocardium (*i.e.*, scarred tissue) for determining the necessity of invasive therapeutic strategy before cardiac catheterization. Particularly in HF patients without known CAD or its prior history, gated stress imaging protocol is useful for differentiating ischemic from non-ischemic etiology in HF patients. without a definitive myocardial perfusion abnormality have a high probability of non-ischemic etiology rather than ischemic with a 100% of negative predictive value and a 63% of positive predictive value [41]. The low positive predictive value indicates the necessity to identify the etiology of fixed perfusion abnormality due to non-ischemic myocardial necrosis or degenerative tissue such post-myocarditis, cardiac sarcoidosis, advanced hypertrophic cardiomyopathy, idiopathic dilated cardiomyopathy, Takotsubo cardiomyopathy and so force. Even before establishment of CAD diagnosis, ischemic perfusion score (SSS) assessed by gated stress MPI is superior to pre-scan clinical information for predicting cardiac mortality risk in patients with HFrEF [42]. In patients with ischemic cardiomyopathy, which is defined as ischemic HFrEF with left ventricular remodeling, gated stress perfusion study can discriminate patients who can benefit from coronary revascularization therapy by evaluating residual myocardial viability (SRS), ischemia (SSS and SDS) and ESV [43]. As mentioned at the previous section, independently of heart failure status, a sufficient ischemic burden together with residual myocardial viability at diseased coronary territories indicates a high probability of improvement in cardiac function and subsequent clinical outcomes. Thus, by combined use of cardiac functional and perfusion data, gated stress MPI can improve differential diagnosis of HF and risk-stratification of patients with ischemic HF, contributing to appropriate selection of therapeutic strategy, including a necessity of invasive coronary interventions, and to better clinical outcomes.

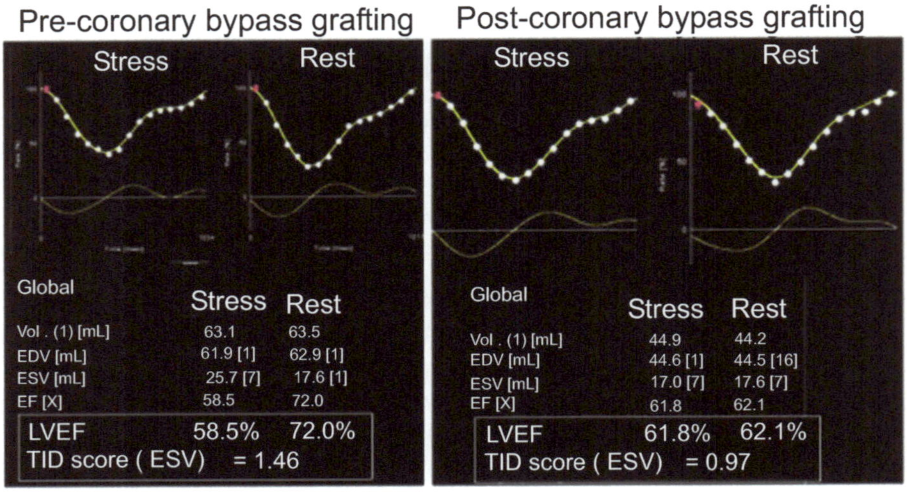

Fig. (2). The quantitative functional analysis of the stress imaging with adenosine shows transient ischemic dilatation (TID) of left ventricle (TID score, 1.46) which apparently disappeared (TID score, 0.97) in association with the ischemia improvement after the coronary revascularization treatment.

Because of recurrent and refractory features of HF, a prophylactic medical management is highly desirable before manifestation or progression of HF symptoms in patients at increased risks for coronary events and ischemic HF. Risks of new-onset HF were revealed using gated stress MPI with quantitative analysis in 3835 patients with suspected or known CAD derived from the J-ACCESS database [44]. ESV index and SSS assessed by gated stress myocardial perfusion study risk-stratified patients into low-, intermediate- and high-risk categories for fatal and non-fatal new-onset HF independently and additively with impaired kidney function. Thus, early risk-stratification of patients with increased clinical risks for HF possibly contributes to cost-saving management strategy for prevention of HF manifestation and improvement in clinical outcomes.

Besides simultaneous assessment of conventional cardiac function and myocardial perfusion, gated MPI can quantify and characterize left ventricular mechanical synchrony using phase analysis of time-volume curves of whole left ventricular segments with a single study. When compared to electrocardiographic or echocardiographic assessment of left ventricular dyssynchrony, this method using gated SPECT data has several advantages. This method is highly reliable, reproducible, objective and repeatable at clinical practice because of recent advances in gated SPECT program and use of three-dimensional SPECT data without a dead corner. A wide-spread phase angles at systole indicate left ventricular mechanical dyssynchrony (LVMD); in other words, dys-synchronized temporal abnormality of the initiation of left ventricular contraction. LVMD assessed by gated SPECT imaging is associated with three-dimensional inhomogeneity in myocardial perfusion abnormality or persistent ischemia, cardiac tissue injury and metabolic impairment (high-energy phosphate depletion), all of which are responsible not only for heterogeneous electrophysiological instability and increased arrhythmogenecity but also for a loss of contractile force. Despite the need of standardization of left ventricular mechanical dyssynchrony, LVMD is defined by several indices such as a standard deviation (SD) of phase angles, a bandwidth of phase histogram or phase entropy. LVMD have significant prognostic values for identifying high cardiac mortality risk and is likely to be superior to conventional prognostic markers such as LVEF, BNP and a wide QRS complex [45 - 53]. LVMD can be a biomarker not only for the indication of synchronization therapy (CRT) but also for predicting patient outcomes following the initiation of CRT in HF patients. In addition to device troubles, this is clinically noted because, despite the definitive efficacies of CRT, CRT is not effective in nearly one third of HFrEF patients who met current CRT criteria using NYHA functional class III/IV, depressed LVEF and prolonged QRS duration (electrical dyssynchrony) in terms of improvement in quality of life and cardiac mortality. LVMD and impairment of cardiac sympathetic innervation assessed by cardiac ^{123}I-metaiodobenzylguanidine (MIBG) activity have independent and additive prognostic values in patients with HRrEF [50, 54].

Thus, gated stress/rest MPI can contribute to improvement in differential diagnosis of HF, risk stratification and selection of therapeutic strategy based on etiology and type of HF, and probably to optimizing clinical benefits of drug and device treatment in HF patients in combination with currently available methods, although a larger-scale multicenter study is still required.

CONSENT FOR PUBLICATION

Not applicable.

CONFLICT OF INTEREST

The authors declare no conflict of interest, financial or otherwise.

ACKNOWLEDGEMENTS

Declared none.

REFERENCES

[1] Klocke FJ, Baird MG, Lorell BH, *et al.* ACC/AHA/ASNC guidelines for the clinical use of cardiac radionuclide imaging--executive summary: a report of the American College of Cardiology/American Heart Association Task Force on Practice Guidelines (ACC/AHA/ASNC Committee to Revise the 1995 Guidelines for the Clinical Use of Cardiac Radionuclide Imaging). Circulation. 2003 Sep 16;108:

1404-18. J Am Coll Cardiol 2003; 42: 1318-33.
[http://dx.doi.org/10.1016/j.jacc.2003.08.011] [PMID: 14522503]

[2] Hendel RC, Berman DS, Di Carli MF, *et al.* ACCF/ASNC/ACR/AHA/ASE/SCCT/SCMR/SNM 2009 Appropriate Use Criteria for Cardiac Radionuclide Imaging: A Report of the American College of Cardiology Foundation Appropriate Use Criteria Task Force. Circulation 2009 Jun 9;119:e561-87. J Am Coll Cardiol 2009; 53: 2201-29.
[http://dx.doi.org/10.1016/j.jacc.2009.02.013] [PMID: 19497454]

[3] Henzlova MJ, Cerqueira MD, Hansen CL, *et al.* ASNC Imaging Guidelines for Nuclear Cardiology Procedures: Stress protocols and tracers. J Nucl Cardiol 2009. http://www.asnc.org/imageuploads/ImagingGuidelinesStressProtocols021109.pdf

[4] JCS Joint Working Group. Guidelines for clinical use of cardiac nuclear medicine (JCS 2010) – digest version –. Circ J 2012; 76(3): 761-7. http://www.j-circ.or.jp/guideline/index.htm
[http://dx.doi.org/10.1253/circj.CJ-88-0019] [PMID: 22293456]

[5] Berman DS, Kang X, Van Train KF, *et al.* Comparative prognostic value of automatic quantitative analysis *versus* semiquantitative visual analysis of exercise myocardial perfusion single-photon emission computed tomography. J Am Coll Cardiol 1998; 32(7): 1987-95.
[http://dx.doi.org/10.1016/S0735-1097(98)00501-4] [PMID: 9857883]

[6] Yoshinaga K, Matsuki T, Hashimoto A, Tsukamoto K, Nakata T, Tamaki N. Validation of automated quantitation of myocardial perfusion and fatty acid metabolism abnormalities on SPECT images. Circ J 2011; 75(9): 2187-95.
[http://dx.doi.org/10.1253/circj.CJ-10-1272] [PMID: 21747199]

[7] Nakata T, Hashimoto A, Matsuki T, Yoshinaga K, Tsukamoto K, Tamaki N. Prognostic value of automated SPECT scoring system for coronary artery disease in stress myocardial perfusion and fatty acid metabolism imaging. Int J Cardiovasc Imaging 2013; 29(1): 253-62.
[http://dx.doi.org/10.1007/s10554-012-0069-6] [PMID: 22782310]

[8] Hashimoto A, Nakata T, Tsuchihashi K, Tanaka S, Fujimori K, Iimura O. Postischemic functional recovery and BMIPP uptake after primary percutaneous transluminal coronary angioplasty in acute myocardial infarction. Am J Cardiol 1996; 77(1): 25-30.
[http://dx.doi.org/10.1016/S0002-9149(97)89129-1] [PMID: 8540452]

[9] Taki J, Nakajima K, Matsunari I, *et al.* Assessment of improvement of myocardial fatty acid uptake and function after revascularization using iodine-123-BMIPP. J Nucl Med 1997; 38(10): 1503-10.
[PMID: 9379183]

[10] DePuey EG, Rozanski A. Using gated technetium-99m-sestamibi SPECT to characterize fixed myocardial defects as infarct or artifact. J Nucl Med 1995; 36(6): 952-5.
[PMID: 7769451]

[11] Taillefer R, DePuey EG, Udelson JE, Beller GA, Latour Y, Reeves F. Comparative diagnostic accuracy of Tl-201 and Tc-99m sestamibi SPECT imaging (perfusion and ECG-gated SPECT) in detecting coronary artery disease in women. J Am Coll Cardiol 1997; 29(1): 69-77.
[http://dx.doi.org/10.1016/S0735-1097(96)00435-4] [PMID: 8996297]

[12] Udelson JE, Coleman PS, Metherall J, *et al.* Predicting recovery of severe regional ventricular dysfunction. Comparison of resting scintigraphy with 201Tl and 99mTc-sestamibi. Circulation 1994; 89(6): 2552-61.
[http://dx.doi.org/10.1161/01.CIR.89.6.2552] [PMID: 8205664]

[13] Gibbons RJ. Myocardial perfusion imaging. Heart 2000; 83(3): 355-60.
[http://dx.doi.org/10.1136/heart.83.3.355] [PMID: 10677421]

[14] Gibbons RJ, Hodge DO, Berman DS, *et al.* Long-term outcome of patients with intermediate-risk exercise electrocardiograms who do not have myocardial perfusion defects on radionuclide imaging. Circulation 1999; 100(21): 2140-5.
[http://dx.doi.org/10.1161/01.CIR.100.21.2140] [PMID: 10571972]

[15] Hachamovitch R, Hayes SW, Friedman JD, Cohen I, Berman DS. Comparison of the short-term survival benefit associated with revascularization compared with medical therapy in patients with no prior coronary artery disease undergoing stress myocardial perfusion single photon emission computed tomography. Circulation 2003; 107(23): 2900-7. [http://dx.doi.org/10.1161/01.CIR.0000072790.23090.41] [PMID: 12771008]

[16] ACCF/AHA/ASE/ASNC/HFSA/HRS/SCAI/SCCT/SCMR/STS 2013. Multimodality appropriate use criteria for the detection and risk assessment of stable ischemic heart disease: A Report of the American College of Cardiology Foundation Appropriate Use Criteria Task Force, American Heart Association, American Society of Echocardiography, American Society of Nuclear Cardiology, Heart Failure Society of America, Heart Rhythm Society, Society for Cardiovascular Angiography and Interventions, Society of Cardiovascular Computed Tomography, Society for Cardiovascular Magnetic Resonance, and Society of Thoracic Surgeons. J Am Coll Cardiol 2013 Dec 10; pii S0735-1097(13)06147-0

[17] Nishimura T, Nakajima K, Kusuoka H, Yamashina A, Nishimura S. Prognostic study of risk stratification among Japanese patients with ischemic heart disease using gated myocardial perfusion SPECT: J-ACCESS study. Eur J Nucl Med Mol Imaging 2008; 35(2): 319-28. [http://dx.doi.org/10.1007/s00259-007-0608-x] [PMID: 17926033]

[18] Hashimoto A, Nakata T, Wakabayashi T, Kusuoka H, Nishimura T. Incremental prognostic value of stress/rest gated perfusion SPECT in patients with coronary artery disease--subanalysis of the J-ACCESS study. Circ J 2009; 73(12): 2288-93. [http://dx.doi.org/10.1253/circj.CJ-09-0212] [PMID: 19797824]

[19] Boden WE, O'Rourke RA, Teo KK, *et al.* COURAGE Trial Research Group. Optimal medical therapy with or without PCI for stable coronary disease. N Engl J Med 2007; 356(15): 1503-16. [http://dx.doi.org/10.1056/NEJMoa070829] [PMID: 17387127]

[20] Hendel RC, Whitfield SS, Villegas BJ, Cutler BS, Leppo JA. Prediction of late cardiac events by dipyridamole thallium imaging in patients undergoing elective vascular surgery. Am J Cardiol 1992; 70(15): 1243-9. [http://dx.doi.org/10.1016/0002-9149(92)90756-O] [PMID: 1442573]

[21] Sharir T, Germano G, Kang X, *et al.* Prediction of myocardial infarction *versus* cardiac death by gated myocardial perfusion SPECT: risk stratification by the amount of stress-induced ischemia and the poststress ejection fraction. J Nucl Med 2001; 42(6): 831-7. [PMID: 11390544]

[22] Sharir T, Germano G, Kavanagh PB, *et al.* Incremental prognostic value of post-stress left ventricular ejection fraction and volume by gated myocardial perfusion single photon emission computed tomography. Circulation 1999; 100(10): 1035-42. [http://dx.doi.org/10.1161/01.CIR.100.10.1035] [PMID: 10477527]

[23] Shaw LJ, Berman DS, Maron DJ, *et al.* COURAGE Investigators. Optimal medical therapy with or without percutaneous coronary intervention to reduce ischemic burden: results from the Clinical Outcomes Utilizing Revascularization and Aggressive Drug Evaluation (COURAGE) trial nuclear substudy. Circulation 2008; 117(10): 1283-91. [http://dx.doi.org/10.1161/CIRCULATIONAHA.107.743963] [PMID: 18268144]

[24] Guenancia C, Cochet A, Humbert O, *et al.* Predictors of post-stress LVEF drop 6 months after reperfused myocardial infarction: a gated myocardial perfusion SPECT study. Ann Nucl Med 2013; 27(2): 112-22. [http://dx.doi.org/10.1007/s12149-012-0661-9] [PMID: 23065422]

[25] Dona M, Massi L, Settimo L, *et al.* Prognostic implications of post-stress ejection fraction decrease detected by gated SPECT in the absence of stress-induced perfusion abnormalities. Eur J Nucl Med Mol Imaging 2011; 38(3): 485-90. [http://dx.doi.org/10.1007/s00259-010-1643-6] [PMID: 21061121]

[26] Kato M, Matsumoto N, Nakano Y, *et al.* Combined assessment of myocardial perfusion and function by ECG-gated myocardial perfusion single-photon emission computed tomography for the prediction of future cardiac events in patients with type 2 diabetes mellitus. Circ J 2011; 75(2): 376-82. [http://dx.doi.org/10.1253/circj.CJ-10-0794] [PMID: 21178295]

[27] Carvalho PA, Aguiar PM, Grossman GB, *et al.* Prognostic implications of the difference between left ventricular ejection fractions after stress and at rest in addition to the quantification of myocardial perfusion abnormalities obtained with gated SPECT. Clin Nucl Med 2012; 37(8): 748-54. [http://dx.doi.org/10.1097/RLU.0b013e31825ae755] [PMID: 22785501]

[28] Candell-Riera J, Ferreira-González I, Marsal JR, *et al.* Usefulness of exercise test and myocardial perfusion-gated single photon emission computed tomography to improve the prediction of major events. Circ Cardiovasc Imaging 2013; 6(4): 531-41. [http://dx.doi.org/10.1161/CIRCIMAGING.112.000158] [PMID: 23766340]

[29] Sharir T, Kang X, Germano G, *et al.* Prognostic value of poststress left ventricular volume and ejection fraction by gated myocardial perfusion SPECT in women and men: gender-related differences in normal limits and outcomes. J Nucl Cardiol 2006; 13(4): 495-506. [http://dx.doi.org/10.1016/j.nuclcard.2006.03.019] [PMID: 16919573]

[30] Shaw LJ, Min JK, Hachamovitch R, Hendel RC, Borges-Neto S, Berman DS. Nomograms for estimating coronary artery disease prognosis with gated stress myocardial perfusion SPECT. J Nucl Cardiol 2012; 19(1): 43-52. [http://dx.doi.org/10.1007/s12350-011-9468-7] [PMID: 22045394]

[31] Afonso L, Mahajan N. Single-photon emission computed tomography myocardial perfusion imaging in the diagnosis of left main disease. Clin Cardiol 2009; 32(12): E11-5. [http://dx.doi.org/10.1002/clc.20534] [PMID: 20014205]

[32] Emmett L, Ng A, Ha L, *et al.* Comparative assessment of rest and post-stress left ventricular volumes and left ventricular ejection fraction on gated myocardial perfusion imaging (MPI) and echocardiography in patients with transient ischaemic dilation on adenosine MPI: myocardial stunning or subendocardial hypoperfusion? J Nucl Cardiol 2012; 19(4): 735-42. [http://dx.doi.org/10.1007/s12350-012-9571-4] [PMID: 22565241]

[33] Xu Y, Arsanjani R, Clond M, *et al.* Transient ischemic dilation for coronary artery disease in quantitative analysis of same-day sestamibi myocardial perfusion SPECT. J Nucl Cardiol 2012; 19(3): 465-73. [http://dx.doi.org/10.1007/s12350-012-9527-8] [PMID: 22399366]

[34] Petretta M, Acampa W, Daniele S, *et al.* Transient ischemic dilation in SPECT myocardial perfusion imaging for prediction of severe coronary artery disease in diabetic patients. J Nucl Cardiol 2013; 20(1): 45-52. [http://dx.doi.org/10.1007/s12350-012-9642-6] [PMID: 23090352]

[35] Kapetanopoulos A, Ahlberg AW, Taub CC, Katten DM, Heller GV. Regional wall-motion abnormalities on post-stress electrocardiographic-gated technetium-99m sestamibi single-photon emission computed tomography imaging predict cardiac events. J Nucl Cardiol 2007; 14(6): 810-7. [http://dx.doi.org/10.1016/j.nuclcard.2007.07.014] [PMID: 18022107]

[36] Travin MI, Heller GV, Johnson LL, *et al.* The prognostic value of ECG-gated SPECT imaging in patients undergoing stress Tc-99m sestamibi myocardial perfusion imaging. J Nucl Cardiol 2004; 11(3): 253-62. [http://dx.doi.org/10.1016/j.nuclcard.2004.02.005] [PMID: 15173772]

[37] Lairez O, Cognet T, Dercle L, *et al.* Prediction of all-cause mortality from gated-SPECT global myocardial wall thickening: comparison with ejection fraction and global longitudinal 2D-strain. J Nucl Cardiol 2014; 21(1): 86-95. [http://dx.doi.org/10.1007/s12350-013-9813-0] [PMID: 24170624]

[38] Muramatsu T, Nishimura S, Yamashina A, Nishimura T. J-ACCESS Investigators. Relation between

prognosis and myocardial perfusion imaging from the difference of end-point criterion for exercise stress testing: a sub-analysis of the J-ACCESS study. J Cardiol 2010; 56(1): 51-8. [http://dx.doi.org/10.1016/j.jjcc.2010.02.005] [PMID: 20381317]

[39] Matsuo S, Nakajima K, Yamasaki Y, Kashiwagi A, Nishimura T. Prognostic value of normal stress myocardial perfusion imaging and ventricular function in Japanese asymptomatic patients with type 2 diabetes--a study based on the J-ACCESS-2 database. Circ J 2010; 74(9): 1916-21. [http://dx.doi.org/10.1253/circj.CJ-10-0098] [PMID: 20631452]

[40] Ferreira MJ, Cunha MJ, Albuquerque A, *et al.* Prognosis of normal stress-only gated-SPECT myocardial perfusion imaging: a single center study. Int J Cardiovasc Imaging 2013; 29(7): 1639-44. [http://dx.doi.org/10.1007/s10554-013-0245-3] [PMID: 23733238]

[41] Udelson JE, Shafer CD, Carrió I. Radionuclide imaging in heart failure: assessing etiology and outcomes and implications for management. J Nucl Cardiol 2002; 9(5) (Suppl.): 40S-52S. [http://dx.doi.org/10.1067/mnc.2002.128461] [PMID: 12271264]

[42] Ahlberg AW, Kazi FA, Azemi T, *et al.* Usefulness of stress gated technetium-99m single photon emission computed tomographic myocardial perfusion imaging for the prediction of cardiac death in patients with moderate to severe left ventricular systolic dysfunction and suspected coronary artery disease. Am J Cardiol 2012; 109(1): 26-30. [http://dx.doi.org/10.1016/j.amjcard.2011.07.066] [PMID: 21943938]

[43] Romero-Farina G, Candell-Riera J, Aguadé-Bruix S, Ferreira-Gonzalez I, Igual A, García-Dorado D. Relationship between myocardial perfusion-gated SPECT and the performance of coronary revascularization in patients with ischemic cardiomyopathy. Clin Nucl Med 2012; 37(10): 965-70. [http://dx.doi.org/10.1097/RLU.0b013e318263907b] [PMID: 22955070]

[44] Nakata T, Hashimoto A, Wakabayashi T, Kusuoka H, Nishimura T. Prediction of new-onset refractory congestive heart failure using stress/rest gated perfusion SPECT imaging in patients with known or suspected coronary artery disease: Sub-analysis of the J-ACCESS. J Am Coll Cardiol Cardiovasc Imaging 2009; 2: 1393-400. [http://dx.doi.org/10.1016/j.jcmg.2009.09.010] [PMID: 20083074]

[45] Friehling M, Chen J, Saba S, *et al.* A prospective pilot study to evaluate the relationship between acute change in left ventricular synchrony after cardiac resynchronization therapy and patient outcome using a single-injection gated SPECT protocol. Circ Cardiovasc Imaging 2011; 4(5): 532-9. [http://dx.doi.org/10.1161/CIRCIMAGING.111.965459] [PMID: 21772007]

[46] Uebleis C, Hellweger S, Laubender RP, *et al.* Left ventricular dyssynchrony assessed by gated SPECT phase analysis is an independent predictor of death in patients with advanced coronary artery disease and reduced left ventricular function not undergoing cardiac resynchronization therapy. Eur J Nucl Med Mol Imaging 2012; 39(10): 1561-9. [http://dx.doi.org/10.1007/s00259-012-2157-1] [PMID: 22752450]

[47] Pazhenkottil AP, Buechel RR, Husmann L, *et al.* Long-term prognostic value of left ventricular dyssynchrony assessment by phase analysis from myocardial perfusion imaging. Heart 2011; 97(1): 33-7. [http://dx.doi.org/10.1136/hrt.2010.201566] [PMID: 20962345]

[48] Wang L, Yang MF, Cai M, Zhao SH, He ZX, Wang YT. Prognostic significance of left ventricular dyssynchrony by phase analysis of gated SPECT in medically treated patients with dilated cardiomyopathy. Clin Nucl Med 2013; 38(7): 510-5. [http://dx.doi.org/10.1097/RLU.0b013e318292eedf] [PMID: 23698460]

[49] Zafrir N, Nevzorov R, Bental T, *et al.* Prognostic value of left ventricular dyssynchrony by myocardial perfusion-gated SPECT in patients with normal and abnormal left ventricular functions. J Nucl Cardiol 2014; 21(3): 532-40. [http://dx.doi.org/10.1007/s12350-014-9852-1] [PMID: 24623397]

[50] Hage FG, Aggarwal H, Patel K, *et al.* The relationship of left ventricular mechanical dyssynchrony

and cardiac sympathetic denervation to potential sudden cardiac death events in systolic heart failure. J Nucl Cardiol 2014; 21(1): 78-85.
[http://dx.doi.org/10.1007/s12350-013-9807-y] [PMID: 24170623]

[51] Chen J, Garcia EV, Bax JJ, Iskandrian AE, Borges-Neto S, Soman P. SPECT myocardial perfusion imaging for the assessment of left ventricular mechanical dyssynchrony. J Nucl Cardiol 2011; 18(4): 685-94.
[http://dx.doi.org/10.1007/s12350-011-9392-x] [PMID: 21567281]

[52] Bhatia RS, Tu JV, Lee DS, *et al.* Outcome of heart failure with preserved ejection fraction in a population-based study. N Engl J Med 2006; 355(3): 260-9.
[http://dx.doi.org/10.1056/NEJMoa051530] [PMID: 16855266]

[53] Hunt SA, Abraham WT, Chin MH, *et al.* American College of Cardiology Foundation; American Heart Association. 2009 Focused update incorporated into the ACC/AHA 2005 Guidelines for the Diagnosis and Management of Heart Failure in Adults A Report of the American College of Cardiology Foundation/American Heart Association Task Force on Practice Guidelines Developed in Collaboration With the International Society for Heart and Lung Transplantation. J Am Coll Cardiol 2009; 53(15): e1-e90.
[http://dx.doi.org/10.1016/j.jacc.2008.11.013] [PMID: 19358937]

[54] Doi T, Nakata T, Yuda S, Hashimoto A. Synergistic prognostic implications of left ventricular mechanical dyssynchrony and impaired cardiac sympathetic nerve activity in heart failure patients with reduced left ventricular ejection fraction. Eur Heart J Cardiovasc Imaging 2018; 19(1): 74-83.
[http://dx.doi.org/10.1093/ehjci/jew334] [PMID: 28158459]

CHAPTER 3

Myocardial Viability Assessment in Predicting Prognosis and Providing Optimal Management for Ischemic Left Ventricular Dysfunction

Tokuo Kasai*

Department of Cardiology, Uonuma Institute of Community Medicine, Niigata University Medical and Dental Hospital, Uonuma Kikan Hospital, 4132 Urasa, Minami-Uonuma, Niigata 949-7302, Japan

Abstract: After the Surgical Treatment for Ischemic Heart Failure (STICH) trial was introduced, it is controversial whether myocardial viability assessment is necessary or not. Myocardial viability assessment has been regarded as an essential element to select candidates for revascularization who will benefit from revascularization. However, viability determination failed to identify the patients with a differential survival benefit from CABG as compared with medical therapy alone from the sub-study of STICH trial. F-18 fluorodeoxyglucose (FDG) positron emission tomography (PET) assisted management for patients with severe left ventricular (LV) dysfunction and suspected coronary artery disease (CAD) also failed to demonstrate a significant reduction in cardiac events compared with standard care (PARR-2 study). However, a significant benefit was observed when there was adherence to PET analysis is limited to PET recommendations. Like this, when the negative report is interpreted carefully, viability assessment can assign the right patients for the right treatment. To assess viability, concomitant myocardial jeopardy is essential to evaluate. Endpoints for viability assessment were regional/global functional recovery, symptom relief, exercise capacity improvement, reduction of re-hospitalization rate, and prevention of LV remodeling after revascularization. Some beneficial effects can be obtained in patients with ischemic LV dysfunction in the presence of viability even if functional recovery was not demonstrated.

The importance of viability assessment and the similarities and differences of imaging modalities are discussed in this chapter.

Keywords: FDG-PET, Functional Recovery, Jeopardy, MRI, Viability.

* **Corresponding author Tokuo Kasai**, Department of Cardiology, Uonuma Institute of Community Medicine, Niigata University Medical and Dental Hospital, Uonuma Kikan Hospital, 4132 Urasa, Minami-Uonuma, Niigata 949-7302, Japan; Tel: +81-25-777-3200; Email: t-kasai@ncmi.or.jp

Shinro Matsuo (Ed.)

INTRODUCTION

Myocardial viability assessment has long been debating whether it is necessary or not prior to revascularization in patients with ischemic left ventricular (LV) dysfunction. Perhaps, it depends upon the definition of viability. Viability is traditionally defined as follows: LV dysfunction secondary to coronary artery disease (CAD) which has the potential for functional recovery with revascularization. The controversy arises when viable myocardium does not demonstrate functional recovery after revascularization. However, some beneficial aspects are reported even absence of functional recovery after revascularization, such as improvement of symptoms, exercise capacity, reduction of cardiac re-hospitalization rate, prevention of remodeling, and long-term prognosis. In addition, even if functional recovery had not been acquainted during the short follow-up period after revascularization, some cases have demonstrated delayed functional recovery in the long-term. With those cases, the better prognosis can be obtained compared to non-responders of revascularization. In this chapter, the impact of myocardial viability assessment on the patient management is reviewed, and importance of the viability assessment is discussed.

Impact of Myocardial Viability on Patient Management

Various studies demonstrated that the prevalence of myocardial viability in patients with chronic ischemic LV dysfunction is about 50-60% [1 - 3]. In the earlier studies, recovery of regional LV dysfunction was used as the criterion for myocardial viability. Subsequently, improvement of LV ejection fraction (EF), heart failure symptoms, and survival were employed for endpoints in assessing myocardial viability. In terms of regional LV functional recovery, 105 viability studies including 3,003 patients demonstrated 7,941 (53%) segments improved its function after revascularization out of 15,045 segments [4]. As for LVEF improvement, 29 viability studies including 758 patients demonstrated that LVEF in patients with viable myocardium improved +8% from before revascularization. On the other hand, no improvement in LVEF was observed in patients without viable myocardium [5]. The most important endpoint is long-term survival. Meta-analysis including 24 viability studies (3,088 patients) demonstrated that revascularization decreased 79.6% annual mortality (16% *vs.* 3.2%, $p < 0.0001$) compared with medical treatment in patients with viability. On the other hand, there was no difference in annual mortality between revascularization and medical treatment in patients without viability (7.7% *vs.* 6.2%, not significant) (Fig. **1**) [6].

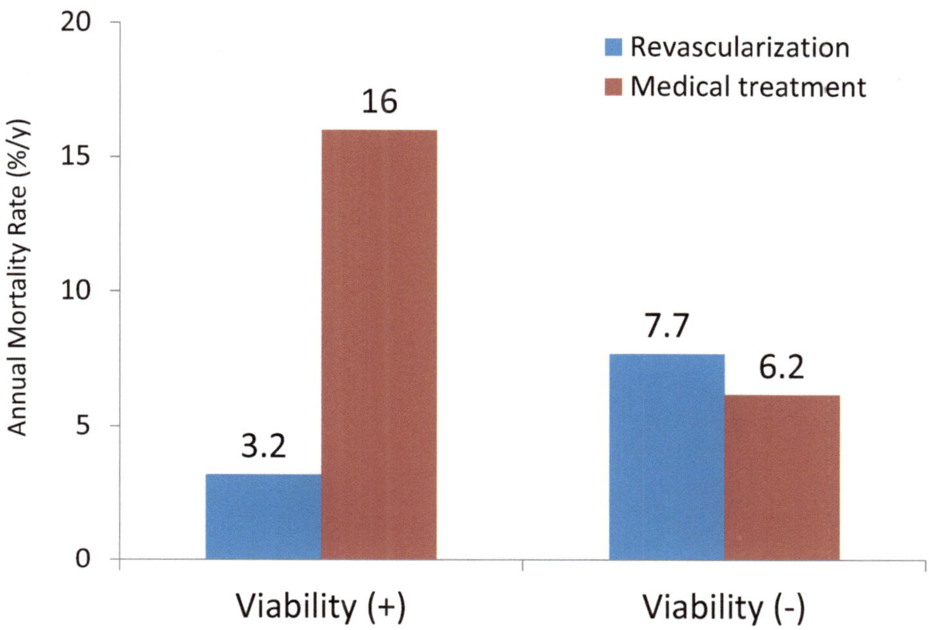

Fig. (1). Meta-analysis demonstrated that revascularization decreased 79.6% annual mortality (16% *vs.* 3.2%, $p < 0.0001$) compared with medical treatment in patients with viability. On the other hand, there was no difference in annual mortality between revascularization and medical treatment in patients without viability (7.7% *vs.* 6.2%, not significant) [6].

Viability studies include thallium-201 (Tl-201) perfusion single photon emission computed tomography (SPECT), F-18 fluorodeoxyglucose (FDG) positron emission tomography (PET) dobutamine stress echocardiography (DSE), and magnetic resonance imaging (MRI). There was no difference for predicting revascularization benefit between these imaging techniques. Therefore, a strong association exists between noninvasive viability testing and improved survival rate after revascularization in patients with chronic ischemic LV dysfunction [6]. Di Carli *et al.* reported that in addition to the survival, angina and heart failure symptoms were improved in patients with severe coronary artery disease and low LVEF who received revascularization when perfusion-metabolism mismatch (reflecting hibernating myocardium) was present [7, 8]. Bax *et al.* also demonstrated similar results using DSE [9]. Exercise capacity is improved more in patients with a larger extent of viable myocardium (Fig. **2**) [8]. Exercise capacity strongly associated with long-term survival. Therefore, these data are consistent, and viability assessment has a pivotal role in predicting prognosis in patients with chronic ischemic LV dysfunction.

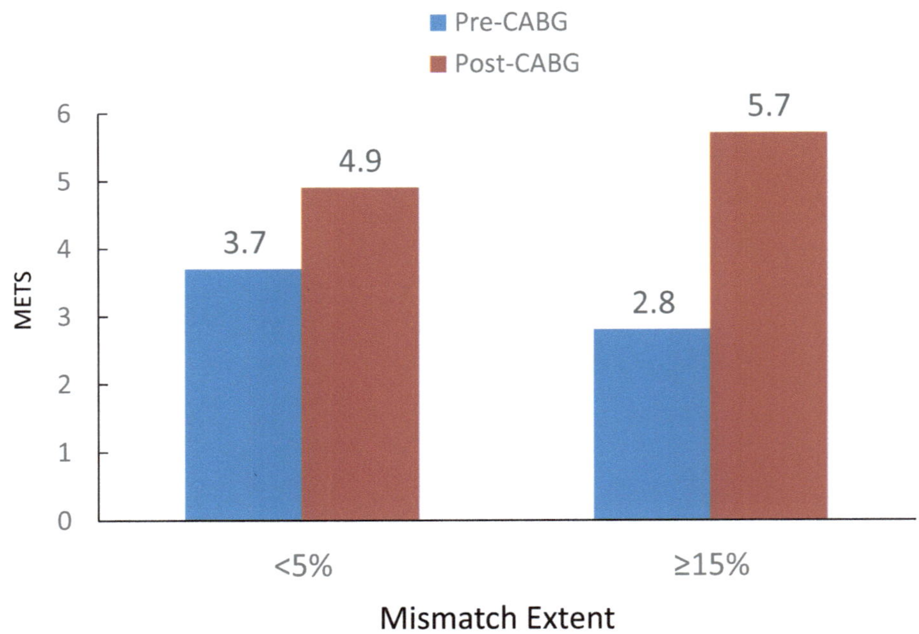

Fig. (2). Changes in exercise capacity (METs) according to the extent of viable myocardium on FDG PET. Large extent of viable myocardium demonstrated high increase in exercise capacity post-CABG [8].

Nonetheless, outcomes after revascularization vary even in the presence of substantial myocardial viability. Controversy has arisen since the STICH trial was introduced. STICH trial was conducted to elucidate the merit of coronary artery bypass grafting (CABG) in patients with heart failure with reduced ejection fraction (HFrEF) and less severe multi-vessel CAD. All-cause mortality was not reduced by CABG, however, cardiovascular death and death from any cause or cardiovascular hospitalization were significantly reduced (relative risk reduction rate was 19% and 26%, respectively) [10]. It has been expected for viability testing to distinguish who is to benefit from CABG. However, the viability determination did not identify the patients with a differential survival benefit from CABG as compared with medical therapy alone from the sub-study of STICH trial [11]. One possible cause for this result was that SPECT or DSE had been recruited for viability determination in the STICH trial. These two modalities are relatively less sensitive in identifying viability, compared with FDG PET which is the most sensitive modality. Therefore, underestimation of viability might have happened, thereby affecting results. However, FDG PET-assisted management for patients with severe LV dysfunction and suspected CAD also failed to demonstrate a significant reduction in cardiac events compared with standard care (PPAR-2 study) [12]. However, rehospitalization rate has been decreased (39%

vs. 46%, p = 0.04). In addition, the patients with adhering to PET recommendations demonstrated less total events than those with the standard care (51% *vs.* 57%, P = 0.042) [13]. Another sub-study of PARR-2 trial revealed that FDG PET-assisted management significantly reduced composite primary endpoint including cardiac death, myocardial infarction, and cardiac hospitalization for revascularization compared with standard care in experienced centers having heart team (19% *vs.* 41%, p=0.005) [14]. Therefore, controversy still exists. However, "benefit" depends upon the endpoints, and cutoff point for defining viability, such as the extent of mismatch between perfusion and metabolism, affects sensitivity of identifying viability. We should carefully interpret these results.

Dysfunctional but viable myocardium, such as stunning and hibernation, can be determined by viability testing and recovers their function with revascularization. In contrast, a mixture of intact myocardium (non-jeopardized) and scar tissue will not recover in function but still be regarded as viable myocardium. Therefore, viability testing requires the simultaneous assessment of myocardial **jeopardy** in terms of functional recovery after revascularization [15].

Pathophysiology of Reversible Ischemic Dysfunction

It had been believed that dysfunctional myocardium, related to coronary artery disease, never recovers its function, *i.e.* scar until 1970's. Thereafter, however, lots of studies demonstrated some functional recovery after revascularization [16 - 18]. This jeopardized dysfunctional but **reversible** myocardium has been known as viable myocardium. This phenomenon resembles hibernation for animals. Rahimtoola's named it "hibernating myocardium" and became prevalent after his report [19]. Resting blood flow in the hibernating myocardium is usually reduced as compared to normal myocardium. Although some studies demonstrated that resting blood flow was not reduced in the hibernating myocardium [20, 21], coronary flow reserve (CFR) is always reduced irrespective of resting blood flow [22, 23]. Animal studies demonstrated that resting myocardial blood flow may be normal or near normal in the early period but regional contraction may already be reduced (stunning) in chronic coronary stenosis probably due to repetitive ischemic episodes. Then, resting myocardial blood flow gradually decreases over time (hibernation) [24, 25]. Based on these observations, reversible ischemic dysfunction temporally progresses from stunning to hibernation probably due to steadily decrease in energy supply. Therefore, stunning and hibernation may coexist in the same patients with multi-vessel disease. This discordance between wall motion abnormality and the absence of myocardial scarring may indicate a protective adaptation of myocardium for hypoperfusion so that energy can be saved and prevent necrosis by reducing contractility (Table **1**) [26]. The absence of functional deterioration or progressive fibrosis suggests that hibernation is an adaptive reaction rather than progressive irreversible injury [27]. Both stunning and hibernation imply compromised flow reserve and require revascularization to regain functional integrity.

Table 1. Physiologic status of chronic ischemic LV dysfunction [26].

	Resting Flow	Flow Reserve	Inotropic Reserve	Metabolism	Structural Change	Reversivility
Chronic Stunning	Normal	Reduced	Yes	Preserved	No	Yes
Transition Phase	Normal	Reduced	Yes	Preserved	Mild	Yes
Chronic Hibernation	Reduced	Severely Reduced	May be absent	Preserved	More severe/fibrosis	Delayed/ incomplete
Infarction	Reduced	Severely Reduced	No	Reduced	Fibrosis	No

Structural Alteration of Hibernating Myocardium

Ultrastructural alteration of myocardium affects functional recovery after revascularization. Segments with less fibrosis and less severe cardiomyocyte alteration are more likely to improve function after revascularization [28]. Cardiomyocyte alteration includes small doughnut-shaped and decreased numbers of cristae with mitochondria, loss of sarcoplasmic reticulum, T tubes, sarcomeres, accumulation and storage of glycogen. The contractile protein, myosin, titin, α-actinin are reduced, and distribution of titin is altered [29, 30]. These structural changes resemble embryonic cells. Altered myocytes re-express contractile proteins that are specific to the fetal heart. In addition, metabolism also resembles the fetal heart which prefers glucose with storage of glycogen. These structural and metabolic alterations suggest cellular adaptation and maladaptation for programmed cell **survival or death (apoptosis)** [28]. These process implies initiation of metabolic and structural remodeling of hibernating myocardium. The severity of structural changes influences on functional recovery after revascularization. The regions with less fibrosis or less alteration of cardiomyocytes and less remodeling are more likely to improve function [31]. The less alteration, the more rapidly function recovers [32]. Delayed functional recovery after revascularization may reflect a persistent reduction in the amount of contractile and metabolic proteins [33]. In addition, **myofibrillar disassembly and myofibrillar loss develop** after a critical decrease in CFR, and these changes also occur in the normally perfused remote area of the chronically dysfunctional heart [34]. This mechanism probably contributes to the advancement of remodeling and progressive heart failure.

Metabolic Alteration in Reversible Ischemic Dysfunction

Chronic hypoperfusion in the hibernating myocardium decreases in oxygen supply, resulting in reduced utilization of Krebs cycle, instead activates anaerobic metabolic circuit (Glycolysis). As a result, ATP production dramatically decreases from 36 to 2 mols from 1 mol of glucose. Insufficient energy (ATP) supply alters major ATP consumption from contraction to viability maintenance. Therefore, hibernating myocardium reveals dysfunctional status but is still alive. In contrast to the Krebs cycle, the anaerobic metabolic circuit can utilize glucose only. Therefore, hibernating myocardium takes up more glucose than normal myocardium, and fluorine-18 deoxyglucose (FDG) uptake is also increased in fasting state in the chronic hibernating myocardium [35]. Chronic hypoxia may be one of the triggers of metabolic alteration which is presumably promoted by structural alteration to adapt hypoxic condition. Glycogen accumulation is frequently observed in hibernating myocardium but it merely happens under transient ongoing ischemia. Therefore, not only activated anaerobic metabolism due to chronic ischemia but also metabolic remodeling induced by structural alteration causes increased glucose/FDG uptake in hibernating myocardium. In fasting state, transmural FDG uptake inversely correlates with regional myocardial flow reserve [36]. Therefore, as far as viability remains, the degree of FDG uptake may correlate with severity of regional perfusion deficit.

Role of Imaging in Assessing Reversible Ischemic Dysfunction

Several imaging modalities, including thallium-201 SPECT, FDG PET, DSE, and MRI are used to assess viability in patients with chronically ischemic LV dysfunction [1, 2, 4, 5]. Each imaging modality has its own strength and limitations (Table **2**) [15, 37]. Sensitivity and specificity of various viability testing in predicting functional recovery after revascularization are reported (Table **3**, Fig. **3**) [38, 39].

Table 2. Application of multi-modality imaging in the diagnosis of viable myocardium. modified from [15, 37].

	Echo	CMR	Nuclear
Remodeling			
LVEDV/ESV	++	+++	++
LVEF	++	+++	++
LV mass	++	+++	
Function			
Systolic	+++	+++	++

(Table 2) cont.....

	Echo	CMR	Nuclear
Diastolic	+++	+++	++
Dyssynchrony	++	+	+
Etiology			
CAD Anatomy		+	
Ischemia	+++	+++	+++
Scar	++	+++	++
Valve Stenosis	+++	+	
Regurgitation	+++	++	
Myocardial tissue characterization	+	+++	+ *
Viability			
Sensitivity	++	++	+++
Specificity	+++	+++	++
Advantage			
	First-line imaging	No radiation	Good availability **
	Excellent availability	Wide application	
	Handy		
	Low cost		
	No radiation		
Disadvantage			
	Poor reproducibility	Limited availability	Radiation
	Echo window needed	Limited image quality with arrhythmia	Limited availability for PET

* Sarcoidosis
** Except for PET

Table 3. Prediction of functional recovery after revascularization. modified from [38, 39].

Modality	No. of Patients (No. of Studies)	Sensitivity (%)	Specificity (%)	PPV (%)
FDG PET	756 (24)	92	63	74
Tl-201 SPECT	1119 (40)	87	54	67
Tc-99m SPECT	721 (25)	83	65	74
DSE	1421 (41)	80	78	75
MRI, CE	178 (5)	84	63	72
Direct Comparison of DSE and Nuclear imaging				
DSE	325 (11)	74	78	84

(Table 3) cont.....

Modality	No. of Patients (No. of Studies)	Sensitivity (%)	Specificity (%)	PPV (%)
Nuclear Imaging	325 (11)	90	57	75

PPV: positive predictive value, FDG: fluodeoxyglucose, PET: positron emission tomography, Tl: Thallium, SPECT: single photon emission computed tomography, Tc: technetium, DSE dobutamine stress echocardiography, MRI: magnetic resonance imaging, CE: contrast enhancement.

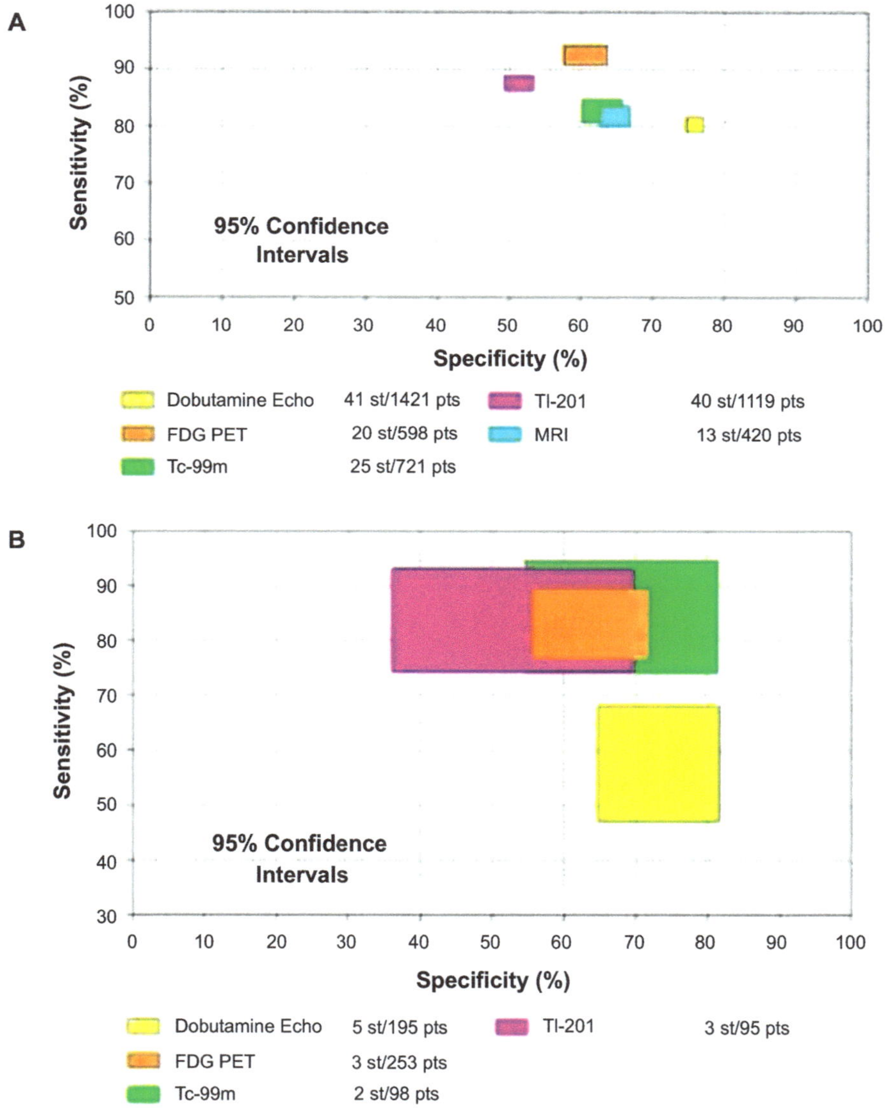

Fig. (3). Sensitivities and specificities with 95% confidence interval of the various viability testing in predicting recovery of regional (A) and global (B) left ventricular function after revascularization [38, 39].

DSE protocol is a stepwise infusion of dobutamine from 5 to 40μg/kg/min while echocardiographic imaging is obtained. The contractile reserve is assessed by wall motion improvement during low-dose phase (5 to 10 μg/kg/min). Ischemia is subsequently evaluated by deterioration of wall motion at high-dose phase (10 to 40 μg/kg/min). Biphasic wall motion response represents viable and ischemic myocardium. However, up to 50% of dysfunctional segments without contractile reserve still have resting perfusion and/or glucose metabolism. This discrepancy means that DSE indicates no viability but FDG PET does. In addition, the sensitivity of DSE for ischemia detection is lower than that of nuclear imaging because "ischemic cascade" demonstrates that perfusion reduces earlier than contraction abnormality appears. Hence, DSE is less sensitive to detect viability compared with nuclear imaging [40, 41]. On the other hand, not all segments with contraction reserve improve in function. About 70% to 80% of the akinetic segments with contractile reserve improved in function, but only 30% to 40% of the hypokinetic segments did [40]. The hypokinetic segments without contractile reserve frequently contain a mixture of normal myocardium and subendocardial scar, which does not improve in function after revascularization because of no jeopardy. Therefore, a low-dose/high-dose protocol has been developed. When segments demonstrate contractile reserve at low-dose followed by worsening of wall motion at high-dose (biphasic response), the likelihood of recovery is high, in contrast to segments with sustained improvement in wall motion during high-dose dobutamine infusion. Rizzello *et al.* reported that 78% of hypokinetic segments with biphasic response improve in function after revascularization, as compared to only 27% of hypokinetic segments [41]. Therefore, not low-dose only but low-dose/high-dose protocol is essential with monophasic response for DSE in predicting functional recovery.

Nuclear imaging has been used widely in assessing viability, and much evidence is available. Tl-201 reflects perfusion and cell membrane integrity. For viability assessment, the conventional stress-rest protocol, rest-redistribution and stress-redistribution-reinjection protocols are feasible. Viability is ascertained when redistribution is demonstrated in a region of dysfunction. Even in the absence of redistribution, ≥50% of the highest uptake (normal region) indicates viability. Between 40% and 50% uptake is so-called "gray zone" for viability assessment, and the likelihood of functional recovery should be anticipated on a case by case basis. With stress-rest protocol, up to 50% of fixed Tl-201 defects improve in function after revascularization [42 - 44]. Thus, the conventional stress-rest protocol has a suboptimal negative predictive value. This technique often underestimates the presence of viable myocardium and the eligibility for revascularization. Fig. (**4A**) demonstrates anteroseptal fixed defects with Tl-201 and apical dyskinesia in patients with prior myocardial infarction. Dyskinesia with no redistribution indicates no viability; however, %uptake maintains >45% in the infarct zone, except at the apex of the left ventricle. After the percutaneous coronary intervention of a severe stenosis of left anterior descending artery, both myocardial perfusion and LV function recovered to normal, including the apex (Fig. **4B**) [15], Underestimation of viability with the stress-rest protocol is confirmed by FDG PET study. Between 38% and 47% of apparent severe fixed Tl-201 defects (considered as scar by Tl-201 imaging) were identified as viable [45 - 48]. Therefore, several modifications in imaging protocols with Tl-201 to detect viability were introduced, including late redistribution imaging, rest redistribution, and stress-redistribution-reinjection protocols.

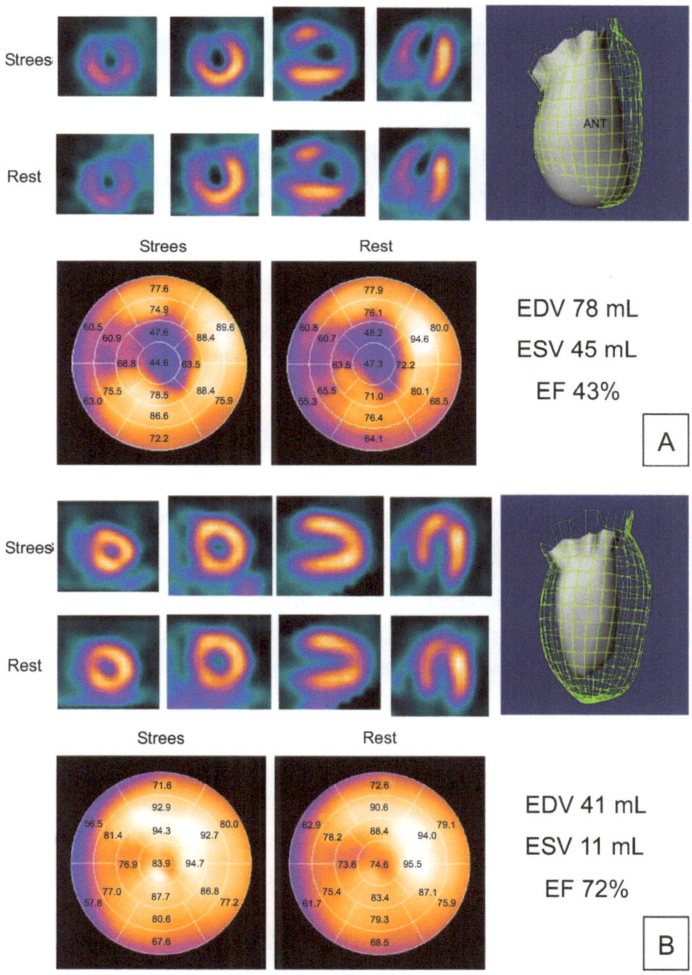

Fig. (4). A, Dyskinetic distal anteroseptal wall without redistribution on Tl-201 SPECT. There is less chance to recover left ventricular function from this information. However, %uptake of dyskinetic region remains > 45%. Therefore, this dyskinetic region is determined viable eventually. B, Both perfusion and function returned normal after percutaneous coronary intervention to proximal tight lesion of left anterior descending artery. Reverse remodeling is also apparent [15].

Late imaging at 18 to 72 hours after administration indicates Tl-201 redistribution in as many as 61% from 22% segments that appear as fixed defects at 3 to 4 hours. This late redistribution was consistent with viable myocardium [43, 49]. Kiat *et al* reported that of all regions that demonstrated fixed defects at 4 hours, 72% showed improvement function after revascularization. Further analysis elucidated that 95% of regions with late redistribution improved function after revascularization, compared with 37% of regions that remained fixed defects on late imaging [43]. Therefore, the conventional stress-redistribution at 3 to 4 hours imaging underestimates the viable myocardium. In contrast, late redistribution demonstrates excellent positive predictive value in predicting improvement after revascularization which is more than 90% [43]. Thus, late redistribution is an excellent marker of viable myocardium. On the other hand, the negative predictive value of late redistribution is still low. As mentioned above, as many as 37% of fixed defect segments at 24 hours demonstrated improvement after revascularization. Besides, nearly 50% of these fixed defect segments demonstrate positive FDG uptake on PET [50]. Therefore, the absence of late redistribution is not suitable for ruling out viability.

The reinjection of Tl-201 at rest following redistribution imaging of the conventional stress-redistribution imaging was introduced to overcome the limitation of the standard protocol. Up to 49% of fixed defects on 3- to 4-hour redistribution images and 39% of fixed defects on 24-hour redistribution images demonstrate improved uptake after Tl-201 reinjection [51 - 53]. Tl-201 uptake after reinjection represents viable myocardium. Two hundred ninety-five patients with ischemic LV dysfunction from 9 studies who were evaluated after revascularization demonstrated improvement in regional function in 69% of segments identified as viable before revascularization [54]. The concordance between data on Tl-201 reinjection and FDG PET were excellent, with 51% of severe fixed defects on 4-hour redistribution studies identified viable by both Tl-201 reinjection and FDG PET [55]. Tl-201 reinjection is a convenient, inexpensive and accurate method in assessing myocardial viability in patients with chronic ischemic LV dysfunction.

Stress-induced ischemia in CAD patients with LV dysfunction is an important prognostic predictor and can stratify the patients who are suitable for medical treatment or eligible for revascularization based on the amount ischemia. Therefore, stress-redistribution-reinjection Tl-201 protocol is an attraction because the most important information, ischemic jeopardy and viability, can be obtained simultaneously. However, not all CAD patients can undergo stress test because of hemodynamic instability and so forth. In those cases, rest-redistribution Tl-201 protocol is an alternative method to stress-redistributio--reinjection protocol because it can provide reliable diagnostic accuracy for viability assessment which is virtually identical to the diagnostic yields with the stress-redistribution-reinjection protocol (Fig. **5**) [54]. Rest-redistribution imaging provides comparable results with FDG PET imaging [56, 57].

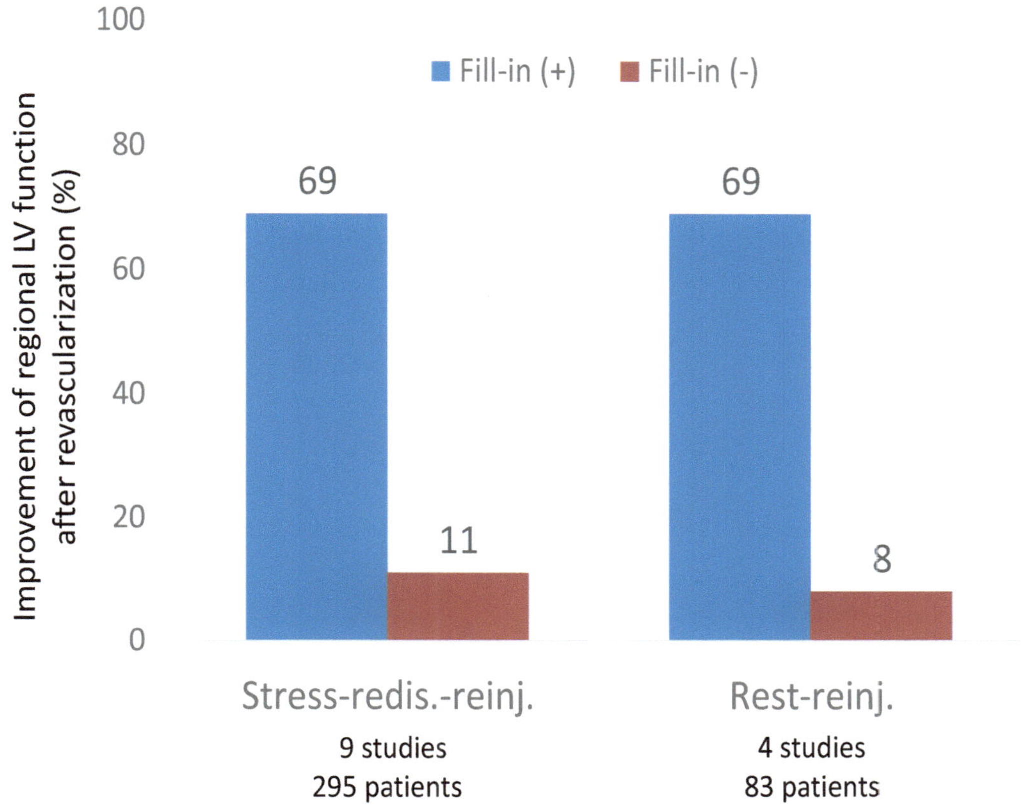

Fig. (5). Improvement of regional LV function after revascularization based on Tl-201 SPECT. Stress-redistribution-reinjection protocol yield high positive predictive value of 69% and low inverse negative predictive value of 11%. Rest-redistribution demonstrated similar good diagnostic yields with stress-redistribution-reinjection protocol [54].

Relative regional uptake of Tl-201 has also been used for viability assessment, and segments indicating >50% uptake of peak myocardial activity is usually regarded as viable myocardium. However, Tl-201 uptake distributes continually rather than a binary function. There is a linear relationship between relative Tl-201 uptake and probability of regional functional recovery after revascularization (Fig. **6**) [58]. Therefore, dysfunctional LV segments indicating <50% uptake may still have a chance to recover in a lesser degree, **especially between 40% and 50%**. Fig. (**4**) demonstrates fixed defects with conventional stress-rest protocol, <50% uptake and dyskinetic wall motion. However, >40% uptake remains and completely recovered its perfusion and function after revascularization. The level of regional Tl-201 activity on delayed redistribution images determines functional recovery after revascularization. Relative regional Tl-201 uptake is a more reliable determinant of functional recovery than regional fill-in from the initial resting images from the delayed redistribution images [58].

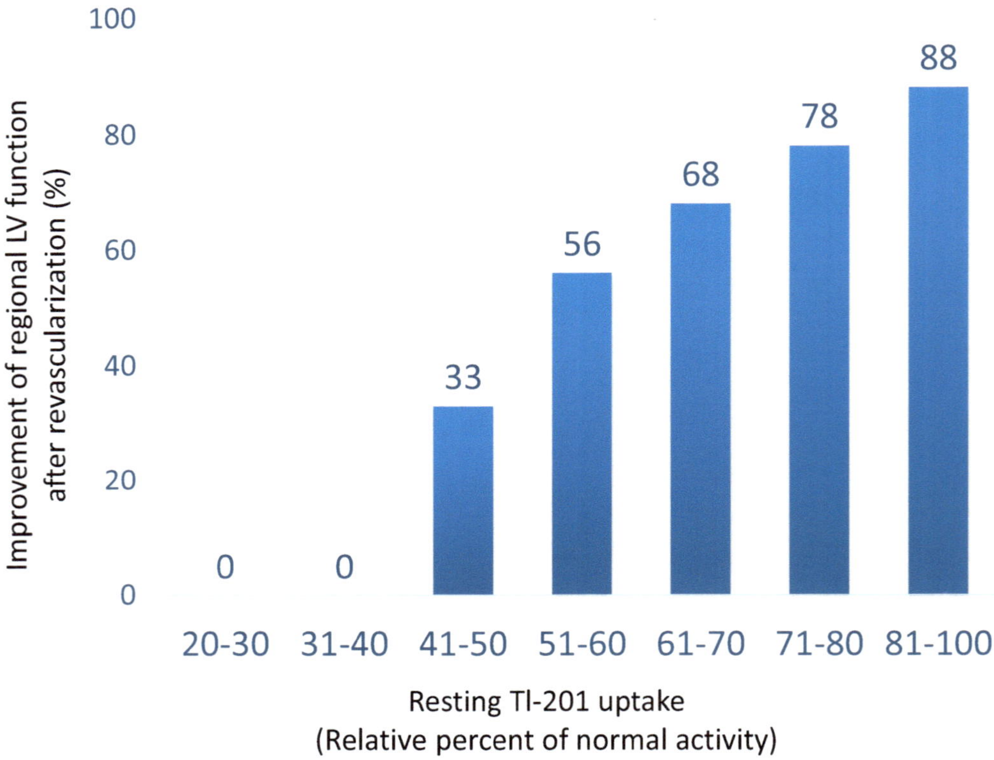

Fig. (6). Linear relationship between the percent Tl-201 uptake to peak activity on rest-redistribution imaging and probability of segmental functional recovery after revascularization [58].

Technetium-99m (Tc-99m) perfusion agents are also available for viability assessment. Retention of the tracers indicates cell membrane integrity and intact mitochondria function. Tc-99m agents have inherent weaknesses for viability assessment when blood supply is severely limited and tracer delivery is restricted [59]. Initial studies reported that Tc-99m-sestamibi underestimates viable myocardium in patients with chronic severe CAD and LV dysfunction [60, 61]. However, subsequent studies demonstrated that Tc-99m-sestamibi provides consistent, nearly identical accuracy for viability assessment compared to rest Tl-201 imaging. Regional Tc-99m-sestamibi activity correlates well with Tl-201 redistribution activity rather than initial resting uptake of Tl-201 [62, 63]. **Similar to the** Tl-201, relative regional Tc-99m sestamibi activity of >60% demonstrated high positive and negative predictive values for functional recovery after revascularization (80% and 96%, respectively [64]. Adding nitroglycerin to Tc-99m sestamibi imaging enhances the detection of viable myocardium [65, 66]. Tc-99m-tetrofosmin can be also used for viability assessment in a similar manner to Tc-99m-sestamibi [67, 68]. Therefore, Tc-99m agents can be used for viability assessment by determining the severity of resting defects with or without nitroglycerin.

FDG PET is the most reliable modality to assess viability and regarded as gold standard. Myocardium uses several energy sources including free fatty acids (FFA), glucose, pyruvate and lactate. In the fasting state, FFA is the dominant source, and glucose is a dominant source in the fed state. FFA metabolism is highly dependent on oxygen. Therefore, it is compromised in the lack of oxygen. During a shortage of oxygen supply, such as ischemia, glucose is the only energy source. Therefore, glucose uptake and metabolism are increased, and FFA metabolism declines during ischemia [69]. This metabolic shift produces much less energy and induces energy consumption switching from LV contraction to keeping myocyte alive in some degree, resulting in LV dysfunction. To evaluate these metabolic adaptations for the ischemic condition, decreased perfusion and increased glucose metabolism should be assessed. FDG is a glucose analog and taken up by myocyte then retains in the cell. Therefore, FDG uptake reflects glucose metabolism and depends on the metabolic circumstances. High blood glucose and low fatty acid with high insulin level are required to obtain maximum uptake. This situation can be achieved by preparation such as simple oral glucose loading or hyperinsulinemic clamping [70]. FDG PET in combination with perfusion studies, such as nitrogen-13-ammonia PET and Tc-99m sestamibi or tetrofosmin SPECT is an important and reliable method in identifying viable myocardium. Perfusion reduction with preserved glucose metabolism reflects hibernating myocardium and is recognized as a "mismatch pattern". Fig. (**7**) demonstrates this mismatch pattern in anteroseptal and inferior regions with Tl-201 SPECT/FDG PET imaging. Diffuse severe hypokinesia was observed with reduced LVEF (24%) and remodeling. These findings predict a poor prognosis. In addition, for a large area of jeopardized but still viable myocardium, revascularization is the preferred option. However, this patient refused reperfusion therapy, which resulted in cardiac death 20 months later [15]. FDG PET is the most sensitive modality in predicting regional functional recovery. (Table **3**, Fig. **3**) [38, 39]. Therefore, in case of questionable viability, such as chronic total occlusion of coronary artery with the absence of collateral circulation or very low LVEF in patients with LV dysfunction, FDG PET is useful to select patients who will most benefit from revascularization [71, 72].

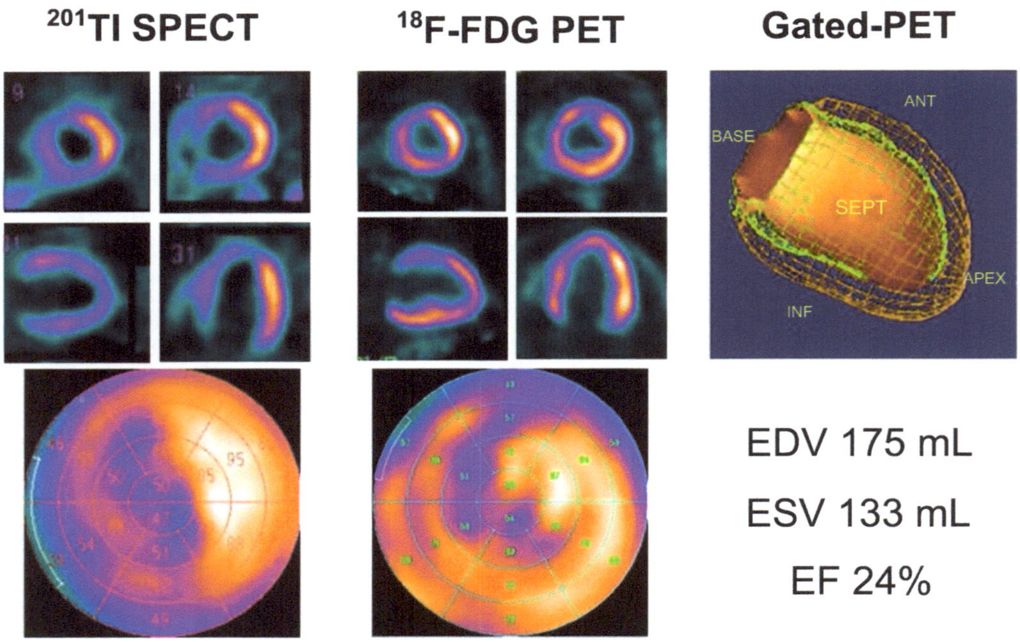

Fig. (7). Severe perfusion defects in anteroseptal and inferior walls on Tl-201 SPECT. Diffuse severe hypokinesis is shown on gated PET imaging. However, preserved uptake was demonstrated in anteroseptal and inferior walls on FDG PET. This mismatch pattern indicates viability and benefit from revascularization. However, this patient refused reperfusion therapy, and then medical treatment was selected. Cardiac death was occurred 20 month later [15].

MRI has been also used for viability assessment. The contractile reserve can be assessed with low dose dobutamine in the same way as DSE and demonstrates similar detectability with DSE (Table **3**, Fig. (**3**) [38, 39]. Gadolinium-based contrast agents accumulate in the interstitial space and reflect nonviable tissue (scar) at a delayed phase. MRI with late gadolinium enhancement imaging is prevalent in predicting functional recovery. Kim *et al.* reported that wall motion recovery can be predicted with an inverse relation to the thickness of myocardial enhancement. As the **depth** of enhancement becomes thicker, there will be a lower success rate for improvement of the wall motion after revascularization. Wall motion recovery cannot be expected in patients with myocardial enhancement exceeding 51% of wall thickness [73]. Although MRI with late contrast enhancement revealed the high sensitivity of 97% to predict functional recovery, a relatively low specificity of 44% should be taken into account [74]. MRI demonstrates a relatively low positive predictive value compared with FDG PET because MRI with delayed enhancement cannot discern ischemic myocardium from non-ischemic one (jeopardy). On the other hand, ^{18}F-FDG PET can identify ischemic (jeopardized) and viable myocardium combined with perfusion imaging. However, FDG PET also has limitations. The spatial resolution of FDG PET is much poorer than that of MRI. Therefore, FDG PET tends to be affected by a partial volume effect. For example, segmental thin myocardium demonstrates a matched defect with perfusion imaging and ^{18}F-FDG PET due to the partial volume effect. However, MRI demonstrates no contrast enhancement in that segmental thin myocardium. For such cases, this inferiority of FDG PET leads to underestimation of myocardial viability [75].

Amount of Residual Ischemic Myocardium

MRI can quantify the "depth" of myocardial scar. Generally, scar thickness $\leq 50\%$ is regarded as viable myocardium [73]. However, even viable myocardium remains > 50% thickness, wall motion would not recover after revascularization in the absence of ischemia.

Another possible determinant of viability is how much amount of myocardium remains in the infarcted zone. LVEF increased after revascularization in patients with three or more viable dysfunctional segments on FDG SPECT. However, LVEF did not increase in patients with less than three viable, dysfunctional segments [76]. Similarly, Mule *et al.* demonstrated that patients with at least 5 jeopardized segments improved LVEF with reverse remodeling, and improved in NYHA class with excellent long-term prognosis after revascularization. Conversely, patients with < 5 jeopardized segments failed to improve in LVEF, and exhibited ongoing remodeling, without improvement in NYHA class, and worse long-term prognosis [77]. These investigations suggest that there is a substantial amount of ischemic viable myocardium in predicting the beneficial effect of revascularization. Bax *et al.* reported that there is the cutoff value of 4 or more dysfunctional but viable segments yielded the highest sensitivity (86%) and specificity (90%) to predict improvement in LVEF [9]. This report suggests that at least 25% of the left ventricle needs to be viable to obtain improvement in LVEF after revascularization.

In the thrombolytic era for acute myocardial infarction, German multicenter trial reported that mortality was reduced from 12.6% in the control (heparin-treated) patients to 5.6% in the thrombolytic treated patients with no effect on LVEF [78]. The portion of salvaged myocardium is more than 20% larger with thrombolytic treated patients than that with placebo-treated patients with only 2% difference of LVEF between 2 groups [79]. Therefore, the effect of reperfusion therapy appears as the amount of salvaged myocardium, leading to better long-term prognosis, which is independent of LVEF. Some studies suggested that 20-30% of ischemic left ventricular myocardium need to be viable to obtain global LVEF improvement [80]. These data were obtained from the studies of acute myocardial infarction. Inaba et al. reported that about 20-40% of viable myocardium required to improve survival with revascularization in patients with chronic ischemic cardiomyopathy (Table **4**) [81]. PARR-2 study was conducted in a randomized fashion to assess the effectiveness of FDG PET-assisted management in patients with severe ventricular dysfunction and suspected CAD. Unfortunately, the PARR-2 study failed to demonstrate the usefulness of FDG PET-assisted management for such patients [12]. However, sub-study of PARR-2 clearly demonstrated that ischemic cardiomyopathy with a larger amount of hibernating myocardium has improved outcomes with revascularization [82].

Table 4. Optimal cutoff values for the extent of viable myocardium in predicting improved survival with revascularization over medical therapy in patients with ischemic cardiomyopathy [81].

Imaging technique (number of studies)	Mean viable myocardium % ± SD	Optimal threshold for viability %, (95% C.I.)
PET overall (7)	21 ± 13	25.8 (16.6-35.0)
PET with FDG/NH3 (3)	20 ± 15	22.5 (10.1-34.8)
PET with FDG/Tc-99m (3)	22 ± 16	29.2 (20.7-37.8)
DSE overall (8)	32 ± 24	35.9 (31.6-40.3)
DSE with LDD (4)	33 ± 28	33.6 (27.4-39.8)
DSE with HDD (2)	35 ± 31	44.1 (37.2-50.9)
SPECT overall (6)	38 ± 25	38.7 (27.7-49.7)
SPECT with Tl-201 (5)	41 ± 35	38.0 (26.2-49.7)

NH3: ammonia, LDD: low dose dobutamine, HDD: high dose dobutamine

In the assessment of viable myocardium using a PET, scar volume can be also quantified. Perfusion/metabolism mismatch is a well-known indicator of viability; however, the extent of scar tissue is negatively correlated with LVEF improvement after revascularization and a stronger predictor of LVEF improvement than perfusion/metabolism mismatch [83].

LV Remodeling

Administration of ACE inhibitors and β-blockers for patients with heart failure and/or acute myocardial infarction can attenuate left ventricular remodeling, resulting in favorable prognosis [84, 85]. Therefore, prevention of LV remodeling is beneficial for prognosis [86]. Revascularization improves not only LV function but also LV geometry (shape and size), leading to better survival in patients with severe chronic ischemic LV dysfunction with viable myocardium [77]. In addition, even in the absence of LVEF improvement, CABG is not associated with poorer outcome in patients with ischemic cardiomyopathy, presumably due to the prevention of (further) LV remodeling [87]. Although the conventional definition of myocardial viability is an improvement of LV function after revascularization, lack of LV functional recovery does not always mean "non-responder". Therefore, the conventional definition of viability may not be the most appropriate definition in terms of long-term prognosis [88].

Based on the law of Laplace, an extremely dilated left ventricle with spherical shape results in a marked increase in wall stress. This stress burden may overwhelm the myocardial contraction reserve, resulting in a lack of functional recovery, *i.e.* non-responder after revascularization. Schinkel *et al.* reported that 67% of 118 consecutive ischemic cardiomyopathy patients (LVEF, 29%±6%) with substantial viability demonstrated improvement in LVEF, whereas 33% did not exhibit the expected improvement. They found that the severity of remodeling was important. The patients with a large LV end-systolic volume tended to be non-responders of revascularization in spite of the presence of viable myocardium [89]. Even for such cases, revascularization would prevent further LV remodeling, leading to better prognosis than without revascularization. Therefore, viability assessment is still important even in the absence of functional recovery after revascularization.

DSE demonstrated that reverse LV remodeling after revascularization correlated with the number of viable segments. Rizzello *et al.* also demonstrated that the likelihood of LV remodeling decreased as the number of viable segments increased. Besides, reverse remodeling was present in patients with > or = 4 viable segments during the follow-up after revascularization [90]. Bax *et al.* reported that the timing of revascularization also affects the outcome in patients with ischemic cardiomyopathy and substantial viability. Early (one month or less after viability testing) revascularization improved LVEF, whereas late (>1 month **after viability testing**) revascularization did not **improve LVEF** after revascularization presumably due to LV remodeling (not only geometrical but metabolic) **progression during "waiting time"** [91]. Bonow *et al.* reported that absence of viability with LV remodeling (end-diastolic volume index > 84 ml/m^2) predicts the highest mortality regardless of treatment. Combination of viability and LV remodeling did not influence the effect of CABG relative to medical therapy in STICH cohort [92]. Therefore, LV remodeling itself is a strong independent predictor of prognosis. Prevention of LV remodeling is another target of revascularization for patients with chronic ischemic LV dysfunction.

Viability and Cardiac Resynchronization Therapy

Cardiac resynchronization therapy (CRT) is effective to improve outcomes of advanced LV dysfunction in patients with chronic heart failure **(especially in the**

presence of wide QRS complex, such as left bundle branch block), regardless of ischemic or non-ischemic etiology [93]. However, about 30% of these patients do not respond to CRT [94]. The magnitude of mechanical dyssynchrony of LV wall motion is one of the potential deterioration factors and also predictor of response to CRT. Dyssynchrony can be assessed by tissue Doppler echocardiography; however, the PROSPECT study, which is a prospective multi-center study including 498 candidates for CRT who fulfilled standard indication for CRT, failed to differentiate between responders and non-responders to CRT using tissue Doppler echocardiography [95]. Boogers *et al.* also demonstrated that dyssynchrony determined by longitudinal and radial strain using echocardiography did not demonstrate survival benefit of CRT [96]. In contrast to echocardiography, nuclear imaging can determine the degree of dyssynchrony with less variability and evaluate viability and dyssynchrony simultaneously [97].

Another predictor of CRT responder is presence of viability. Large scar was associated with unfavorable outcomes [96, 97]. Therefore, identification of CRT candidate is a new target of viability assessment for nuclear imaging [15].

CONCLUSION

Is viability assessment is essential before revascularization or not? This issue is still controversial. Even if functional recovery has not been demonstrated after revascularization in the presence of viability, most of the patients will obtain some favorable effect, such as improvement of symptoms, exercise capacity, prevention of LV remodeling and reduction of rehospitalization **as long as coexisting myocardial jeopardy**. Non-responders of revascularization with viable myocardium may have a large scar, or may not have jeopardized myocardium. Viability assessment should be performed before the decision of treatment strategy and focus on the endpoints. A large amount of hibernating myocardium likely to demonstrate apparent functional recovery after revascularization. On the other hand, large scar with a small amount of jeopardized myocardium less likely to demonstrate functional recovery but prevent LV remodeling after revascularization. Less than 50% thickness of late contrast enhancement on MRI without jeopardy indicate viability but will not demonstrate favorable outcomes after revascularization. Therefore, before revascularization for patients with ischemic LV dysfunction, integrated assessment of viability, concomitant myocardial jeopardy, and scar burden is demanding to accurate prediction whether the patients obtain benefit from revascularization [15].

CONSENT FOR PUBLICATION

Not applicable.

CONFLICT OF INTEREST

The authors declare no conflict of interest, financial or otherwise.

ACKNOWLEDGEMENTS

Declared none.

REFERENCES

[1] Scinkel AFL, Bax JJ, Sozzi FB, *et al.* Prevalence of myocardial viability assessed by single photon emission computed tomography in patients with chronic ischemic left bentricular dysfunction. Heart 2002; 88: 125-30.
[http://dx.doi.org/10.1136/heart.88.2.125]

[2] Auerbach MA, Schoder H, Hoh C, *et al.* Prevalence of myocardial viability as detected by positron emission tomography in patients with ischemic cardiomyopathy. Cieculation 1999; 99: 2921-6.
[http://dx.doi.org/10.1161/01.CIR.99.22.2921]

[3] Scinkel AFL, Bax JJ, Boersma E, *et al.* Assessment of residual myocardial viability in regions with chronic electrocardiographic Q-wave infarction. Am Heart J 2002; 144: 865-9.
[http://dx.doi.org/10.1067/mhj.2002.125627]

[4] Bax JJ, Poldermans D, Eihendy A, Boersma E, Rahimtoola S. Sensitivity, specificity, and predictive accuracies of various noninvasive techniques for detecting hibernating myocardium. Curr Probl Cardiol 2001; 26: 142-86.
[http://dx.doi.org/10.1067/mcd.2001.109973]

[5] Bax JJ, van der Wall EE, Harbinson M. Radionuclide techniques for the assessment of myocardial viability and hibernation. Heart 2004; 90: V26-33.
[http://dx.doi.org/10.1136/hrt.2002.007575]

[6] Allman KC, Shaw LJ, Hachamovitch R, Udelson JE. Myocardial viability testing and impact of revascularization on prognosis inpatients with coronary artery disease and left ventricular dysfunction: a meta-analysis. J Am Coll Cardiol 2002; 39: 1151-8.
[http://dx.doi.org/10.1016/S0735-1097(02)01726-6]

[7] Di Carli MF, Maddahi J, Rokhsar S, *et al.* Long-term survival of patients with coronary artery disease and left ventricular dysfunction: implications for the role of myocardial viability assessment in management decisions. J Thorac Cardiovasc Surg 1998; 116: 997-1004.
[http://dx.doi.org/10.1016/S0022-5223(98)70052-2]

[8] Di Carli MF, Asgarzadie F, Schelbert HR, *et al.* Quantitative relation between myocardial viability and improvement in heart failure symptoms after revascularization in patients with ischemic cardiomyopathy. Circulation 1995; 92: 3436-44.
[http://dx.doi.org/10.1161/01.CIR.92.12.3436]

[9] Bax JJ, Poldermans D, Elhendy A, *et al.* Improvement of left ventricular ejection fraction, heart failure symptoms and prognosis after revascularization in patients with chronic coronary artery disease and viable myocardium detected by dobutamine stress echocardiography. J Am Coll Cardiol 1999; 34: 163-9.
[http://dx.doi.org/10.1016/S0735-1097(99)00157-6]

[10] Velazquez EJ, Lee KL, Deja MA, *et al.* Coronary-artery bypass surgery in patients with left ventricular dysfunction. N Engl J Med 2011; 364: 1607-16.
[http://dx.doi.org/10.1056/NEJMoa1100356]

[11] Bonow RO, Maurer G, Lee KL, *et al.* Myocardial viability and survival in ischemic left ventricular dysfunction. N Engl J Med 2011; 354: 1617-25.

[http://dx.doi.org/10.1056/NEJMoa1100358]

[12] Beanlands RS, Nichol G, Huszti E, *et al.* F-18-fluorodeoxyglucose positron emission tomography imaging-assisted management of patients with severe left ventricular dysfunction and suspected coronary disease: a randomized, controlled trial (PARR-2). J Am Coll Cardiol 2007; 50: 2002-12. [http://dx.doi.org/10.1016/j.jacc.2007.09.006]

[13] McArdle B, Shukla T, Nichol G, *et al.* PARR-2 investigators. Long-term follow-up of outcomes with F-18-Fluorodeoxyglucose positron emission tomography imaging-assisted management of patients with severe left ventricular dysfunction secondary to coronary disease. Circ Cardiovasc Imaging 2016; 9: e004331.

[14] Abraham A, Nichol G, Williams KA, Guo A, deKemo RA, Garrard L, *et al.* 18F-FDG PET imaging of myocardial viability in an experienced center with access to 18F-FDG and integration with clinical management teams: the Ottawa-FIVE substudy of the PARR-2 trial. J Nucl Med 2010; 51: 567-74. [http://dx.doi.org/10.2967/jnumed.109.065938]

[15] Kasai T. Myocardial viability assessment is still alive and an important element in predicting prognosis and providing optimal management for ischemic heart failure. Int J Radiol Med Imag 2016; 2: 110-9.
[http://dx.doi.org/10.15344/2456-446X/2016/110]

[16] Tillisch J, Brunken R, Marchall R, *et al.* Reversibility of cardiac wall-motion abnormalities predicted bt positron tomography. N Engl J Med 1986; 31: 884-8.
[http://dx.doi.org/10.1056/NEJM198604033141405]

[17] Braunwald E, Rutherford JD. Reversible ischemic left ventricular dysfunction: evidence for the "hibernating myocardium". J Am Coll Cardiol 1986; 8: 1467-70.
[http://dx.doi.org/10.1016/S0735-1097(86)80325-4]

[18] Bonow RO. Identification of viable myocardium. Circulation 1996; 94: 2674-80.
[http://dx.doi.org/10.1161/01.CIR.94.11.2674]

[19] Rahimtoola SH. The hibernating myocardium. Am Heart J 1989; 117: 211-21.
[http://dx.doi.org/10.1016/0002-8703(89)90685-6]

[20] Depre C, Vanoverschelde JL, Gerber B, *et al.* Correlation of functional recovery with myocardial blood flow, glucose uptake, and morphologic features in patients with chronic left ventricular ischemic dysfunction undergoing coronary artery bypass grafting. J Thorac Cardiovasc Surg 1997; 113: 371-8. [http://dx.doi.org/10.1016/S0022-5223(97)70335-0]

[21] Vanoverschelde JL, Melin JA. The pathophysiology of myocardial hibernation: current controversies and future directions. Prog Cardiovasc Dis 2001; 43: 387-98.
[http://dx.doi.org/10.1053/pcad.2001.20655]

[22] Vanoverschelde JL, Wijns W, Depré C, *et al.* Mechanisms of chronic regional postischemic dysfunction in humans. New insights from the study of noninfarcted collateral-dependent myocardium. Circulation 1993; 87: 1513-23.
[http://dx.doi.org/10.1161/01.CIR.87.5.1513]

[23] Marzullo P, Parodi O, Sambuceti G, *et al.* Residual coronary reserve identifies segmental viability in patients with wall motion abnormalities. J Am Coll Cardiol 1995; 26: 342-50.
[http://dx.doi.org/10.1016/0735-1097(95)80005-2]

[24] Heusch G, Schulz R, Rahimtoola SH. Myocardial hibernation: a delicate balance. Am J Physiol Heart Circ Physiol 2005; 288: H984-99.
[http://dx.doi.org/10.1152/ajpheart.01109.2004]

[25] Fallavollita JA, Canty JM. Differential F-18-2-deoxyglucose uptake in viable dysfunctional myocardium with normal resting perfusion – evidence for chronic stunning in pigs. Circulation 1999; 99: 2798-805.
[http://dx.doi.org/10.1161/01.CIR.99.21.2798]

[26] Vanoverschelde JJ, Gerbere B, Pasquet A, Melin JA. Physiologic and metabolic basis of myocardial viability imaging.Clinical nuclear cardiology State of the art and future direction. 3rd ed. Philadelphia: Elsevier 2005; pp. 495-501.

[27] Fallavollita JA, Logue M, Canty JM Jr. Stability of hibernating myocardium in pigs with a chronic left anterior descending coronary artery stenosis: absence of progressive fibrosis in the setting of stable reductions in flow, function and coronary flow reserve. J Am Coll Cardiol 2001; 37: 1989-95. [http://dx.doi.org/10.1016/S0735-1097(01)01250-5]

[28] Depré C, Vanoverschelde JL, Melin JA, *et al.* Structural and metabolic correlates of the reversibility of chronic left ventricular ischemic dysfunction in humans. Am J Physiol 1995; 268: H1265-75.

[29] Borgers M, Thone F, Wouters L, *et al.* Structural correlates of regional myocardial dysfunction in patients with critical coronary artery stenosis: Chronic hibernation? Cardiovasc Pathol 1993; 2: 237-45. [http://dx.doi.org/10.1016/1054-8807(93)90030-6]

[30] Ausma J, Furst D, Thone F, *et al.* Molecular changes of titin in left ventricular dysfunction as a result of chronic hibernation. J Mol Cell Cardiol 1995; 27: 1203-12. [http://dx.doi.org/10.1016/0022-2828(95)90056-X]

[31] Depre C, Taegtmeyer H. Metabolic aspects of programmed cell survival and cell death in the heart. Cardiovasc Res 2000; 45: 538-48. [http://dx.doi.org/10.1016/S0008-6363(99)00266-7]

[32] Vanoverschelde J-L, Depre C, Gerber BL, *et al.* Time-course of functional recovery after coronary bypass surgery in patients with chronic left ventricular ischemic dysfunction. Am J Cardiol 2000; 85: 1432-9. [http://dx.doi.org/10.1016/S0002-9149(00)00790-6]

[33] Page BJ, Banas MD, Suzuki G, *et al.* Revascularization of chronic hibernating myocardium stimulates myocyte proliferation and partially reverses chronic adaptations to ischemia. J Am Coll Cardiol 2015; 65: 684-97. [http://dx.doi.org/10.1016/j.jacc.2014.11.040]

[34] Thomas SA, Fallavollita JA, Suzuki G, *et al.* Discussion of regional adaptation to ischemia and global myolysis in an accelerated swine model of chronic hibernating myocardium. Circ Res 2002; 91: 970-7. [http://dx.doi.org/10.1161/01.RES.0000040396.79379.77]

[35] Maki M, Luotolahti M, Nuutila P, *et al.* Glucose uptake in the chronically dysfunctional but viable myocardium. Circulation 1996; 93: 1658-66. [http://dx.doi.org/10.1161/01.CIR.93.9.1658]

[36] Fallavollita JA. Spatial heterogeneity in fasting and insulin-stimulated 18F-deoxyglucose uptake in pigs with hibernating myocardium. Circulation 2000; 102: 908-14. [http://dx.doi.org/10.1161/01.CIR.102.8.908]

[37] McMurray JJ, Adamopoulos S, Anker SD, Auricchio A, Bohm M, Dickstein K, *et al.* ESC Guidelines for the diagnosis and treatment of acute and chronic heart failure 2012: The Task Force for the Diagnosis and Treatment of Acute and Chronic Heart Failure 2012 of the European Society of Cardiology. Developed in collaboration with the Heart Failure Association (HFA) of the ESC. Eur Heart J 2012; 33: 1787-847. [http://dx.doi.org/10.1093/eurheartj/ehs104]

[38] Schinkel AF, Bax JJ, Poldermans D, Elhendy A, Ferrari R, Rahimtoola SH. Hibernating myocardium: Diagnosis and patient outcomes. Curr Probl Cardiol 2007; 32: 375-410. [http://dx.doi.org/10.1016/j.cpcardiol.2007.04.001]

[39] Bax JJ, Delgado V. Myocardial viability as integral part of the diagnostic and therapeutic approach to ischemic heart failure. J Nucl Cardiol 2015; 22: 229-45. [http://dx.doi.org/10.1007/s12350-015-0096-5]

[40] Cornel JH, Bax JJ, Elhendy A, *et al.* Predictive accuracy of echocardiographic response of mildly dyssynergic myocardial segments to low-dose dubutamine. Am J Cardiol 1997; 80: 1484-4. [http://dx.doi.org/10.1016/S0002-9149(97)00721-2]

[41] Rizzello V, Biagini E, Schinkel AFL, *et al.* Comparison of functional recovery of mildly hypokinetic versus severly dysfunctional left ventricular segments after revascularization in patients with ischemic cardiomyopathy. Am J Cardiol 2004; 93: 394-8. [http://dx.doi.org/10.1016/j.amjcard.2003.10.030]

[42] Gibons RS, Watson DD, Taylor GJ, *et al.* Prospective assessment of regional myocardial perfusion before and after coronary revascularization surgery by quantitative thallium-201 scintigrapgy. J Am Coll Cardiol 1983; 1: 804-15. [http://dx.doi.org/10.1016/S0735-1097(83)80194-6]

[43] Kiat H, Berman DS, Maddahi J, *et al.* Late reversibility of tomographic myocardial thallium-201 defects: An accurate marker of myocardial viability. J Am Coll Cardiol 1988; 12: 1456-63. [http://dx.doi.org/10.1016/S0735-1097(88)80009-3]

[44] Manyari DE, Knudtson M, Kloiber R, *et al.* Sequential thallium-201 myocardial perfusion studies after successful percutaneous transluminal coronary artery angioplasty: Delayed resolution of exercise induced scintigraphic abnormalities. Circulation 1988; 77: 86-95. [http://dx.doi.org/10.1161/01.CIR.77.1.86]

[45] Brunken R, Schwaiger M, Grover-Mckay M, *et al.* Positron emission tomography detects tissue metabolic activity in myocardial segments with persistent thallium perfusion defects. J Am Coll Cardiol 1987; 10: 557-67. [http://dx.doi.org/10.1016/S0735-1097(87)80198-5]

[46] Tamaki N, Yonekura Y, Yamashita K, *et al.* Relation of left ventricular perfusion and wall motion with metabolic activity in persistent defects on thallium-201 tomography in healed myocardial infarction. Am J Cardiol 1988; 62: 202-8. [http://dx.doi.org/10.1016/0002-9149(88)90212-3]

[47] Tamaki N, Yonekura Y, Yamashita K, *et al.* SPECT thallium-201 tomography and positron tomography using N-13 ammonia and F-18 fluorodeoxyglucose in coronary artery disease. Am J Card Imaging 1989; 3: 3-9.

[48] Brunken RC, Kottou S, Nienaber CA, *et al.* PET detection of viable tissue in myocardial segments with persistent defects at Tl-201 SPECT. Radiology 1989; 65: 65-73. [http://dx.doi.org/10.1148/radiology.172.1.2787037]

[49] Yang LD, Berman DS, Kiat H, *et al.* The frequency of late reversibility in SPECT thallium-201 stress-redistribution studies. J Am Coll Cardiol 1990; 15: 334-40. [http://dx.doi.org/10.1016/S0735-1097(10)80057-9]

[50] Brunken RC, Mody FV, Hawkins RA, *et al.* Positron emission tomography detects metabolic activity in myocardium with persistent 24-hour single photon emission computed tomography 201Tl defects. Circulation 1992; 86: 1357-69. [http://dx.doi.org/10.1161/01.CIR.86.5.1357]

[51] Dilsizian V, Rocco TP, Freedman NM, *et al.* Enhanced detection of ischemic but viable myocardium by the reinjection of thallium after stress-redistribution imaging. N Engl J Med 1990; 323: 141-6. [http://dx.doi.org/10.1056/NEJM199007193230301]

[52] Rocco TP, Disizian V, McKusick KA, *et al.* Comparison of thallium redistribution with rest "reinjection" imaging for detection of viable myocardium. Am J Cardiol 1990; 66: 158-63. [http://dx.doi.org/10.1016/0002-9149(90)90580-T]

[53] Mori T, Minamiji K, Kurogane H, *et al.* Rest-injected thallium-201 imaging for assessing viability of severe asynergic regions. J Nucl Med 1991; 32: 1718-24.

[54] Holly TA, Bonow RO. Assessment of myocardial viability with thallium-201 and technetium-based

agents.Clinical nuclear cardiology State of the art and future direction. 3rd ed. Philadelphia: Elsevier 2005; pp. 503-17.

[55] Bonow RO, Dilsizian V, Cuocolo A, *et al.* Identification of viable myocardium in patients with chronic coronary artery disease and left ventricular dysfunction: Comparison of thallium scintigraphy with reinjection and PET imaging with 18F-fluorodeoxyglucose. Circulation 1991; 83: 26-37. [http://dx.doi.org/10.1161/01.CIR.83.1.26]

[56] Bax JJ, Cornel JH, Visser FC, *et al.* Comparison of fluorine-18-FDG with rest-redistribution thallium-201 SPECT to delineate viable myocardium and predict functional recovery after revascularization. J Nucl Med 1998; 39: 1481-6.

[57] Dilsizian V, Perrone-Filardi P, Arrighi JA, *et al.* Concordance and discordance between stress-redistribution-reinjection and rest-redistribution thallium imaging for assessing viable myocardium: Comparison with metabolic activity by positron emission tomography. Circulation 1993; 88: 941-52. [http://dx.doi.org/10.1161/01.CIR.88.3.941]

[58] Perrone-Filardi P, Pace L, Prastaro M, *et al.* Assessment of myocardial viability in patients with chronic coronary artery disease. Rest-4-hour-24-hour 201Tl tomography versus dobutamine echocardiography. Circulation 1996; 94: 2712-9. [http://dx.doi.org/10.1161/01.CIR.94.11.2712]

[59] Bonow RO, Dilsizian V. Thallium-201 and technetium-99m-sestamibi for assessing viable myocardium. J Nucl Med 1992; 33: 815-8.

[60] Cuocolo A, Pace L, Ricciardelli B, *et al.* Identification of viable myocardium in patients with chronic coronary artery disease: Comparison of thallium-201 scintigraphy with reinjection and technetium-99m-methoxyisobutyl isonitrile. J Nucl Med 1992; 33: 505-11.

[61] Sawada SG, Allman KC, Muzik O, *et al.* Positron emission tomography detects viability in rest technetium-99m-sestamibi defects. J Am Coll Cardiol 1994; 23: 92-8. [http://dx.doi.org/10.1016/0735-1097(94)90506-1]

[62] Sansoy V, Glover DK, Watson DD, *et al.* Comparison of thallium-201 resting redistribution with technetium-99m-sestamibi uptake and functional response to dobutamine for assessment of myocardial viability. Circulation 1995; 92: 994-1004. [http://dx.doi.org/10.1161/01.CIR.92.4.994]

[63] Kauffman GJ, Boyne TS, Watson DD, *et al.* Comparison of rest thallium-201 imaging and rest technetium-99m sestamibi for assessment of myocardial viability in patients with coronary artery disease and severe left ventricular dysfunction. J Am Coll Cardiol 1996; 27: 1592-7. [http://dx.doi.org/10.1016/0735-1097(96)00090-3]

[64] Udelson JE, Coleman PS, Metherall J, *et al.* Predicting recovery of severe regional ventricular dysfunction: Comparison of resting scintigraphy with 201Tl and 99mTc-sestamibi. Circulation 1994; 89: 2552-61. [http://dx.doi.org/10.1161/01.CIR.89.6.2552]

[65] Bisi G, Sciagra R, Santoro GM, *et al.* Rest technetium-99m sestamibi in combination with short-term administration of nitrates: Feasibility and reliability for prediction of postrevascularization outcome of asynergic territories. J Am Coll Cardiol 1994; 24: 1282-9. [http://dx.doi.org/10.1016/0735-1097(94)90110-4]

[66] Maurea S, Cuocolo A, Soricelli A, *et al.* Enhanced detection of viable myocardium by technetium-99m-MIBI imaging after nitrate administration in chronic coronary artery disease. J Nucl Med 1995; 36: 1945-52.

[67] Acampa W, Cuocolo A, Petretta M, *et al.* Tetrofosmin imaging in the detection of myocardial viability in patients with previous myocardial infarction: Comparison with sestamibi and Tl-201 scintigraphy. J Nucl Cardiol 2002; 9: 33-40. [http://dx.doi.org/10.1067/mnc.2002.118122]

[68] He w. Tc-99m tetrofosmin tomography after nitrate administration in patients with ischemic left ventricular dysfunction: Relation to metabolic imaging by PET. J Nucl Cardiol 2003; 10: 599-606. [http://dx.doi.org/10.1016/S1071-3581(03)00649-4]

[69] Opie LH. Effects of regional ischemia on metabolism of glucose and fatty acids. Circ Res 1976; 38: 152-74.

[70] Knuuti MJ, Nuutila P, Ruotsalainen U, *et al.* Euglycemic hyperinsulinemic clamp and oral glucose load in stimulating myocardial glucose utilization during positron emission tomography. J Nucl Med 1992; 33: 1255-62.

[71] Dong W, Li J, Mi H, Song X, Jiao J, Li Q. Relationship between collateral circulation and myocardial viability of 18F-FDG PET/CT subtended by chronic total occluded coronary arteries. Ann Nucl Med 2018; 32: 197-205. [http://dx.doi.org/10.1007/s12149-018-1234-3]

[72] Srinvasan G, Kitsiou AN, Bacharach SL, *et al.* 18F-Deoxyglucose SPECT: Can it replace PET and thalliu-201 SPECT for the assessment of myocardial viability? Circulation 1998; 97: 843-50. [http://dx.doi.org/10.1161/01.CIR.97.9.843]

[73] Kim RJ, Wu E, Rafael A, Chen EL, Parker MA, Simonetti O, *et al.* The use of contrast-enhanced magnetic resonance imaging to identify reversible myocardial dysfunction. N Engl J Med 2000; 343: 1445-53. [http://dx.doi.org/10.1056/NEJM200011163432003]

[74] Bax JJ, Poldermans D, Elhendy A, *et al.* Sensitivity, specificity, and predictive accuracies of various noninvasive techniques for detecting hibernating myocardium. Curr Probl Cardiol 2001; 26: 144-73. [http://dx.doi.org/10.1067/mcd.2001.109973]

[75] Maddahi J. Viability assessment with MRI is superior to FDG-PET for viability: Pro. J Nucl Cardiol 2010; 17: 292-7. [http://dx.doi.org/10.1007/s12350-010-9201-y]

[76] Bax JJ, Cornel JH, Visser FC, *et al.* Prediction of improvement of contractile function in patients with ischemic ventricular dysfunction after revascularization by fluorine-18 fluorodeoxyglucose single-photon emission computed tomography. J Am Coll Cardiol 1997; 30: 377-83. [http://dx.doi.org/10.1016/S0735-1097(97)00174-5]

[77] Mule JD, Bax JJ, Zingone B, *et al.* The beneficial effect of revascularization on jeopardized myocardium: reverse remodeling and improved long-term prognosis. Eur J Cardiothorac Surg 2002; 22: 426-30. [http://dx.doi.org/10.1016/S1010-7940(02)00359-7]

[78] Meinertz T, Kasper W, Schumacher M, *et al.* The German multicenter trial of anisoylated plasminogen streptokinase activator complex versus heparin for acute myocardial infarction. Am J Cardiol 1988; 62: 347-51. [http://dx.doi.org/10.1016/0002-9149(88)90956-3]

[79] Bax JJ, Poldermans D. Clinical value of assessment of perfusion and function for the evaluation of myocardial viability in patients with ischemic left ventricular dysfunction.Clinical Gated Cardiac SPECT. 2nd ed. New York: Blackwell Publishing 2006; pp. 257-63. [http://dx.doi.org/10.1002/9780470987520.ch10]

[80] Mortelmans L, Vanhaecke J, Lesaffre E, *et al.* Evaluation of the effect of thrombolytic treatment on infarct size and left ventricular function by enzymatic, scintigraphic, and angiographic methods. The European Cooperative Study Group for Recombinant Tissue Type Plasminogen Activator. Am Heart J 1990; 119: 1231-7. [http://dx.doi.org/10.1016/S0002-8703(05)80169-3]

[81] Inaba Y, Chen JA, Bergmann SR. Quantity of viable myocardium required to improve survival with revascularization in patients with ischemic cardiomyopathy: A meta-analysis. J Nucl Cardiol 2010; 17:

646-54.
[http://dx.doi.org/10.1007/s12350-010-9226-2]

[82] D'Egidio G, Nichol G, Whillams KA, *et al.* Increasing benefit from revascularization is associated with increasing amount of myocardial hibernation: a substudy of the PARR-2 trial. JACC Cardiovasc Imaging 2009; 2: 1060-8.
[http://dx.doi.org/10.1016/j.jcmg.2009.02.017]

[83] Beanlands RSB, Ruddy TD, She L, *et al.* Positron emission tomography and recovery following revascularization (PARR-1): The importance of scar and the development of a prediction rule for the degree of recovery of left ventricular function. J Am Coll Cardiol 2002; 40: 1735-43.
[http://dx.doi.org/10.1016/S0735-1097(02)02489-0]

[84] Konstam MA, Rousseau MF, Kronenberg MW, *et al.* Effects of the angiotensin converting enzyme inhibitor enalapril on the long-term progression of left ventricular dysfunction in patients with heart failure. SOLVD Investigators. Circulation 1992; 86: 431-8.
[http://dx.doi.org/10.1161/01.CIR.86.2.431]

[85] St John Sutton M, Pfeffer MA, Moye L, *et al.* Cardiovascular death and left ventricular remodeling two years after myocardial infarction: baseline predictors and impact of long-term use of captopril: information from the Survival and Ventricular Enlargement (SAVE) trial. Circulation 1997; 96: 3294-9.
[http://dx.doi.org/10.1161/01.CIR.96.10.3294]

[86] Udelson JE, Konstam MA. Relation between left ventricular remodeling and clinical outcomes in heart failure patients with left ventricular systolic dysfunction. J Card Fail 2002; 6 (Suppl.): S465-71.
[http://dx.doi.org/10.1054/jcaf.2002.129289]

[87] Senior R, Lahiri A, Kaul S. Effect of revascularization on left ventricular remodeling in patients with heart failure from severe chronic ischemic left ventricular dysfunction. Am J Cardiol 2001; 88: 624-9.
[http://dx.doi.org/10.1016/S0002-9149(01)01803-3]

[88] Samady H, Elefteriades JA, Abbott BG, *et al.* Failure to improve left ventricular function after coronary revascularization for ischemic cardiomyopathy is not associated with worse outcome. Circulation 1999; 100: 1298-304.
[http://dx.doi.org/10.1161/01.CIR.100.12.1298]

[89] Schinkel AF, Poldermans D, Rizzello V, *et al.* Why do patients with ischemic cardiomyopathy and a substantial amount of viable myocardium not always recover in function after revascularization? J Thorac Cardiovasc Surg 2004; 127: 385-90.
[http://dx.doi.org/10.1016/j.jtcvs.2003.08.005]

[90] Rizzello V, Poldermans D, Boersma E, *et al.* Opposite patterns of left ventricular remodeling after coronary revascularization in patients with ischemic cardiomyopathy: role of myocardial viability. Circulation 2004; 110: 2383-8.
[http://dx.doi.org/10.1161/01.CIR.0000145115.29952.14]

[91] Bax JJ, Schinkel AF, Boersma E, *et al.* Early versus delayed revascularization in patients with ischemic cardiomyopathy and substantial viability: impact on outcome. Circulation 2003; 108: 1954-9.
[http://dx.doi.org/10.1161/01.cir.0000089041.69175.9d]

[92] Bonow RO, Castelvecchio S, Panza JA, *et al.* Severity of remodeling, myocardial viability, and survival in ischemic LV dysfunction after surgical revascularization. JACC Cardiovasc Imaging 2015; 8: 1121-9.
[http://dx.doi.org/10.1016/j.jcmg.2015.03.013]

[93] Chen Y, Duan C, Liu F, Shen S, Chen P, Bin J. Impact of etiology on the outcomes in heart failure patients treated with cardiac resynchronization therapy: A meta-analysis. Plos ONE 2014; 9(4): e94614.
[http://dx.doi.org/10.1371/journal.pone.0094614]

[94] Abraham WT, Fisher WG, Smith AL, *et al.* Cardiac resynchronization in chronic heart failure. N Engl

J Med 2002; 346: 1845-53.
[http://dx.doi.org/10.1056/NEJMoa013168]

[95] Chung ES, Leon AR, Tavazzi L, *et al.* Results of the Predictors of Response to CRT (PROSPECT) trial. Circulation 2008; 117: 2608-16.
[http://dx.doi.org/10.1161/CIRCULATIONAHA.107.743120]

[96] Boogers MM, Van Kriekinge SD, Henneman MM, *et al.* Quantitative gated SPECT-derived phase analysis on gated myocardial perfusion SPECT detects left ventricular dyssynchrony and predicts response to cardiac resynchronization therapy. J Nucl Med 2009; 50: 718-25.
[http://dx.doi.org/10.2967/jnumed.108.060657]

[97] Adelstein EC, Tanaka H, Soman P, *et al.* Impact of scar burden by single-photon emission computed tomography myocardial perfusion imaging on patient outcomes following cardiac resynchronization therapy. Eur Heart J 2011; 32: 93-103.
[http://dx.doi.org/10.1093/eurheartj/ehq389]

CHAPTER 4

Cardiac Hybrid or Fusion Imaging and Future Prospective

Shinro Matsuo*

Department of Nuclear Medicine, Kanazawa University Hospital, Kanazawa, Japan

Graduate School of Advanced Preventive Medical Sciences, Kanazawa, Japan

Abstract: Cardiac single photon emission computed tomography (SPECT) / computed tomography (CT) has been introduced to provide anatomical information on such as coronary calcification combined with functional information of myocardial perfusion imaging. Fusion imaging provides accurate co-registration of coronary stenosis and perfusion abnormalities, and allows identification of reduced coronary flow reserve. This chapter shows an overview of relevant literature including clinical value in SPECT/CT.

Keywords: CT Angiography, Hybrid Imaging, Ischemia, SPECT.

INTRODUCTION

Ischemic heart disease is a multifactorial entity that can be diagnosed through non-invasive tests such as nuclear cardiology examination and computed tomography (CT) [1]. The stress myocardial perfusion imaging plays an important role in the risk-stratification of the patients with suspected coronary artery disease, diagnosing the extent and severity of infarction and ischemia induced by both epicardial coronary arteries and resistance vessels [2]. CT coronary angiography can help identify morphological features of coronary arteries [3, 4]. If the ischemia-causing coronary stenosis is identified by non-invasive imaging, the culprit lesion can be determined as a therapeutic target of coronary intervention [5]. The relationship between ischemia and coronary artery narrowing can be accurately diagnosed by fusion imaging between single photon emission computed tomography (SPECT) and CT coronary angiography [5 - 6]. Additional information on vessel calcification and inflammation can be identified by the CT

* **Corresponding author Shinro Matsuo:** Department of Nuclear Medicine, Kanazawa University Hospital, 13-1 Takara-machi, Kanazawa 920-8641, Japan, Advanced Preventive Medical Sciences, Kanazawa University Graduate School, 13-1 Takara-machi, Kanazawa, Japan 920-8641; Tel: 81-76-265-2333; Fax: 81-76-234-4257; E-mail: smatsuo@med.kanazawa-u.ac.jp

and the ^{18}F-fluorodeoxyglucose-positron emission tomography (FDG-PET) in the process of coronary artery disease, as well as ischemia and infarction [7].

Recently, non-invasive imaging has advanced recently in the field of the nuclear cardiology, including of SPECT / CT with multifocal collimator and semi-conductor detectors, enabling a short acquisition time [8, 9]. The SPECT/CT also becomes available and quantifies calcification and cardiac function. This chapter describes a method of diagnosing through hybrid information from multiple modalities in characterizing the pathophy- siology of coronary artery disease.

Anatomic and Physiological Stenosis

Anatomical information of the coronary arteries can be easily obtained by CT angiography [3, 4]. Accurate documenting coronary stenosis is critical target in a strategy of coronary intervention therapy [5]. However, not all of these pathophysiological conditions can be diagnosed by CT information, since small arteries and arterioles level as well as the epicardial coronary artery plays an important role in controlling the coronary circulation at the same time [10]. Actually coronary stenosis on CT may not induce ischemia on SPECT images [11, 12]. Reduced coronary flow reserve might be observed in patients without stenosis [10, 13]. Myocardial perfusion tracers as ^{201}Tl or ^{99m}Tc agents will be distributed according to the antegrade blood flow and the amount of coronary flow, and also depends on the blood flow of the collateral circulation. Understanding of these physiologies is essential in order to interpret well a hybrid or fusion imaging.

In addition to the detection of coronary stenosis, important information such as coronary plaque, vascular remodeling, micro-calcifications and the myocardial wall thickness could be obtained by the CT scan. Coronary plaque morphology had been intensively investigated [14, 15]. There was a good agreement between CT angiography plaque and intravascular ultrasound [16]. Low density CT density or napkin ring sign plaque, and thin cap fibroatheroma are considered to be suggestive feature for the unstable condition [17, 18]. However, there might be a long way to use CT plaque information as a clinical indicator for evaluating the prognosis of the patients with stable angina pectoris.

Quantitative Evaluation of Myocardial Ischemia

The Courage trial nuclear sub-study showed that the subjects with improved perfusion had better prognosis than those without, by using myocardial perfusion imaging [19]. And, the beneficial prognostic result was observed in the patients especially with more than 5% ischemic improvement through coronary intervention. The incidence of cardiac events for the patients with coronary artery disease becomes higher according to the degree of perfusion defect in stress myocardial perfusion scan [2]. The prognosis of the subjects with coronary artery disease is reportedly improved by performing coronary intervention in patients with more than 10% ischemia. Therefore, the quantification of the degree of ischemia or infarction is so important in selecting subjects to treat for improving the prognosis. Without using invasive methods such as fractional flow reserve (FFR) measurement by cardiac catheterization, a recent study demonstrated that myocardial perfusion imaging could identify the lesion to be accurately evaluated by non-invasive stress SPECT [20, 21]. Recent advancements of nuclear cardiology techniques support this analysis by novel software. The neural network software called cardioREPO (Fuji Film RI Pharma, Tokyo, Japan), which was developed in collaboration with Exini Co., Sweden. This software can identify the blood flow abnormalities and myocardial ischemia in quantified analysis [21]. Since the amount of ischemia is closely related to the subsequent cardiac death, the precise analysis of myocardial ischemic area would become so important (Fig. **3**). Only patients with decreased ischemia demonstrated in myocardial imaging have the benefits of revascularization, including bypass surgery [19]. Meanwhile, when the subject with suspected ischemic heart disease is diagnosed as having normal SPECT, annual hard cardiac events of the patients with normal SPECT images is 0.6% / per year [22]. The annual hard event rate in patients asymptomatic of type 2 diabetes is 0.8% / year [23]. The patients with normal myocardial perfusion imaging can be managed as having a low risk of cardiac event [22, 23]. Coronary intervention to the patient without ischemia further may become harmful results in terms of the prognosis. Cardiac event risk could be estimated using myocardial perfusion imaging defect score and left ventricular ejection fraction in conjunction of other clinical information [24]. Thus, myocardial perfusion imaging is to help physicians in risk stratification of each patient rather than identifying a per-coronary artery lesion. And we should treat invasively the particular patient with reduced myocardial blood flow reserve [25].

Fusion Imaging of CT Angiography and SPECT

Contrast CT coronary angiography is widely used in clinical setting. A multi-slice CT with eight-detector-low had emerged in early 2000, the diagnostic sensitivity of coronary CT angiography was 75% when compared to the standard invasive coronary angiography as a reference [4]. CT coronary angiography had advanced then from 16, 32, and 64 to 320 detectors. The diagnostic performance of coronary CT angiography when compared to invasive coronary angiography has been has been proved to be eligible in many studies with a high specificity. By extracting the coronary arteries obtained from the CT coronary angiography, it is possible to create a fused image of the myocardial perfusion SPECT and CT coronary angiography even if the manufacturers of the SPECT and CT were different [8, 26]. Organic narrowing lesions of a right coronary artery caused a mild ischemia in the basal inferior wall area of the left ventricle in the case of Fig. (**1**). Culprit coronary artery lesions can be determined to be the middle right coronary artery in a definitive diagnosis. The perfusion abnormalities in an 83-year-old male with coronary artery bypass surgery could be demonstrated to be due to high lateral branch of the left anterior descending coronary artery, by the fusion imaging (Fig. **2**). Thus, the fusion image enabled the diagnosis of the dominant region of the blood vessel, even after bypass surgery [8].

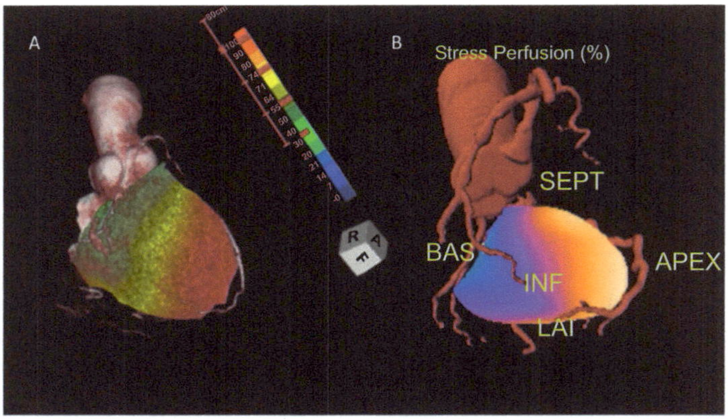

Fig. (1). Fusion imaging in patients with organic stenosis in right coronary artery. Culprit lesions of ischemia were determined in both A and B.

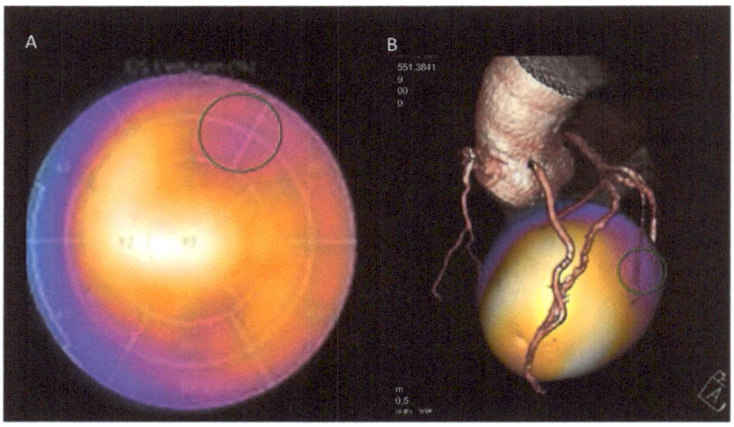

Fig. (2). Fusion imaging in a patient with coronary bypass graft. High lateral branch was diagnosed as a culprit lesion. A, polar map. B, fusion imaging.

The Benefits of Fusion Imaging

Fused SPECT/CT imaging provides an additional clinical value in deciding the strategy of the treatment for the patients with coronary artery disease, as well as inflammatory disease. The matched finding of ischemia and stenosis indicates a higher incidence of major adverse cardiac events (MACE) [26]. The incidence of MACE in subjects with the unmatched findings was significantly lower than that in matched subjects. Furthermore, when both perfusion and anatomical coronary arteries were normal, the MACE incidence of subjects is the lowest [27, 28]. Performing a coronary intervention treatment to the stenotic vessels responsible for ischemia, which were identified by fusion imaging, has a merit of reducing the occurrence of the patient's MACE and improving the prognosis. The fusion imaging is proved to have the advantage that allows the identification of a side-branch ischemia in patients with ischemic heart disease [8, 26]. However, it is important to read the fusion imaging is familiar with divergence and microcirculation disorders of the coronary arteries of form and function, as previously described. The assessment that ischemia is associated with coronary stenosis by the fusion imaging matching, is extremely important in considering the coronary intervention treatment strategy (Fig. **3**).

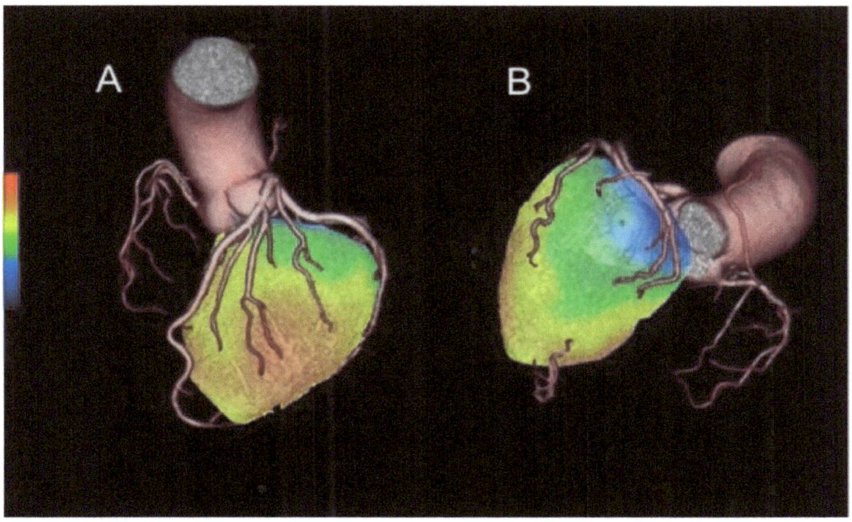

Fig. (3). Fusion imaging in a patient without apparent coronary stenosis. There was no significant stenosis in left anterior descending coronary artery and left circumflex. However, sight hypo-perfusion in basal infero-lateral area was observed.

The Coronary Artery Calcification Evaluation by SPECT / CT

Recently a hybrid SPECT / CT has been introduced and available in clinical evaluation of perfusion and coronary calcification [11, 29]. The coronary calcification score can be used to estimate the total magnitude of atherosclerotic burden of the coronary arteries. A hybrid SPECT/CT system provides subclinical information of the risk of the patients. The higher the calcification score, the more possibilities of ischemia or infarction exist.

Since myocardial perfusion by SPECT can display a relative perfusion image, balanced ischemia such as multi-vessel coronary arteries may be determined to as ischemia and considered to be normal as false negative. However, coronary calcification evaluation may provide additional information. Coronary artery calcification could suggest that the inflammatory lesions had been present previously in the coronary arteries. If severe calcification were observed in patients with Agatston score more than 1000 in even normal SPECT, the patients would be considered to have the risk of coronary artery disease. Previous studies demonstrated that it would become possible to carry out improved effective screening by using a combination calcification score and myocardial perfusion SPECT [7, 29]. The study showed that the subjects with higher calcium score more than 1000 had a trend toward ischemia and infarction [11]. The documentation of coronary calcification as a marker of coronary atherosclerosis can be used to manage the patients with coronary risk factors. Coronary active inflammation observed from the information of FDG-PET may indicate unstable plaque leading to plaque rapture and acute coronary syndrome.

Fusion Diagnosis of Functional Information and Blood Flow

The exercise or pharmacological stress induces the ischemia, resulting in transient left ventricular cavity dilatation, left ventricular systolic or diastolic function [30]. Gated SPECT detects these functional changes of left ventricular volumes and ejection fraction. Post-stress dysfunction provides us a diagnostic clue in patients with multi-vessel disease [30, 31]. Utilizing this functional information as well as myocardial perfusion, diagnosis of balanced ischemia would become possible. And the transient ischemic dilatation and post-stress dysfunction are the clinical indicators for poor prognosis of ischemic heart disease patients [30].

Multifocal collimators with dedicated reconstruction software and CT have been introduced [9]. This IQ-SPECT system with ^{99m}Tc or ^{201}Tl shortens acquisition times and is clinically applicable in diagnosing patients with high image quality [9]. The cadmium zink-telluride (CZT) cameras provide shorter scan times and higher temporal and spatial resolution than Anger camera [32, 33]. An experimental pig model reported that the quantification of absolute myocardial blood flow (MBF) measurement could become possible using ^{99m}Tc agents and ^{201}Tl [32]. Fractional flow reserve (FFR) is a clinical indicator for the decision-making of coronary intervention. It may provide better information than angiography alone [34]. Dynamic SPECT (D-SPECT) imaging during first pass of a tracer was attained with the use of CZT camera [33]. Although PET plays a major role in precise evaluation of myocardial flow reserve using ^{13}N-ammonia, ^{82}Rb, ^{15}O-water and ^{18}F-flupiridaz [35, 36], myocardial perfusion can be measured in many facilities and enhance the quantitative properties. SPECT quantification may really improve the diagnostic accuracy including the detection of balanced ischemia. The main disadvantage of SPECT in quantification may be underestimation of myocardial flow reserve when compared to that with PET. This limitation of underestimation comes from the lower extraction of ^{99m}Tc agents at high flow.

CONCLUSION

In the past few years, nuclear cardiology techniques made a great advancement, including fusion images and SPECT / CT, and have greatly been changed by the appearance of a short time acquisition time. The novel hybrid system and fusion imaging to diagnose together anatomical information and functional information provides essential information in considering the therapeutic strategy of coronary intervention.

CONSENT FOR PUBLICATION

Not applicable.

CONFLICT OF INTEREST

The author declares no conflict of interest, financial or otherwise.

ACKNOWLEDGEMENTS

Declared none.

REFERENCES

[1] Hachamovitch R, Nutter B, Hlatky MA, *et al.* Patient management after noninvasive cardiac imaging results from SPARC (Study of myocardial perfusion and coronary anatomy imaging roles in coronary artery disease). J Am Coll Cardiol 2012; 59(5): 462-74. [http://dx.doi.org/10.1016/j.jacc.2011.09.066] [PMID: 22281249]

[2] Nishimura T, Nakajima K, Kusuoka H, Yamashina A, Nishimura S. Prognostic study of risk stratification among Japanese patients with ischemic heart disease using gated myocardial perfusion SPECT: J-ACCESS study. Eur J Nucl Med Mol Imaging 2008; 35(2): 319-28. [http://dx.doi.org/10.1007/s00259-007-0608-x] [PMID: 17926033]

[3] Matsuo S, Horie M. Cardiovascular imaging by means of multi-slice CT in cardiology. Nippon Hoshasen Gijutsu Gakkai Zasshi 2005; 61(9): 1309-17. [http://dx.doi.org/10.6009/jjrt.KJ00004028547] [PMID: 16192918]

[4] Matsuo S, Nakamura Y, Matsumoto T, *et al.* Visual assessment of coronary artery stenosis with electrocardiographically-gated multislice computed tomography. Int J Cardiovasc Imaging 2004; 20(1): 61-6. [http://dx.doi.org/10.1023/B:CAIM.0000013159.01950.7c] [PMID: 15055822]

[5] Koo BK, Erglis A, Doh JH, *et al.* Diagnosis of ischemia-causing coronary stenoses by noninvasive fractional flow reserve computed from coronary computed tomographic angiograms. Results from the prospective multicenter DISCOVER-FLOW (Diagnosis of Ischemia-Causing Stenoses Obtained Via Noninvasive Fractional Flow Reserve) study. J Am Coll Cardiol 2011; 58(19): 1989-97. [http://dx.doi.org/10.1016/j.jacc.2011.06.066] [PMID: 22032711]

[6] Gaemperli O, Schepis T, Valenta I, *et al.* Functionally relevant coronary artery disease: comparison of 64-section CT angiography with myocardial perfusion SPECT. Radiology 2008; 248(2): 414-23. [http://dx.doi.org/10.1148/radiol.2482071307] [PMID: 18552310]

[7] Uebleis C, Becker A, Griesshammer I, *et al.* Stable coronary artery disease: prognostic value of myocardial perfusion SPECT in relation to coronary calcium scoring--long-term follow-up. Radiology 2009; 252(3): 682-90. [http://dx.doi.org/10.1148/radiol.2531082137] [PMID: 19703866]

[8] Matsuo S, Nakajima K, Akhter N, *et al.* Clinical usefulness of novel cardiac MDCT/SPECT fusion image. Ann Nucl Med 2009; 23(6): 579-86. [http://dx.doi.org/10.1007/s12149-009-0279-8] [PMID: 19572098]

[9] Matsuo S, Nakajima K, Onoguchi M, Wakabayash H, Okuda K, Kinuya S. Nuclear myocardial perfusion imaging using thallium-201 with a novel multifocal collimator SPECT/CT: IQ-SPECT versus conventional protocols in normal subjects. Ann Nucl Med 2015; 29(5): 452-9. [http://dx.doi.org/10.1007/s12149-015-0965-7] [PMID: 25821018]

[10] Matsuo S, Nakamura Y, Matsumoto T, Takahashi M, Kinoshita M. Detection of coronary microvascular disease by means of cardiac scintigraphy. Can J Cardiol 2002; 18(2): 183-6. [PMID: 11875588]

[11] Matsuo S, Nakajima K, Okuda K, Kinuya S. The relationship between stress-induced myocardial ischemia and coronary artery atherosclerosis measured by hybrid SPECT/CT camera. Ann Nucl Med 2011; 25(9): 650-6. [http://dx.doi.org/10.1007/s12149-011-0517-8] [PMID: 21779962]

[12] Matsuo S, Matsumoto T, Takashima H, *et al.* The relationship between flow-mediated brachial artery vasodilation and coronary vasomotor responses to bradykinin: comparison with those to acetylcholine. J Cardiovasc Pharmacol 2004; 44(2): 164-70. [http://dx.doi.org/10.1097/00005344-200408000-00004] [PMID: 15243296]

[13] Mohri M, Koyanagi M, Egashira K, *et al.* Angina pectoris caused by coronary microvascular spasm. Lancet 1998; 351(9110): 1165-9. [http://dx.doi.org/10.1016/S0140-6736(97)07329-7] [PMID: 9643687]

[14] Matsumoto N, Sato Y, Yoda S, *et al.* Prognostic value of non-obstructive CT low-dense coronary artery plaques detected by multislice computed tomography. Circ J 2007; 71(12): 1898-903. [http://dx.doi.org/10.1253/circj.71.1898] [PMID: 18037743]

[15] Rozanski A, Gransar H, Wong ND, *et al.* Clinical outcomes after both coronary calcium scanning and exercise myocardial perfusion scintigraphy. J Am Coll Cardiol 2007; 49(12): 1352-61. [http://dx.doi.org/10.1016/j.jacc.2006.12.035] [PMID: 17394969]

[16] Matsuo S, Nakamura Y, Matsumoto T, Nakae I, Koh T, Horie M. Noninvasive evaluation of coronary artery plaque with ECG-gated multislice computed tomography. J Am Coll Cardiol 2004; 43: 363-4. [http://dx.doi.org/10.1016/S0735-1097(04)91537-9]

[17] Maurovich-Horvat P, Schlett CL, Alkadhi H, *et al.* The napkin-ring sign indicates advanced atherosclerotic lesions in coronary CT angiography. JACC Cardiovasc Imaging 2012; 5(12): 1243-52. [http://dx.doi.org/10.1016/j.jcmg.2012.03.019] [PMID: 23236975]

[18] Otsuka K, Fukuda S, Tanaka A, *et al.* Napkin-ring sign on coronary CT angiography for the prediction of acute coronary syndrome. JACC Cardiovasc Imaging 2013; 6(4): 448-57. [http://dx.doi.org/10.1016/j.jcmg.2012.09.016] [PMID: 23498679]

[19] Shaw LJ, Berman DS, Maron DJ, *et al.* Optimal medical therapy with or without percutaneous coronary intervention to reduce ischemic burden: results from the Clinical Outcomes Utilizing Revascularization and Aggressive Drug Evaluation (COURAGE) trial nuclear substudy. Circulation 2008; 117(10): 1283-91. [http://dx.doi.org/10.1161/CIRCULATIONAHA.107.743963] [PMID: 18268144]

[20] Takx RA, Blomberg BA, El Aidi H, *et al.* Diagnostic accuracy of stress myocardial perfusion imaging compared to invasive coronary angiography with fractional flow reserve meta-analysis. Circ Cardiovasc Imaging 2015; 8(1): e002666. [http://dx.doi.org/10.1161/CIRCIMAGING.114.002666] [PMID: 25596143]

[21] Edenbrandt L, Höglund P, Frantz S, *et al.* Area of ischemia assessed by physicians and software packages from myocardial perfusion scintigrams BMC Medical imaging 2014 Jan; 14: 5.

[22] Matsuo S, Nakajima K, Horie M, Nakae I, Nishimura T. Prognostic value of normal stress myocardial perfusion imaging in Japanese population. Circ J 2008; 72(4): 611-7. [http://dx.doi.org/10.1253/circj.72.611] [PMID: 18362434]

[23] Matsuo S, Nakajima K, Yamasaki Y, Kashiwagi A, Nishimura T. Prognostic value of normal stress myocardial perfusion imaging and ventricular function in Japanese asymptomatic patients with type 2 diabetes--a study based on the J-ACCESS-2 database. Circ J 2010; 74(9): 1916-21. [http://dx.doi.org/10.1253/circj.CJ-10-0098] [PMID: 20631452]

[24] Nakajima K, Matsuo S, Okuyama C, *et al.* Cardiac event risk in Japanese subjects estimated using gated myocardial perfusion imaging, in conjunction with diabetes mellitus and chronic kidney disease. Circ J 2012; 76(1): 168-75. [http://dx.doi.org/10.1253/circj.CJ-11-0857] [PMID: 22104035]

[25] Taqueti VR, Hachamovitch R, Murthy VL, *et al.* Global coronary flow reserve is associated with adverse cardiovascular events independently of luminal angiographic severity and modifies the effect of early revascularization. Circulation 2015; 131(1): 19-27. [http://dx.doi.org/10.1161/CIRCULATIONAHA.114.011939] [PMID: 25400060]

[26] Gaemperli O, Schepis T, Valenta I, *et al.* Cardiac image fusion from stand-alone SPECT and CT: clinical experience. J Nucl Med 2007; 48(5): 696-703. [http://dx.doi.org/10.2967/jnumed.106.037606] [PMID: 17475956]

[27] Pazhenkottil AP, Nkoulou RN, Ghadri JR, *et al.* Impact of cardiac hybrid single-photon emission computed tomography/computed tomography imaging on choice of treatment strategy in coronary artery disease. Eur Heart J 2011; 32(22): 2824-9. [http://dx.doi.org/10.1093/eurheartj/ehr232] [PMID: 21804107]

[28] Pazhenkottil AP, Benz DC, Gräni C, *et al.* Hybrid SPECT Perfusion Imaging and Coronary CT Angiography: Long-term Prognostic Value for Cardiovascular Outcomes. Radiology 2018; 288(3): 694-702. [http://dx.doi.org/10.1148/radiol.2018171303] [PMID: 29969066]

[29] Slart RH, Tio RA, Zijlstra F, Dierckx RA. Diagnostic pathway of integrated SPECT/CT for coronary artery disease. Eur J Nucl Med Mol Imaging 2009; 36(11): 1829-34. [http://dx.doi.org/10.1007/s00259-009-1179-9] [PMID: 19526236]

[30] Matsuo S, Matsumoto T, Nakae I, *et al.* Prognostic value of ECG-gated thallium-201 single-photon emission tomography in patients with coronary artery disease. Ann Nucl Med 2004; 18(7): 617-22. [http://dx.doi.org/10.1007/BF02984584] [PMID: 15586636]

[31] Matsuo S. Phase analysis using gated myocardial perfusion single-photon emission computed tomography imaging for evaluating cardiac dyssynchrony. Circ J 2012; 76(8): 1832-3. [http://dx.doi.org/10.1253/circj.CJ-12-0636] [PMID: 22664418]

[32] Wells RG, Timmins R, Klein R, *et al.* Dynamic SPECT measurement of absolute myocardial blood flow in a porcine model. J Nucl Med 2014; 55(10): 1685-91. [http://dx.doi.org/10.2967/jnumed.114.139782] [PMID: 25189340]

[33] Ben-Haim S, Murthy VL, Breault C, *et al.* Quantification of Myocardial Perfusion Reserve Using Dynamic SPECT Imaging in Humans: A Feasibility Study. J Nucl Med 2013; 54(6): 873-9. [http://dx.doi.org/10.2967/jnumed.112.109652] [PMID: 23578996]

[34] Zimmermann FM, De Bruyne B, Pijls NH, *et al.* Rationale and design of the Fractional Flow Reserve

versus Angiography for Multivessel Evaluation (FAME) 3 Trial: a comparison of fractional flow reserve-guided percutaneous coronary intervention and coronary artery bypass graft surgery in patients with multivessel coronary artery disease. Am Heart J 2015; 170(4): 619-626.e2. [http://dx.doi.org/10.1016/j.ahj.2015.06.024] [PMID: 26386784]

[35] Hagemann CE, Ghotbi AA, Kjær A, Hasbak P. Quantitative myocardial blood flow with Rubidium-82 PET: a clinical perspective. Am J Nucl Med Mol Imaging 2015; 5(5): 457-68. [PMID: 26550537]

[36] Berman DS, Maddahi J, Tamarappoo BK, *et al.* Phase II safety and clinical comparison with single-photon emission computed tomography myocardial perfusion imaging for detection of coronary artery disease: flurpiridaz F 18 positron emission tomography. J Am Coll Cardiol 2013; 61(4): 469-77. [http://dx.doi.org/10.1016/j.jacc.2012.11.022] [PMID: 23265345]

CHAPTER 5

Positron Emission Tomography Myocardial Perfusion Imaging

Keiichiro Yoshinaga[1,*] and **Osamu Manabe**[2]

[1] *Diagnostic and Therapeutic Nuclear Medicine, National Institute of Radiological Sciences, Chiba, Japan*

[2] *Department of Nuclear Medicine, Hokkaido University Graduate School of Medicine, Sapporo, Japan*

Abstract: With the increasing availability of positron emission tomography (PET) myocardial perfusion imaging (MPI), PET MPI and the absolute quantification of myocardial blood flow (MBF) have become popular in clinical settings [1]. PET MPI shows higher diagnostic accuracy than that of single-photon emission computed tomography (SPECT) and shows predictive value for cardiac events [2, 3]. Quantitative MBF assessment also provides important additional diagnostic or prognostic information over that attained through conventional visual assessment [4]. The success of MBF quantification using PET/computed tomography (CT) has increased demand for this quantitative diagnostic approach to be more accessible. In this regard, MBF quantification approaches have been developed using several other diagnostic imaging modalities including SPECT, dynamic CT perfusion imaging, and cardiac magnetic resonance (CMR). In the United States (US), the Food and Drug Administration (FDA) has approved ^{13}N-ammonia ($^{13}N-NH_3$) and ^{82}rubidium (^{82}Rb) for clinical use [5]. The Japanese Ministry of Health, Labour and Welfare (JMHLW) approved $^{13}N-NH_3$ PET MPI for diagnosis of coronary artery disease (CAD) in March 2012 but has not approved other PET MPI tracers [6, 7]. Since $^{13}N-NH_3$ PET MPI will be addressed elsewhere in this e-book, this review will address the clinical aspects of PET/CT MPI using other PET flow tracers.

Keywords: Blood Flow, Coronary Artery Disease, Endothelial Function, Flow Reserve, Positron Emission Tomography, Quantification.

TRACERS FOR PET MYOCARDIAL PERFUSION IMAGING

PET MPI tracers can be divided into (a) inert freely diffusible tracers such as O-15-labeled water ($^{15}O-H_2O$) and (b) physiologically retained tracers such as

* **Corresponding author Keiichiro Yoshinaga:** Diagnostic and Therapeutic Nuclear Medicine, National Institutes for Quantum and Radiological Science and Technology, National Institute of Radiological Sciences 4-9-1 Anagawa, Inage-Ku, Chiba, 263-8555, Japan; Tel: 81 (43) 206 3429; Fax: 81 (43) 206 4079; E-mail: yoshinaga.keiichiro@qst.go.jp

Shinro Matsuo (Ed.)

^{13}N-NH$_3$, ^{82}Rb, and ^{18}F-flurpiridaz [8]. The basic characteristics of commonly used PET MPI tracers are listed in (Table **1**).

Among these commonly used tracers, physically retained tracers can be used to produce standard tomographic images similar to those with SPECT MPI. Therefore, these tracers can be used in clinical settings. The FDA has approved these tracers for clinical use. On the other hand, it is difficult to create static images using freely diffusible tracers, and these tracers are therefore used mainly in research settings [9].

Rubidium-82

^{82}Rb is produced from a ^{82}strontium (^{82}Sr) /^{82}Rb generator which can be eluted every 10 minutes (Fig. **1**) [10, 11]. Since ^{82}Rb production does not require an on-site cyclotron, ^{82}Rb is the most widely used tracer in PET centers [12, 13]. The physical half-life of the parent isotope is 25.5 days. Thus, the shelf life of the generator is 4 to 6 weeks. In 2016, the FDA granted additional approval of a different pharmaceutical company's ^{82}Sr/^{82}Rb generator. The more recently approved generator can be used for 6 to 8 weeks and has a longer shelf life [14].

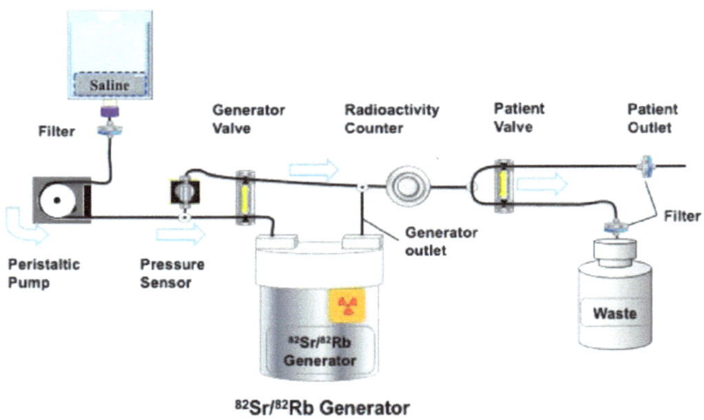

Fig. (1). A conceptual diagram of a ^{82}Rb infusion system that can control the ^{82}Rb activity infusion profile. The generator valve is modulated to control the concentration of ^{82}Rb activity administered to the patient. The radioactivity counter is used by the control system and for QA. The system can also flush the activity from the patient line at the end of the infusion. (Permission pending from Yoshinaga K, *et al.* J Cardiol 2009;55:63-73).

^{82}Rb has received FDA approval in the US [5] and is currently under investigation in some European countries and Canada. There has been some use of ^{82}Rb in Japan for clinical research purposes [15, 16].

The short physical half-life of 76 seconds makes ^{82}Rb suitable for consecutive rest and stress perfusion studies (Fig. **2A**). With a PET/CT scanner with CT attenuation correction, the total rest and stress data acquisition can be done within 30 minutes (Fig. **2**). This short acquisition time is one of the great advantages of ^{82}Rb PET MPI in clinical settings.

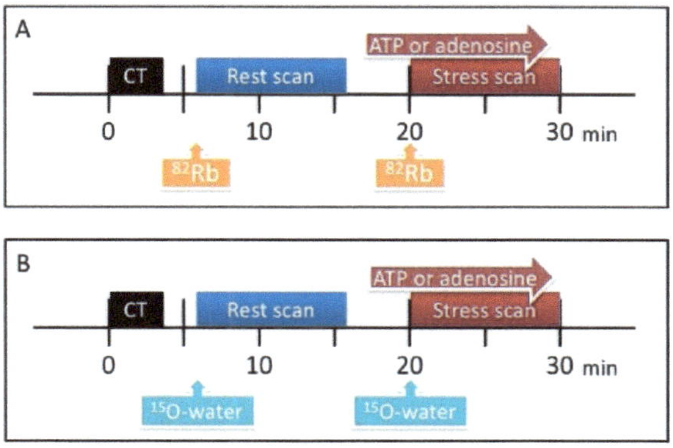

Fig. (2). (**A**) Imaging protocol of adenosine/adenosine triphosphate (ATP) stress ^{82}Rb PET/CT myocardial perfusion imaging. (**B**) Imaging protocol of ATP stress ^{15}O-labeled water PET/CT myocardial perfusion.

The relatively high positron energy of ^{82}Rb of 3.15 MeV is associated with a positron range averaging 7.5 mm and may contribute to relatively lower spatial resolution than that seen with ^{13}N-NH_3 with a positron range of 2.5 mm.

^{82}Rb is an analog of potassium and has biological kinetics similar to those of ^{201}thallium (^{201}Tl) [8, 17, 18]. ^{82}Rb is rapidly extracted from the blood and concentrated by the myocardium. In animal models, the first-pass extraction fraction (EXF – I prefer another abbreviation since this is already reserved for ejection fraction) is 50% to 60% at rest and decreases to 25% to 30% at peak stress flow (Fig. **3**) [17, 19, 20].

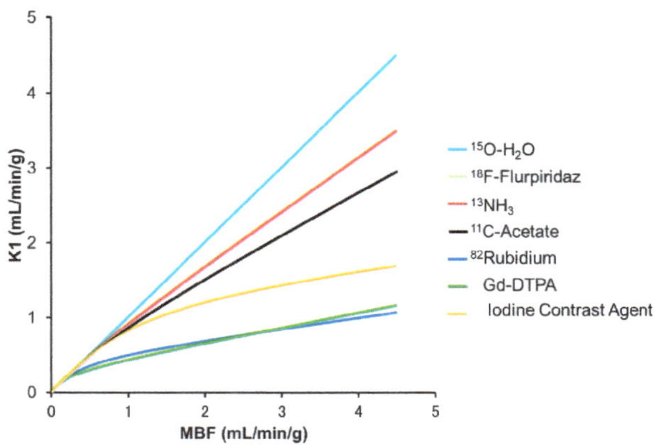

Fig. (3). Correlation between MBF and Extraction. Reproduced with permission from Yoshinaga K (author) and the *J Nucl Cardiol* 2018;25(2):635-51 (PERMISSION PENDING).

Due to its short physical half-life, ^{82}Rb presents low risk of radiation exposure to personnel and patients (Table **1**) [10]. The 3D PET/CT system currently in use presents even lower radiation exposure [21].

Table 1. PET Tracers for Myocardial Perfusion Imaging.

Pharmaceutical	Radioisotopes	Half-life	Positron Energy (MeV)	Effective Dose (mSv/MBq)
Rubidium	Rb-82	76 sec	3.15	0.0048
Water	O-15	120 sec	1.72	0.0011
Potassium [68]	K-38	7.6 min	2.7	0.0187
PTSM [69]	Cu-62	9.8 min	2.94	0.0036
Ammonia	N-13	10 min	1.19	0.0022
Acetate [70]	C-11	20 min	0.96	0.0049
Flurpiridaz	F-18	110 min	0.63	0.019

MBF quantification is quite feasible and clinically practical with this generator as compared to with cyclotron-produced compounds [22 - 27]. ^{82}Rb MBF quantification has been validated using other standard measurement techniques including $^{13}N\text{-}NH_3$ and $^{15}O\text{-}H_2O$ PET [28, 29].

^{15}O-labeled Water

$^{15}O\text{-}H_2O$ was one of the first radiopharmaceuticals developed for PET. Among PET flow tracers, $^{15}O\text{-}H_2O$ has the highest EF (Fig. **3**) and thus is considered to be the gold standard for quantification of MBF [4, 8]. $^{15}O\text{-}H_2O$ is usually obtained from O-15 O_2 gas combined with hydrogen gas. The ^{15}O gas is produced either through $^{14}N(d,n)$ ^{15}O reaction or through the $^{15}N(p,n)$ ^{15}O method. $^{15}O\text{-}H_2O$ has a short physical half-life (110 seconds) and must therefore be produced using an on-site cyclotron. The short physical half-life of $^{15}O\text{-}H_2O$ makes it suitable for various stress study protocols such as pharmacological stress and the cold pressor test (Fig. **2B**) [30].

Although it is difficult to create static myocardial perfusion images, one of the major advantages of $^{15}O\text{-}H_2O$ is its feasibility for quantitative assessment of MBF.

^{18}Fluorine-labeled Myocardial Perfusion Agents

^{18}Fluorine-(^{18}F)-labeled compounds have a relatively long physical half-life (110 minutes) and can be delivered to PET centers from pharmaceutical companies in the same manner as is ^{18}F-fluorodeoxyglucose (^{18}F-FDG). ^{82}Rb is suitable for PET centers in which many cardiac PET studies are performed [31]. In contrast, for

PET centers doing limited numbers of PET MPI studies per day, it may be convenient to use ^{18}F-labeled PET MPI tracers.

There are two categories of ^{18}F-labeled PET MPI tracers, namely, analogs of mitochondrial complex-1 (MC-1) inhibitors and lipophilic cations [32]. Among ^{18}F-labeled radiotracers, ^{18}F-fluorobenzyl triphenyl phosphonium (^{18}F-FBnTP) initially showed promise [33]. However, recent developments of ^{18}F-labeled PET MPI have shifted from using ^{18}F-FBnTP to using ^{18}F-flurpiridaz (^{18}F-BM--747158-02) [34]. This tracer is a structural analog of pyridaben, a known mitochondria complex one (MC-1), most complicated component of the respiratory chain, inhibitor. Mitochondria constitute 20% to 30% of the myocardial intracellular volume. Consequently, molecules that target mitochondrial proteins will be accumulated and retained selectively in the myocardium.

^{18}F-flurpiridaz showed a high first-pass EF by the myocardium, greater than 90%, in isolated rat hearts [35]. Such a high EF would certainly increase the level of the accuracy of MBF quantification attainable through static perfusion images, a significant characteristic for ^{18}F-flurpiridaz.

A phase 3 study in the US showed the usefulness of ^{18}F-flurpiridaz in diagnosing CAD in specific subpopulations, namely, women and obese people. One Japanese radiopharmaceutical company has announced that it is considering introducing ^{18}F-flurpiridaz in Japan. ^{18}F-flurpiridaz still requires thorough investigation and the establishment of suitable protocols but definitely shows promise as a new PET MPI agent.

C-11-labeled PET Agents

Some ^{11}C-labeled cardiac PET tracers originally designed for evaluating myocardial metabolism or sympathetic nervous function can also be used to estimate MBF through a suitable kinetic model. These include ^{11}C-acetate and ^{11}C-hydroxyephedrine (^{11}C-HED) [8].

^{11}C-acetate

^{11}C-acetate is a PET tracer used to evaluate myocardial oxygen consumption. Injected ^{11}C-acetate is taken up by the heart, rapidly converted to acetyl coenzyme A (CoA), and readily metabolized to CO_2 through the tricarboxylic acid (TCA) cycle with oxidative phosphorylation [36]. The K1 inflow rate of ^{11}C-acetate is largely dependent on MBF (Sun KT, J Nucl Med. 1998;39:272–80.) [37]. Several methods such as measuring net myocardial uptake of the tracer (Chan SY, J Nucl Med. 1991;32:665–72.) [38], using a two-tissue compartment model or using a one-tissue compartment model have been reported for assessing MBF using ^{11}C-acetate. The estimated EF is higher than that associated with ^{82}Rb but lower than with ^{13}N-NH_3 [37, 39]. ^{11}C-acetate PET is increasingly used both to assess regional myocardial oxygen consumption and to quantify MBF.

^{11}C-HED

^{11}C-HED is a noradrenaline analog PET tracer that reflects mainly the activity of the sarcolemmal norepinephrine transporter (uptake-1) of the heart and is used to visualize the sympathetic nervous system (SNS). The risk of ventricular arrhythmias has been estimated by evaluating the mismatch between areas of reduced MBF and reduced myocardial innervation [40, 41]. The inflow rate of ^{11}C-HED (K1) from the one-tissue compartment model can be converted to assess MBF using the Renkin-Crone model, which allows for simultaneous MBF quantification and SNS function measurement. However, the EF is lower than that associated with ^{82}Rb, a factor that may lead to relatively high variability in MBF estimates [42].

CLINICAL INDICATION AND IMAGING PROTOCOLS

Clinical Indication

ACC/AHA/ASNC clinical guidelines and a joint position statement by CCS/CAR/CANM/CNCS/CanSCMR provide indications of intermediate likelihood of CAD when a patient has had non-diagnostic or equivocal SPECT MPI or other non-invasive imaging tests. For such patients, indications for PET MPI for diagnosis and detection of myocardial ischemia are considered class I (level of evidence B) [43, 44]. The Japanese Ministry of Health Labour and Welfare (JMHLW) indication and reimbursement policy for ^{13}N-NH_3 PET MPI also stipulates the same condition [6, 7]. In addition to this indication, for patients who are unable to exercise or who have left bundle branch block (LBBB) or ventricular paced rhythm PET MPI may be appropriate for diagnosing CAD (ACC/AHA/ASNC class IIa) [43, 44].

Imaging Protocol

Patient Preparation

Patients scheduled for PET MPI should fast for at least 6 hours and abstain from caffeine-containing products (*i.e.*, coffee, tea, chocolate, and soft drinks containing caffeine) for at least 12 hours but ideally 24 hours [45]. Patients should also avoid theophylline-containing medications for 48 hours prior to pharmacological stress tests employing adenosine, adenosine triphosphate (ATP), dipyridamole, or regadenoson [46, 47]. Patients undergoing dobutamine stress tests should stop beta-blockers 48 hours before the PET MPI studies if the goal is diagnosis of CAD.

Stress Protocol

Since PET MPI tracers have very short physical half-lives, the current PET MPI stress protocol involves pharmacological stress [4].

Pharmacological Vasodilator Stress

Adenosine, adenosine triphosphate, and dipyridamole stress have been used for PET MPI studies in clinical settings. These vasodilator agents inhibit transport of adenosine into the cells and/or increase extracellular levels of adenosine resulting in coronary vasodilatation due to the interaction with adenosine A_2 receptors in the smooth muscle cell membrane. Activation of A_2 receptors dilates the coronary vasculature *via* the production of adenylate cyclase and cyclic adenosine monophosphate stimulation of potassium channels. These agents increase MBF and permit measurement of MBF reserve (MFR). Vasodilator agents such as adenosine, ATP and dipyridamole increase MBF threefold to fivefold in normal coronary territories without increasing oxygen demand. In contrast, myocardial regions supplied by stenotic coronary arteries already have dilated coronary arterioles at rest to maintain resting blood supply to the myocardium. Therefore, the hyperemic response and MFR can be reduced [4, 48, 49].

Recently the highly specific adenosine A2A receptor agonist regadenoson has been used for MPI in clinical settings [50]. Regadenoson may also induce maximal vasodilation similar to that with dipyridamole as demonstrated by ^{82}Rb PET study [51]. Use of regadenoson for PET MPI is expected to increase in clinical settings in the near future.

Dobutamine Stress

Dobutamine stress is an alternative approach in patients with severe reactive airway disease or caffeine intake [52]. Dobutamine increases regional MBF based on the physiological principles of MFR. MBF increases to meet increasing oxygen demand. However, this response is attenuated during high-dose dobutamine administration (20-40 μg/kg/min) in segments supplied by diseased vessels.

Dobutamine dosing can start at 5 to 10 μg/kg/min and be increased by 5μg/kg/min at 3-minute intervals up to a maximum dose of 40 μg/kg/min to achieve >85% of the target heart rate [0.85 × (220 - age)].

Image Acquisition and Processing

^{82}Rubidium

After a CT transmission scan, approximately 20-40 mCi (740-1480 MBq) of ^{82}Rb can be injected as a bolus dose for ≤30 seconds followed by serial dynamic acquisition using PET/CT with a data acquisition time of less than 10 minutes (Fig. **2**) [11, 46]. After 70 to 150 seconds of tracer injection, images are acquired for 3 to 7.5 minutes [3, 46].

A two-compartment model has been used for quantitative assessment of regional MBF including showing activity in the vascular space and within the tissue compartment [27, 53]. In a canine model, regional MBF can be accurately estimated using ^{82}Rb [54]. MBF quantification using ^{82}Rb has also been validated using ^{13}N-NH_3 PET [28].

^{15}O-labeled Water

Participants are instructed to abstain from caffeine-containing products for at least 24 h prior to the PET scan. After a low-dose CT scan during free breathing for attenuation and scatter correction, about 370-740 MBq (10-20 mCi) of ^{15}O-H_2O is slowly administered intravenously with simultaneous list-mode acquisition. The short half-life (2.04 min) enables consecutive rest/stress PET acquisition (Fig. **2B**). Pharmacological stress is induced through intravenous injection of ATP or adenosine before stress emission scanning.

After the reconstruction of the attenuation-corrected radioactivity images, the MBF is calculated using a one-tissue-compartment tracer kinetic model. The MFR is calculated as the ratio of MBF during stress to MBF at rest.

Assessment of Absolute Myocardial Blood Flow

A tracer kinetics model makes absolute measurement of physiological or biochemical function possible. A parametric physical model uses the time course of radioactivity of the arterial blood input function Ca (t), which can measure blood radioactivity in the left ventricular (LV) cavity through PET/CT scanners, and myocardial response function Cm (t) to estimate a quantitative rate constant [55, 56].

The compartments represent tissue volumes which include physical factors (arterial blood and intracellular fluid) or biochemical factors (tracer compound and labeled metabolite). A mathematical model is constructed with parameters such as flux of radioactivity between the compartments. The compartment model approach is used mainly for $^{13}N\text{-}NH_3$, $^{15}O\text{-}H_2O$, and, more recently, ^{82}Rb MBF quantification [57 - 59].

CLINICAL APPLICATIONS

Diagnosis in Coronary Artery Disease

Similar to the case with SPECT MPI, standard visual perfusion imaging assessment is applied for CAD diagnosis with ^{82}Rb (Fig. **4**) and $^{13}N\text{-}NH_3$. The ability to diagnose CAD through advanced MBF quantification assessed using $^{15}O\text{-}H_2O$ has also been reported [60].

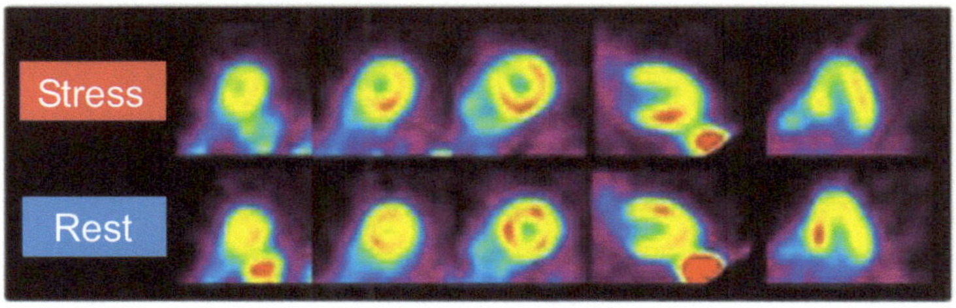

Fig. (4). Representative images from a woman in her 60s with coronary artery disease. The ^{82}Rb PET images show reversible perfusion defect in antero-septum, indicating myocardial ischemia in LAD territory.

Visual Assessment

The Canadian Cardiovascular Society (CCS) and colleagues conducted a systematic literature review for ^{82}Rb and $^{13}N\text{-}NH_3$ PET MPI in the diagnosis of CAD. The mean sensitivity and specificity of PET MPI are 89% and 89% with ranges from 83% to 100% and 73% to 100% based on 14 studies involving a total 1460 patients [43].

Some studies have compared the diagnostic accuracy of PET MPI and SPECT MPI in the same patient population for detecting CAD. Bateman *et al.* compared the diagnostic accuracy of ECG-gated ^{82}Rb PET MPI and ECG-gated ^{99m}Tc sestamibi SPECT in 112 MPI studies. With 50% coronary artery stenosis being used as the diagnostic standard, the diagnostic accuracy of PET was higher than that of SPECT [2].

As would be expected, current PET/CT scanners also have high diagnostic accuracy in the detection of CAD (sensitivity 93%, specificity 85% and accuracy 87%) using ^{82}Rb PET/CT MPI (Table **2**) [61].

The phase 2 trial of ^{18}F-flupiridaz PET MPI showed that it had higher diagnostic sensitivity for detecting CAD than did ^{99m}Tc SPECT MPI (78.8% *vs.* 61.5%) and no significant difference in specificity (76.5% *vs.* 73.5%) [34].

Table 2. PET CAD Diagnosis.

Author	Year	Number	Stress	Tracer	Reference CAG	Sensitivity			Specificity		
						+ve test	Pt. w. CAD	%	-ve test	Pt. w.o. CAD	%
Gould L (@) [71]	1986	50	dipyridamole	^{82}Rb/^{13}NH$_3$	QCA SFR < 3	21	22	95%	9	9	100%
Demer L (@) [72]	1989	193	dipyridamole	^{82}Rb/^{13}NH$_3$	QCA SFR < 4	126	152	83%	39	41	95%
Go RT [73]	1990	202	dipyridamole	^{82}Rb	>50%	142	152	93%	39	50	78%
Stewart RE [74]	1991	81	dipyridamole	^{82}Rb	QCA >50%*	50†	60	84%	18†	21	88%
Marwick T [75]	1992	74	dipyridamole	^{82}Rb	>50%	63	70	90%	4	4	100%
Grover McKay [76]	1992	31	dipyridamole	^{82}Rb	>50%	16	16	100%	11	15	73%
Bateman TM†† [2]	2006	112	dipyridamole	^{82}Rb	>50%*	64	74	86%	38	38	100%
Williams BR** [12]	1994	287	dipyridamole	^{82}Rb	>67%	88	101	87%	99	112	88%
Simone GL** [77]	1992	225	dipyridamole	^{82}Rb	>67%	**	**	83%	**	**	91%
Chow BJ [78]	2007	26	dipyridamole	^{82}Rb	>50%	18	19	95%	3	5	60%
Dorbala S [79]	2007	68	adenosine or dipyridamole	^{82}Rb	≥70% and ≥50% for LMT	53	48	92%	15	15	100%
Esteves FP [80]	2008	52		^{82}Rb	≥70% and ≥50% for LMT			86%			100%
Esteves FP [81]	2010	57	adenosine	^{82}Rb	>50%	36	39	90%	13	18	72%
Groves AM [82]	2009	33	adenosine	^{82}Rb	>50%	21	23	91%	9	10	90%
Nakazato R [83]	2012	83	adenosine	^{82}Rb	>50%	53	62	85%	18	21	86%
Sampson UK [61]	2007	102	adenosine or dipyridamole	^{82}Rb	≥70% and ≥50% for LMT	41	44	93%	48	58	83%
Non-weighted Mean								**89.6%**			**87.8%**

@ -Study reported that 50 pts in Gould *et al.* 1986 were included. Thus Gould *et al.* not included in mean calculations.

** - Retrospective study; MPI influenced CAG decision; mixed patient and region method for sensitivity / specificity;

patients with disease could not be easily determined in one study.

* - Other cut-offs reported; >50% noted here

† - derived from reported sensitivity and specificity

††- Electronic database, matched cohort design; values derived from reported population, sensitivity and specificity.
N/R = Not reported
R/S = Retrospective
CAG = Coronary Angiogram
QCA = Quantitative Coronary Angiography
SFR = Stenosis Flow Reserve Based on QCA Data

Based on those previous data, PET MPI is considered to be the most well-balanced diagnostic tool for CAD [62].

MBF Assessment

Quantitative MBF assessment has been performed mainly as part of research studies (Fig. **5**) [30, 63]. For patients with CAD, Yoshinaga *et al.* reported the additional diagnostic value of regional MBF quantification using ^{82}Rb PET over conventional visual analysis [16]. Conventional visual analysis relies on relative perfusion imaging and therefore has an inherent weakness in terms of the detection of multi-vessel CAD. In this regard, a quantitative approach to MBF assessment may have a role in accurately diagnosing such multi-vessel CAD [64].

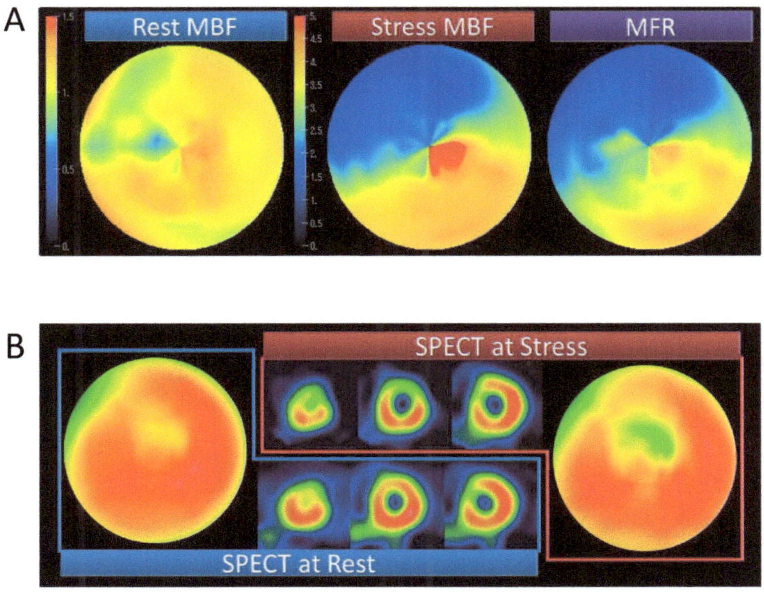

	Rest MBF	Stress MBF	MFR
Whole	1.1	2.7	2.4
LAD	1.1	1.9	1.7
RCA	1.1	3.6	3.2
LCX	1.1	3.5	3.1

Fig. (5). Representative images from a man in his 70s with chest pain. ^{99m}Tc SPECT MPI shows reversible perfusion defect in anterior, indicating myocardial ischemia in LAD territory. ^{15}O-H_2O labeled water PET/CT MBF show reduced hyperemic MBF and reduced MFR? in anterior.

Recently, Danad *et al.* estimated the diagnostic value of MBF and MFR? using ^{15}O-H_2O PET. The study used functional flow reserve (FFR) rather than classic morphological coronary stenosis as the diagnostic standard for CAD. This is the significant strength of this study [60]. With an MFR cut-off value of 2.5, the sensitivity of CAD was 86%, specificity was 72%, and accuracy was 78%. This should be a landmark study for establishing the role of MBF quantification for the diagnosis of CAD.

Prognosis in Coronary Artery Disease

Visual Analysis

Early reports using ^{82}Rb PET showed independent predictors of cardiac death and total cardiac events. PET MPI provided incremental prognostic information over clinical and angiographic findings (Table **3**) [65]. Yoshinaga *et al.* reported the low hard cardiac event rate in normal stress imaging as 0.4%/year and found that PET-determined perfusion defect was a significant predictor for hard cardiac events (Table **3**). ^{82}Rb PET also seems to have prognostic value for patients whose diagnosis remains uncertain after SPECT MPI and for obese patients [3]. Following this study, Dorbala *et al.* conducted multi-center observational analysis using ^{82}Rb PET. The study included a total of 7061 patients from 4 PET centers [66]. This study confirmed the findings of the previous study by Yoshinaga *et al.* and established the role of ^{82}Rb PET as a prognostic marker in patients with known or suspected CAD.

Table 3. PET CAD Prognosis.

Author	Year	Patient Number	Stress	Tracer	Outcomes	Follow-up Time (Years)	Normal Scan-Annual Event Rate (%/yr)		Abnormal Scan-Annual Event Rate (%/yr)	
							Hard Events	Total Events	Hard Events	Total Events
Yoshinaga [84]	2004	367	dipyridamole	^{82}Rb	death, MI, Rev, Hosp	3.1	0.4	1.7	mild: 2.3 mod/sev: 7.0	mild: 12.9 mod/sev: 13.2
Chow [85]	2005	629	dipyridamole	^{82}Rb	death, MI, Rev, CAG	2.3	0.09	0.98	ECG +ve NormalMP:0.6	ECG +ve Normal MP: 1.9
Marwick T [65]	1997	581	dipyridamole	^{82}Rb	death, MI, Rev, UAP	3.4	0.9	4	4	7
Kay J [86]	2013	6037	Adenosine, dipyridamole	^{82}Rb	death	3.3	0.9 (women) 1.5 (men)		12.9 (women) 17.5 (men)	

(Table 3) cont.....

Author	Year	Patient Number	Stress	Tracer	Outcomes	Follow-up Time (Years)	Normal Scan-Annual Event Rate (%/yr)		Abnormal Scan-Annual Event Rate (%/yr)	
							Hard Events	Total Events	Hard Events	Total Events
Farhad H [87]	2013	318	adenosine	^{82}Rb	death, MI,Rev, Hosp, UAP	1.7		SSS <3: 2.3		SSS 3–8: 4.8 SSS ≥9: 18

MI = Myocardial Infarction
Rev = Revascularization
CAG = Coronary Angiogram
UAP = Unstable Angina

Quantitative Analysis

The prognostic value of ^{82}Rb PET for patients with suspected or known CAD has been established. However, visual analysis has limited value since it may lead to underestimation of multi-vessel CAD [64]. In this regard, Ziadi *et al.* further investigated the role of ^{82}Rb PET using a visual approach and a quantitative MBF approach [67]. Importantly, visual analysis identified that even with normal stress perfusion, patients with reduced MFR had increased risk of major cardiac events. This was also a landmark study showing the predictive value of PET MBF quantification (Table **4**).

Table 4. MFR Prognosis.

Author	Year	Patient Number	MFR Cut-off	Tracer	Outcomes	Follow-up (Median Years)	Events	Univariate Hazard Ratio (95% Confidence Interval)	Adjusted Multivariate Hazard Ratio (95% Confidence Interval)
Ziadi [67]	2011	677	2.0	^{82}Rb	cardiac death,MI,Rev,Hosp	1.1	71	-	2.4 (1.4 to 4.4)
Fukushima [88]	2011	224	2.11	^{82}Rb	cardiac death,MI,Hosp,CAG	1.2	33	-	2.93 (1.30–6.65)
Murthy [89]	2011	2783	Tertiles (1.5, 2.0)	^{82}Rb	cardiac death	1.4	137	Lower *vs.* upper: 15.68 (7.27-33.82) Middle *vs.* upper: 5.71 (2.54-12.8)	Lower vs. upper: 5.55 (2.49-12.4) Middle vs. upper: 3.40 (1.50-7.72)
Farhad [87]	2013	318	Tertiles (1.8, 2.4)	^{82}Rb	cardiac death,MI,Rev,Hosp	1.7	35	0.27 (0.15–0.50)	Not significant

CONSENT FOR PUBLICATION

Not applicable.

CONFLICT OF INTEREST

The authors declare no conflict of interest, financial or otherwise.

ACKNOWLEDGEMENTS

The authors thank Natsue Ito, MT, Eriko Suzuki, MT, and Mariko Yamazaki, MA, for their help in preparing this chapter. Prior to submission the manuscript was reviewed by a North American English-language professional editor, Holly Beanlands. The authors thank her for critical reading of the manuscript.

REFERENCES

[1] Bateman TM, Dilsizian V, Beanlands RS, DePuey EG, Heller GV, Wolinsky DA. American Society of Nuclear Cardiology and Society of Nuclear Medicine and Molecular Imaging Joint Position Statement on the Clinical Indications for Myocardial Perfusion PET. J Nucl Med 2016; 57(10): 1654-6.
[http://dx.doi.org/10.2967/jnumed.116.180448] [PMID: 27561879]

[2] Bateman TM, Heller GV, McGhie AI, *et al.* Diagnostic accuracy of rest/stress ECG-gated Rb-82 myocardial perfusion PET: comparison with ECG-gated Tc-99m sestamibi SPECT. J Nucl Cardiol 2006; 13(1): 24-33.
[http://dx.doi.org/10.1016/j.nuclcard.2005.12.004] [PMID: 16464714]

[3] Yoshinaga K, Chow BJ, Williams K, *et al.* What is the prognostic value of myocardial perfusion imaging using rubidium-82 positron emission tomography? J Am Coll Cardiol 2006; 48(5): 1029-39.
[http://dx.doi.org/10.1016/j.jacc.2006.06.025] [PMID: 16949498]

[4] Yoshinaga K, Manabe O, Tamaki N. Absolute quantification of myocardial blood flow. J Nucl Cardiol 2018; 25(2): 635-51.
[http://dx.doi.org/10.1007/s12350-016-0591-3] [PMID: 27444500]

[5] Bengel FM, Higuchi T, Javadi MS, Lautamäki R. Cardiac positron emission tomography. J Am Coll Cardiol 2009; 54(1): 1-15.
[http://dx.doi.org/10.1016/j.jacc.2009.02.065] [PMID: 19555834]

[6] Yoshinaga K. Current Japanese ministry of health, labor, and welfare approval of cardiac positron emission tomography. Ann Nucl Cardiol 2015; 1: 106-7.
[http://dx.doi.org/10.17996/ANC.01.01.106]

[7] Yoshinaga K, Tamaki N. Current status of nuclear cardiology in Japan: Ongoing efforts to improve clinical standards and to establish evidence. J Nucl Cardiol 2015; 22(4): 690-9.
[http://dx.doi.org/10.1007/s12350-015-0136-1] [PMID: 25896679]

[8] Manabe O, Kikuchi T, Scholte A, *et al.* Radiopharmaceutical tracers for cardiac imaging. J Nucl Cardiol 2017; 25(4): 1204-36.
[http://dx.doi.org/10.1007/s12350-017-1131-5] [PMID: 29196910]

[9] Tomiyama Y, Manabe O, Oyama-Manabe N, *et al.* Quantification of myocardial blood flow with dynamic perfusion 3.0 Tesla MRI: Validation with (15) O-water PET. J Magn Reson Imaging 2015; 42(3): 754-62.
[http://dx.doi.org/10.1002/jmri.24834] [PMID: 25557072]

[10] Alvarez-Diez TM, deKemp R, Beanlands R, Vincent J. Manufacture of strontium-82/rubidium-82 generators and quality control of rubidium-82 chloride for myocardial perfusion imaging in patients using positron emission tomography. Appl Radiat Isot 1999; 50(6): 1015-23. [http://dx.doi.org/10.1016/S0969-8043(98)00170-5] [PMID: 10355104]

[11] Yoshinaga K, Klein R, Tamaki N. Generator-produced rubidium-82 positron emission tomography myocardial perfusion imaging-From basic aspects to clinical applications. J Cardiol 2010; 55(2): 163-73. [http://dx.doi.org/10.1016/j.jjcc.2010.01.001] [PMID: 20206068]

[12] Williams BR, Mullani NA, Jansen DE, Anderson BA. A retrospective study of the diagnostic accuracy of a community hospital-based PET center for the detection of coronary artery disease using rubidium-82. J Nucl Med 1994; 35(10): 1586-92. [PMID: 7931654]

[13] Yoshinaga K, Chow BJ, dekemp RA, *et al.* Application of cardiac molecular imaging using positron emission tomography in evaluation of drug and therapeutics for cardiovascular disorders. Curr Pharm Des 2005; 11(7): 903-32. [http://dx.doi.org/10.2174/1381612053381800] [PMID: 15777243]

[14] Moody JB, Hiller KM, Lee BC, Corbett JR, Ficaro EP, Murthy VL. Limitations of Rb-82 weight-adjusted dosing accuracy at low doses. J Nucl Cardiol 2017; 24(4): 1395-401. [http://dx.doi.org/10.1007/s12350-016-0531-2] [PMID: 27184903]

[15] Manabe O, Yoshinaga K, Katoh C, Naya M, deKemp RA, Tamaki N. Repeatability of rest and hyperemic myocardial blood flow measurements with 82Rb dynamic PET. J Nucl Med 2009; 50(1): 68-71. [http://dx.doi.org/10.2967/jnumed.108.055673] [PMID: 19091892]

[16] Yoshinaga K, Katoh C, Manabe O, *et al.* Incremental diagnostic value of regional myocardial blood flow quantification over relative perfusion imaging with generator-produced rubidium-82 PET. Circ J 2011; 75(11): 2628-34. [http://dx.doi.org/10.1253/circj.CJ-11-0502] [PMID: 21873801]

[17] Mullani NA, Gould KL. First-pass measurements of regional blood flow with external detectors. J Nucl Med 1983; 24(7): 577-81. [PMID: 6602868]

[18] Nishiyama H, Sodd VJ, Adolph RJ, Saenger EL, Lewis JT, Gabel M. Intercomparison of myocardial imaging agents: 201Ti, 129Cs, 43K, and 81Rb. J Nucl Med 1976; 17(10): 880-9. [PMID: 966055]

[19] Mullani NA, Goldstein RA, Gould KL, *et al.* Myocardial perfusion with rubidium-82. I. Measurement of extraction fraction and flow with external detectors. J Nucl Med 1983; 24(10): 898-906. [PMID: 6619960]

[20] Ziegler WH, Goresky CA. Kinetics of rubidium uptake in the working dog heart. Circ Res 1971; 29(2): 208-20. [http://dx.doi.org/10.1161/01.RES.29.2.208] [PMID: 4935841]

[21] deKemp RA, Yoshinaga K, Beanlands RS. Will 3-dimensional PET-CT enable the routine quantification of myocardial blood flow? J Nucl Cardiol 2007; 14(3): 380-97. [http://dx.doi.org/10.1016/j.nuclcard.2007.04.006] [PMID: 17556173]

[22] deKemp RA, Ruddy TD, Hewitt T, Dalipaj MM, Beanlands RS. Detection of serial changes in absolute myocardial perfusion with 82Rb PET. J Nucl Med 2000; 41(8): 1426-35. [PMID: 10945537]

[23] Parkash R, deKemp RA, Ruddy TD, *et al.* Potential utility of rubidium 82 PET quantification in patients with 3-vessel coronary artery disease. J Nucl Cardiol 2004; 11(4): 440-9. [http://dx.doi.org/10.1016/j.nuclcard.2004.04.005] [PMID: 15295413]

[24] Scott NS, Le May MR, de Kemp R, Ruddy TD, Labinaz M, Marquis JF, *et al.* Evaluation of myocardial perfusion using rubidium-82 positron emission tomography after myocardial infarction in patients receiving primary stent implantation or thrombolytic therapy. Am J Cardiol 2001; 88: 886-9.

[25] Yoshida K, Mullani N, Gould KL. Coronary flow and flow reserve by PET simplified for clinical applications using rubidium-82 or nitrogen-13-ammonia. J Nucl Med 1996; 37(10): 1701-12. [PMID: 8862316]

[26] Yoshinaga K, Beanlands RS, Dekemp RA, Lortie M, Morin J, Aung M, *et al.* Effect of exercise training on myocardial blood flow in patients with stable coronary artery disease. Am Heart J 2006; 151(1324): e11-8.

[27] Katoh C, Yoshinaga K, Klein R, *et al.* Quantification of regional myocardial blood flow estimation with three-dimensional dynamic rubidium-82 PET and modified spillover correction model. J Nucl Cardiol 2012; 19(4): 763-74. [http://dx.doi.org/10.1007/s12350-012-9558-1] [PMID: 22527800]

[28] Lortie M, Beanlands RS, Yoshinaga K, Klein R, Dasilva JN, DeKemp RA. Quantification of myocardial blood flow with 82Rb dynamic PET imaging. Eur J Nucl Med Mol Imaging 2007; 34(11): 1765-74. [http://dx.doi.org/10.1007/s00259-007-0478-2] [PMID: 17619189]

[29] Yoshinaga K, Manabe O, Katoh C, *et al.* Quantitative analysis of coronary endothelial function with generator-produced 82Rb PET: comparison with 15O-labelled water PET. Eur J Nucl Med Mol Imaging 2010; 37(12): 2233-41. [http://dx.doi.org/10.1007/s00259-010-1541-y] [PMID: 20625721]

[30] Yoshinaga K, Manabe O, Tamaki N. Assessment of coronary endothelial function using PET. J Nucl Cardiol 2011; 18(3): 486-500. [http://dx.doi.org/10.1007/s12350-011-9370-3] [PMID: 21448758]

[31] Bateman TM. Current Status of Myocardial Perfusion PET in the United States. Ann Nucl Cardiol 2017; 3: 157-62. [http://dx.doi.org/10.17996/anc.17-00047]

[32] Higuchi T, Nekolla SG, Huisman MM, *et al.* A new 18F-labeled myocardial PET tracer: myocardial uptake after permanent and transient coronary occlusion in rats. J Nucl Med 2008; 49(10): 1715-22. [http://dx.doi.org/10.2967/jnumed.108.053967] [PMID: 18794259]

[33] Madar I, Ravert HT, Du Y, *et al.* Characterization of uptake of the new PET imaging compound 18F-fluorobenzyl triphenyl phosphonium in dog myocardium. J Nucl Med 2006; 47(8): 1359-66. [PMID: 16883017]

[34] Berman DS, Maddahi J, Tamarappoo BK, *et al.* Phase II safety and clinical comparison with single-photon emission computed tomography myocardial perfusion imaging for detection of coronary artery disease: flurpiridaz F 18 positron emission tomography. J Am Coll Cardiol 2013; 61(4): 469-77. [http://dx.doi.org/10.1016/j.jacc.2012.11.022] [PMID: 23265345]

[35] Huisman MC, Higuchi T, Reder S, *et al.* Initial characterization of an 18F-labeled myocardial perfusion tracer. J Nucl Med 2008; 49(4): 630-6. [http://dx.doi.org/10.2967/jnumed.107.044727] [PMID: 18344426]

[36] Brown MA, Myears DW, Bergmann SR. Validity of estimates of myocardial oxidative metabolism with carbon-11 acetate and positron emission tomography despite altered patterns of substrate utilization. J Nucl Med 1989; 30(2): 187-93. [PMID: 2786932]

[37] Sun KT, Yeatman LA, Buxton DB, *et al.* Simultaneous measurement of myocardial oxygen consumption and blood flow using [1-carbon-11]acetate. J Nucl Med 1998; 39(2): 272-80. [PMID: 9476935]

[38] Chan SY, Brunken RC, Phelps ME, Schelbert HR. Use of the metabolic tracer carbon-11-acetate for

evaluation of regional myocardial perfusion. J Nucl Med 1991; 32(4): 665-72.
[PMID: 2013805]

[39] van den Hoff J. Methodologic aspects of myocardial blood flow quantification with 1-11C-acetate PET. J Nucl Med 2001; 42(9): 1438-9.
[PMID: 11535737]

[40] Bulow HP, Stahl F, Lauer B, *et al.* Alterations of myocardial presynaptic sympathetic innervation in patients with multi-vessel coronary artery disease but without history of myocardial infarction. Nucl Med Commun 2003; 24(3): 233-9.
[http://dx.doi.org/10.1097/00006231-200303000-00002] [PMID: 12612463]

[41] Harms HJ, Lubberink M, de Haan S, *et al.* Use of a Single 11C-Meta-Hydroxyephedrine Scan for Assessing Flow-Innervation Mismatches in Patients with Ischemic Cardiomyopathy. J Nucl Med 2015; 56(11): 1706-11.
[http://dx.doi.org/10.2967/jnumed.115.154377] [PMID: 26229146]

[42] Mori Y, Manabe O, Naya M, *et al.* Improved spillover correction model to quantify myocardial blood flow by 11C-acetate PET: comparison with 15O-H 2O PET. Ann Nucl Med 2015; 29(1): 15-20.
[http://dx.doi.org/10.1007/s12149-014-0904-z] [PMID: 25209232]

[43] Beanlands R, Chow BJ, Dick A, *et al.* CCS / CAR / CANM / CNCS / CanSCMR Joint Position Statement on Advanced Non-invasive Cardiac Imaging using Positron Emission Tomography, Magnetic Resonance Imaging and Multi-Detector Computed Tomographic Angiography in the Diagnosis and Evaluation of Ischemic Heart Disease Abbreviated Report. Can J Cardiol in press

[44] Klocke FJ, Baird MG, Lorell BH, *et al.* ACC/AHA/ASNC guidelines for the clinical use of cardiac radionuclide imaging--executive summary: a report of the American College of Cardiology/American Heart Association Task Force on Practice Guidelines (ACC/AHA/ASNC Committee to Revise the 1995 Guidelines for the Clinical Use of Cardiac Radionuclide Imaging). J Am Coll Cardiol 2003; 42(7): 1318-33.
[http://dx.doi.org/10.1016/j.jacc.2003.08.011] [PMID: 14522503]

[45] Powles KE, Hessian RC, Ruddy TD. Practicing safe SPECT: caffeine abstinence in nuclear myocardial perfusion imaging. J Nucl Cardiol 2008; 15(5): 709-18.
[http://dx.doi.org/10.1016/j.nuclcard.2008.02.038] [PMID: 18761274]

[46] Machac J, Bacharach SL, Bateman TM, *et al.* Positron emission tomography myocardial perfusion and glucose metabolism imaging. J Nucl Cardiol 2006; 13(6): e121-51.
[http://dx.doi.org/10.1016/j.nuclcard.2006.08.009] [PMID: 17174789]

[47] Brinkert M, Reyes E, Walker S, *et al.* Regadenoson in Europe: first-year experience of regadenoson stress combined with submaximal exercise in patients undergoing myocardial perfusion scintigraphy. Eur J Nucl Med Mol Imaging 2014; 41(3): 511-21.
[http://dx.doi.org/10.1007/s00259-013-2619-0] [PMID: 24265072]

[48] Camici PG. Positron emission tomography and myocardial imaging. Heart 2000; 83(4): 475-80.
[http://dx.doi.org/10.1136/heart.83.4.475] [PMID: 10722554]

[49] Gould KL, Schelbert HR, Phelps ME, Hoffman EJ. Noninvasive assessment of coronary stenoses with myocardial perfusion imaging during pharmacologic coronary vasodilatation. V. Detection of 47 percent diameter coronary stenosis with intravenous nitrogen-13 ammonia and emission-computed tomography in intact dogs. Am J Cardiol 1979; 43(2): 200-8.
[http://dx.doi.org/10.1016/S0002-9149(79)80005-3] [PMID: 760474]

[50] Reyes E. Regadenoson stress for myocardial perfusion imaging. Future Cardiol 2016; 12(1): 59-67.
[http://dx.doi.org/10.2217/fca.15.70] [PMID: 26639775]

[51] Goudarzi B, Fukushima K, Bravo P, Merrill J, Bengel FM. Comparison of the myocardial blood flow response to regadenoson and dipyridamole: a quantitative analysis in patients referred for clinical 82Rb myocardial perfusion PET. Eur J Nucl Med Mol Imaging 2011; 38(10): 1908-16.
[http://dx.doi.org/10.1007/s00259-011-1853-6] [PMID: 21656246]

[52] Imaging guidelines for nuclear cardiology procedures, part 2. J Nucl Cardiol 1999; 6(2): G47-84. [http://dx.doi.org/10.1016/S1071-3581(99)90088-0] [PMID: 10327112]

[53] Herrero P, Markham J, Shelton ME, Bergmann SR. Implementation and evaluation of a two-compartment model for quantification of myocardial perfusion with rubidium-82 and positron emission tomography. Circ Res 1992; 70(3): 496-507. [http://dx.doi.org/10.1161/01.RES.70.3.496] [PMID: 1537087]

[54] Herrero P, Markham J, Shelton ME, Weinheimer CJ, Bergmann SR. Noninvasive quantification of regional myocardial perfusion with rubidium-82 and positron emission tomography. Exploration of a mathematical model. Circulation 1990; 82(4): 1377-86. [http://dx.doi.org/10.1161/01.CIR.82.4.1377] [PMID: 2401071]

[55] Iida H, Rhodes CG, de Silva R, *et al.* Use of the left ventricular time-activity curve as a noninvasive input function in dynamic oxygen-15-water positron emission tomography. J Nucl Med 1992; 33(9): 1669-77. [PMID: 1517842]

[56] Weinberg IN, Huang SC, Hoffman EJ, *et al.* Validation of PET-acquired input functions for cardiac studies. J Nucl Med 1988; 29(2): 241-7. [PMID: 3258026]

[57] Hutchins GD, Schwaiger M, Rosenspire KC, Krivokapich J, Schelbert H, Kuhl DE. Noninvasive quantification of regional blood flow in the human heart using N-13 ammonia and dynamic positron emission tomographic imaging. J Am Coll Cardiol 1990; 15(5): 1032-42. [http://dx.doi.org/10.1016/0735-1097(90)90237-J] [PMID: 2312957]

[58] Iida H, Kanno I, Takahashi A, *et al.* Measurement of absolute myocardial blood flow with H215O and dynamic positron-emission tomography. Strategy for quantification in relation to the partial-volume effect. Circulation 1988; 78(1): 104-15. [http://dx.doi.org/10.1161/01.CIR.78.1.104] [PMID: 3260151]

[59] Nesterov SV, Deshayes E, Sciagrà R, *et al.* Quantification of myocardial blood flow in absolute terms using (82)Rb PET imaging: the RUBY-10 Study. JACC Cardiovasc Imaging 2014; 7(11): 1119-27. [http://dx.doi.org/10.1016/j.jcmg.2014.08.003] [PMID: 25306543]

[60] Danad I, Uusitalo V, Kero T, *et al.* Quantitative assessment of myocardial perfusion in the detection of significant coronary artery disease: cutoff values and diagnostic accuracy of quantitative [(15)O]H2O PET imaging. J Am Coll Cardiol 2014; 64(14): 1464-75. [http://dx.doi.org/10.1016/j.jacc.2014.05.069] [PMID: 25277618]

[61] Sampson UK, Dorbala S, Limaye A, Kwong R, Di Carli MF. Diagnostic accuracy of rubidium-82 myocardial perfusion imaging with hybrid positron emission tomography/computed tomography in the detection of coronary artery disease. J Am Coll Cardiol 2007; 49(10): 1052-8. [http://dx.doi.org/10.1016/j.jacc.2006.12.015] [PMID: 17349884]

[62] Jaarsma C, Leiner T, Bekkers SC, *et al.* Diagnostic performance of noninvasive myocardial perfusion imaging using single-photon emission computed tomography, cardiac magnetic resonance, and positron emission tomography imaging for the detection of obstructive coronary artery disease: a meta-analysis. J Am Coll Cardiol 2012; 59(19): 1719-28. [http://dx.doi.org/10.1016/j.jacc.2011.12.040] [PMID: 22554604]

[63] Schindler TH, Schelbert HR, Quercioli A, Dilsizian V. Cardiac PET imaging for the detection and monitoring of coronary artery disease and microvascular health. JACC Cardiovasc Imaging 2010; 3(6): 623-40. [http://dx.doi.org/10.1016/j.jcmg.2010.04.007] [PMID: 20541718]

[64] Ziadi MC, Dekemp RA, Williams K, *et al.* Does quantification of myocardial flow reserve using rubidium-82 positron emission tomography facilitate detection of multivessel coronary artery disease? J Nucl Cardiol 2012; 19(4): 670-80. [http://dx.doi.org/10.1007/s12350-011-9506-5] [PMID: 22415819]

[65] Marwick TH, Shan K, Patel S, Go RT, Lauer MS. Incremental value of rubidium-82 positron emission tomography for prognostic assessment of known or suspected coronary artery disease. Am J Cardiol 1997; 80(7): 865-70.
[http://dx.doi.org/10.1016/S0002-9149(97)00537-7] [PMID: 9381999]

[66] Dorbala S, Di Carli MF, Beanlands RS, *et al.* Prognostic value of stress myocardial perfusion positron emission tomography: results from a multicenter observational registry. J Am Coll Cardiol 2013; 61(2): 176-84.
[http://dx.doi.org/10.1016/j.jacc.2012.09.043] [PMID: 23219297]

[67] Ziadi MC, Dekemp RA, Williams KA, *et al.* Impaired myocardial flow reserve on rubidium-82 positron emission tomography imaging predicts adverse outcomes in patients assessed for myocardial ischemia. J Am Coll Cardiol 2011; 58(7): 740-8.
[http://dx.doi.org/10.1016/j.jacc.2011.01.065] [PMID: 21816311]

[68] Pagani M, Stone-Elander S, Larsson SA. Alternative positron emission tomography with non-conventional positron emitters: effects of their physical properties on image quality and potential clinical applications. Eur J Nucl Med 1997; 24(10): 1301-27.
[http://dx.doi.org/10.1007/s002590050156] [PMID: 9323273]

[69] Williams HA, Robinson S, Julyan P, Zweit J, Hastings D. A comparison of PET imaging characteristics of various copper radioisotopes. Eur J Nucl Med Mol Imaging 2005; 32(12): 1473-80.
[http://dx.doi.org/10.1007/s00259-005-1906-9] [PMID: 16258764]

[70] Seltzer MA, Jahan SA, Sparks R, *et al.* Radiation dose estimates in humans for (11)C-acetate whole-body PET. J Nucl Med 2004; 45(7): 1233-6.
[PMID: 15235071]

[71] Gould KL, Goldstein RA, Mullani NA, *et al.* Noninvasive assessment of coronary stenoses by myocardial perfusion imaging during pharmacologic coronary vasodilation. VIII. Clinical feasibility of positron cardiac imaging without a cyclotron using generator-produced rubidium-82. J Am Coll Cardiol 1986; 7(4): 775-89.
[http://dx.doi.org/10.1016/S0735-1097(86)80336-9] [PMID: 3485669]

[72] Demer LL, Gould KL, Goldstein RA, *et al.* Assessment of coronary artery disease severity by positron emission tomography. Comparison with quantitative arteriography in 193 patients. Circulation 1989; 79(4): 825-35.
[http://dx.doi.org/10.1161/01.CIR.79.4.825] [PMID: 2784361]

[73] Go RT, Marwick TH, MacIntyre WJ, *et al.* A prospective comparison of rubidium-82 PET and thallium-201 SPECT myocardial perfusion imaging utilizing a single dipyridamole stress in the diagnosis of coronary artery disease. J Nucl Med 1990; 31(12): 1899-905.
[PMID: 2266384]

[74] Stewart RE, Schwaiger M, Molina E, *et al.* Comparison of rubidium-82 positron emission tomography and thallium-201 SPECT imaging for detection of coronary artery disease. Am J Cardiol 1991; 67(16): 1303-10.
[http://dx.doi.org/10.1016/0002-9149(91)90456-U] [PMID: 2042560]

[75] Marwick TH, Nemec JJ, Stewart WJ, Salcedo EE. Diagnosis of coronary artery disease using exercise echocardiography and positron emission tomography: comparison and analysis of discrepant results. J Am Soc Echocardiogr 1992; 5(3): 231-8.
[http://dx.doi.org/10.1016/S0894-7317(14)80342-8] [PMID: 1622613]

[76] Grover-McKay M, Ratib O, Schwaiger M, *et al.* Detection of coronary artery disease with positron emission tomography and rubidium 82. Am Heart J 1992; 123(3): 646-52.
[http://dx.doi.org/10.1016/0002-8703(92)90502-M] [PMID: 1539516]

[77] Simone GL, Mullani NA, Page DA, Anderson BA Sr. Utilization statistics and diagnostic accuracy of a nonhospital-based positron emission tomography center for the detection of coronary artery disease using rubidium-82. Am J Physiol Imaging 1992; 7(3-4): 203-9.

[PMID: 1343217]

[78] Chow BJ, Dennie C, Hoffmann U, *et al.* Comparison of computed tomographic angiography *versus* rubidium-82 positron emission tomography for the detection of patients with anatomical coronary artery disease. Can J Cardiol 2007; 23(10): 801-7.
[http://dx.doi.org/10.1016/S0828-282X(07)70831-0] [PMID: 17703259]

[79] Dorbala S, Vangala D, Sampson U, Limaye A, Kwong R, Di Carli MF. Value of vasodilator left ventricular ejection fraction reserve in evaluating the magnitude of myocardium at risk and the extent of angiographic coronary artery disease: a 82Rb PET/CT study. J Nucl Med 2007; 48(3): 349-58.
[PMID: 17332611]

[80] Esteves FP, Sanyal R, Nye JA, Santana CA, Verdes L, Raggi P. Adenosine stress rubidium-82 PET/computed tomography in patients with known and suspected coronary artery disease. Nucl Med Commun 2008; 29(8): 674-8.
[http://dx.doi.org/10.1097/MNM.0b013e328301a614] [PMID: 18753818]

[81] Esteves FP, Nye JA, Khan A, *et al.* Prompt-gamma compensation in Rb-82 myocardial perfusion 3D PET/CT. J Nucl Cardiol 2010; 17(2): 247-53.
[http://dx.doi.org/10.1007/s12350-009-9170-1] [PMID: 19937169]

[82] Groves AM, Speechly-Dick ME, Kayani I, *et al.* First experience of combined cardiac PET/64-detector CT angiography with invasive angiographic validation. Eur J Nucl Med Mol Imaging 2009; 36(12): 2027-33.
[http://dx.doi.org/10.1007/s00259-009-1213-y] [PMID: 19618180]

[83] Nakazato R, Berman DS, Dey D, *et al.* Automated quantitative Rb-82 3D PET/CT myocardial perfusion imaging: normal limits and correlation with invasive coronary angiography. J Nucl Cardiol 2012; 19(2): 265-76.
[http://dx.doi.org/10.1007/s12350-011-9496-3] [PMID: 22203445]

[84] Yoshinaga K, Chow BJ. Prognostic value of Rubidium-82 perfusion positron emission tomography in patients referred after SPECT imaging. J Nucl Cardiol 2005; 12: S43.
[http://dx.doi.org/10.1016/j.nuclcard.2004.12.138]

[85] Chow BJ, Wong JW, Yoshinaga K, *et al.* Prognostic significance of dipyridamole-induced ST depression in patients with normal 82Rb PET myocardial perfusion imaging. J Nucl Med 2005; 46(7): 1095-101.
[PMID: 16000277]

[86] Kay J, Dorbala S, Goyal A, *et al.* Influence of sex on risk stratification with stress myocardial perfusion Rb-82 positron emission tomography: Results from the PET (Positron Emission Tomography) Prognosis Multicenter Registry. J Am Coll Cardiol 2013; 62(20): 1866-76.
[http://dx.doi.org/10.1016/j.jacc.2013.06.017] [PMID: 23850903]

[87] Farhad H, Dunet V, Bachelard K, Allenbach G, Kaufmann PA, Prior JO. Added prognostic value of myocardial blood flow quantitation in rubidium-82 positron emission tomography imaging. Eur Heart J Cardiovasc Imaging 2013; 14(12): 1203-10.
[http://dx.doi.org/10.1093/ehjci/jet068] [PMID: 23660750]

[88] Fukushima K, Javadi MS, Higuchi T, *et al.* Prediction of short-term cardiovascular events using quantification of global myocardial flow reserve in patients referred for clinical 82Rb PET perfusion imaging. J Nucl Med 2011; 52(5): 726-32.
[http://dx.doi.org/10.2967/jnumed.110.081828] [PMID: 21498538]

[89] Murthy VL, Naya M, Foster CR, *et al.* Improved cardiac risk assessment with noninvasive measures of coronary flow reserve. Circulation 2011; 124(20): 2215-24.
[http://dx.doi.org/10.1161/CIRCULATIONAHA.111.050427] [PMID: 22007073]

CHAPTER 6

Myocardial Perfusion Imaging and other Modalities

Yasuyo Taniguchi*

Hyogo Brain and Heart Center, Himeji, Hyogo, Japan

Abstract: Rapid technological advance has brought many myocardial perfusion imaging (MPI) modalities other than myocardial single-photon emission computed tomography (SPECT) imaging. Cardiac magnetic resonance (CMR) and cardiac computer tomography (CCT) myocardial imaging give us more precise imaging with an improved special resolution which can depict subendocardial ischemia. As for CMR, T2 weighted imaging demonstrated edematous region without enhancement. Recent advances in CMR of parametric mapping technique now permit the visualization and quantification of the tissue characteristics and also give us the opportunity to guess disease process. On the other hand, SPECT fusion imaging with a coronary artery from CCT or CMR also gives us useful territorial information of coronary artery disease. In this chapter, recent advances and status of CMR and CCT imaging surrounding SPECT MPI are described.

Keyword: Cardiac Computed Tomography, Cardiac Magnetic Resonance Imaging, Functional Flow Reserve, Myocardial Viability, Myocardial Tissue Imaging, Myocardial Perfusion Imaging, Parametric Mapping Imaging.

CARDIAC MAGNETIC RESONANCE IMAGING (CMR) IMAGING

CMR has been applied in a wide variety of indications in clinical cardiology and depicts the heart from three different views, including functionally or physiologically, anatomically or morphologically, and histologically. Aside from functional imaging data such as four chamber motion and volumetric or valvular functions, CMR also gives us useful information on the relationships between the heart and pericardial organs and takes on an important role in the diagnostic evaluation and pre-procedural planning for patients with congenital heart disease [1]. Recently developed four-dimensional (4D) flow techniques offer the visualization and quantification of flow and can estimate hemodynamic effects at

* **Corresponding author Yasuyo Taniguchi:** Hyogo Brain and Heart Center, Himeji, Hyogo, Japan, Tel: +81792933131; E-mail: ytaniguchi0@gmail.com

Shinro Matsuo (Ed.)

the vessel wall and myocardium, as well as provide visualization of flow pathways in the heart and great vessels [2].

For evaluating myocardial perfusion, the gadolinium enhancement stress first-pass perfusion and late gadolinium enhancement (LGE) technique can visualize myocardial ischemia and infarction, respectively, which is the same manner as stress and rest SPECT MPI [1]. Coronary MR angiography allows the assessment of coronary arteries without the use of ionizing radiation or iodinated contrast enhancement and can assess the coronary artery lumen in the presence of severe calcification. Comprehensive assessment of ventricular wall motion and myocardial perfusion combined with coronary anatomy is a powerful tool for diagnosing cardiac disease.

Assessment of Myocardial Perfusion

Myocardial stress imaging using a vasodilator such as adenosine or dipyridamole may reveal various states of myocardial perfusion and amounts of ischemia. Using a T1-weighted (T1W) sequence with gadolinium contrast agent, myocardial perfusion imaging may visualize the myocardium as the first pass imaging. From signal intensity correlated with the passing contrast agent, the state of myocardial perfusion is evaluated in a semi-quantitative and qualitative manner [3]. Diagnostic accuracy of CMR perfusion for each segment and territory of patient based meta analyses showed good diagnostic performance with sensitivity values of over 0.85 and specificity values over 0.70 (the area under the curve (AUC) of the receiver operator curve (ROC) over 0.85) [4]. In Magnetic Resonance Imaging for Myocardial Perfusion Assessment in Coronary artery diseases Trial II, a multicenter, multivendor trial of perfusion-CMR as an alternative to SPECT as for coronary artery disease (CAD) detection, showed equal performance in the head-to-head comparison [5]. A CMR-based management strategy for patients with stable CAD was safe and reduced revascularization procedures and resulted in a better quality of life at the 12-month follow-up examination [5, 6]. In this trial, the sensitivity of perfusion of CMR to detect CAD was superior to that of SPECT, although its specificity was inferior to that of SPECT. Cardiac magnetic resonance is a safe alternative to SPECT to detect perfusion deficits in CAD. In patients of known and suspected CAD, an ischemic burden over 1.5 of ischemic segments on stress-perfusion CMR was the strongest predictor of major cardiac events (Fig. **1**) [7]. In the three most commonly used modalities for MPI, SPECT, CMR, and positron emission tomography (PET) all yielded a high sensitivity, while a broad range of specificity was observed. SPECT is widely available and most extensively validated; PET achieved the highest diagnostic performance; CMR may provide an alternative without ionizing radiation and a similar diagnostic accuracy as PET [8].

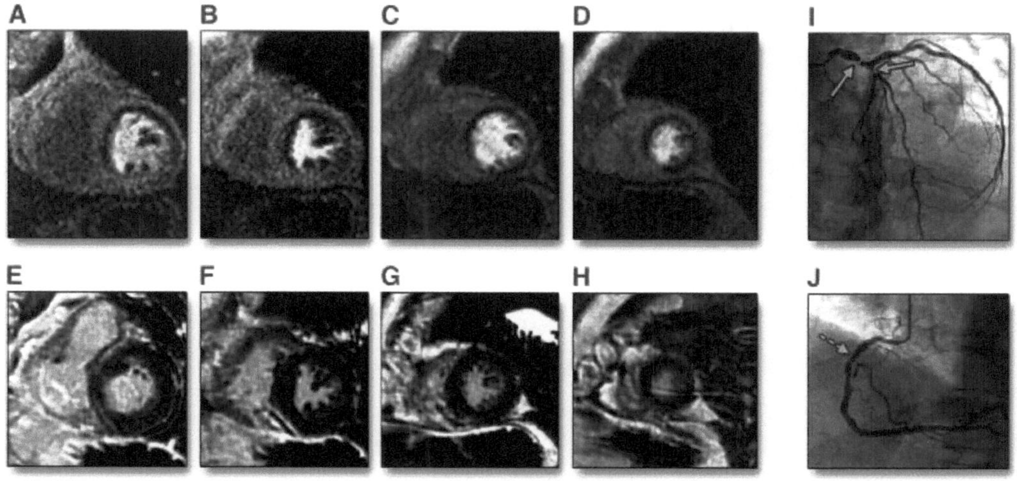

Fig. (1). With a large perfusion deficit (14 segments) in the (A to D) territory of the left main artery (E to H) without scar on late gadolinium enhancement imaging. Coronary angiography shows a severe stenosis of the left main artery (90% to 99%) and the proximal circumflex artery (I, arrows); mild nonsignificant right coronary wall irregularities (<50%). Cited [7].

Pharmacological stress with CMR is a Class IIa indication for patients with an intermediate to high pretest probability of obstructive ischemic heart disease, with an uninterpretable ECG, and with at least moderate physical functioning or no disabling comorbidity [9].

Assessment of Area at Risk in AMI

Myocardial salvage is an important prognostic factor in patients with acute myocardial infarction [10]. To assess the efficacy of reperfusion therapy, it is necessary to determine the area by measuring both the final infarct size and the initial damaged myocardium size at risk. Myocardial perfusion imaging with SPECT is the technique most widely practiced for directly measuring the myocardial salvage area [11]. The assessed salvage area determined by CMR using T2-weighted (T2W) and LGE imaging also correlates with the data which have already been reported on the established modality; SPECT [12, 13]. T2W imaging allows for the visualization of infarct-related edema and area at risk after reperfusion was defined as a region of hyper enhanced myocardium with signal intensity above 2 standard deviations (SD) of the healthy remote myocardium [14]. The microvascular obstruction which was identified in LGE images as hypointense recesses within the hyper enhanced myocardium was a highly anatomical correlation with hypointense areas on T2w-images which was thought to be intramyocardial hemorrhage [14]. Intramyocardial hemorrhage from T2W imaging and microvascular obstruction are useful imaging for establishing a prognosis [14, 15]. For this assessment, CMR has advantages over SPECT which

CMR study is not associated with radiation exposure and only once examination about after early phase after reperfusion therapy. But there are clear drawbacks too. Adding to the contraindication about CMR study, the T2W imaging sequence has a low contrast-to-noise ratio, necessitating a quite low threshold of 2 SD for edema detection and is prone to artifacts that may necessitate individual sequence adjustments. Especially tachycardia, arrhythmias, and pleural effusion limit the image quality or prevent a valid image analysis at all. Sometimes the exclusion rate accumulates to 13% because of insufficient image quality [16].

In both the guidelines of American College of Cardiology (ACC) and American Heart Association (AHA) and European Society for Cardiology (ESC), imaging with ventriculography, echocardiography, or CMR imaging is class I indication for the diagnosis of stress (Takotsubo) cardiomyopathy [9, 17].

Assessment of Myocardial Viability

Additional information about myocardial perfusion, viability, and fibrosis can help to identify heart failure etiology and assess prognostic information. In normal myocardium, the myocytes are densely packed, and gadolinium is unable to penetrate intact sarcolemma membranes. In pathophysiologic states that cause a reduced density of viable myocytes, such as acute and chronic AMI and non-ischemic cardiomyopathies, CMR imaging shows a higher concentration and increased volume of distribution for gadolinium in the interstitial space. In AMI, ruptured myocyte membranes allow gadolinium to passively diffuse into the intracellular space, resulting in an increased volume of distribution for gadolinium and increased tissue concentration when compared with normal myocardium (Fig. **2**) [18].

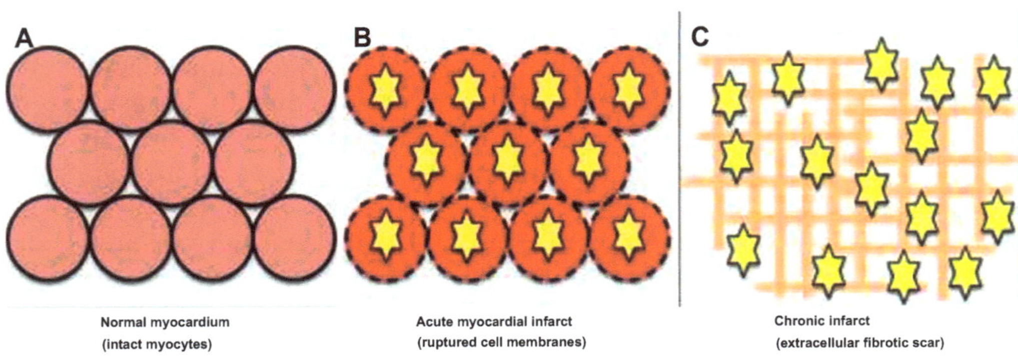

Fig. (2). Mechanism of late gadolinium enhancement. Gadolinium is extracellular. A: In normal myocardium, gadolinium washes out approximately 10 min post administration and there is no late gadolinium enhancement (LGE); B: In acute infarct, gadolinium (stars) enters ruptured cell membranes and causes LGE; C: In chronic infarct, LGE results from increased extracellular space due to fibrotic scar deposition. Cited [18].

In chronic infarction, as the necrotic tissue is replaced by collagenous scar, the interstitial space is expanded, and gadolinium tissue concentration is increased. T1W sequences with LGE enhancement depict infarcted regions as bright or *hyper-enhanced* areas, whereas viable regions appear as black or *null* areas. LGE CMR is a highly effective imaging technique as it reveals the obvious presence, location, and extent of myocardial damage in both acute and chronic settings. The transmural extent of infarction (TEI) measured by LGE was found to be inversely related to an improvement in segmental function in a stepwise fashion [19]. In addition to predicting improvement in regional function, LGE CMR also provides the best predictors of improvement in global function. Important findings include the following:

- The percentage of the left ventricle (LV) defined as dysfunctional but viable (TEI $\leq$ 25%) is directly related to future changes in the LV wall thickening score (r = 0.87, p = 0.002) [18, 20].
- Where the TEI $\leq$ 75%, determination of the extent of LGE and functional recovery in AMI had a sensitivity of 98% but a specificity of 66% for predicting viability at follow-up. There exists the possibility of underestimating viability in the acute phase of MI [19].
- Where the TEI is 50-75% in ischemic cardiomyopathy, administration of inotropic reserve (IR) during low-dose dobutamine (LDD) is a better prediction of segmental recovery than LGE and scar rim evaluation [22].
- In heart failure management including revascularization, for ischemia detection and viability assessment, MPI (stress SPECT/CMR imaging) is the Class IIa recommendation in AHA/ACC and ESC guideline [9, 17].
- In the management of functional ischemic mitral valve regurgitation, stress MPI (SPECT, CMR) is a useful diagnostic aid and a Class I indication.
- In the ESC guideline, the evaluation of CMR viability imaging is conservative: The guideline rates its ability to detect viability and predict functional recovery as being no better than that achieved with other imaging techniques.

Tissue Characterization

LGE imaging is a useful tool for direct visualization of myocardial injury and depicts fibrosis. The distribution of gadolinium enhancement may differentiate ischemic cardiomyopathy from non-ischemic cardiomyopathy [23, 24]. In the setting of diffuse fibrosis, the presence of LGE has been shown to correlate poorly with collagen volume calculated from endomyocardial biopsies.

Recent rapid advances in parametric mapping techniques provide improved non-invasive quantifying of myocardial tissue characterization. The parametric mapping method is useful for imaging diffuse myocardial fibrosis or diffuse deposition of iron or specific lipid because of the absence of normal reference myocardium. Native T1 (noncontrast) reflects myocardial disease involving the myocyte and interstitium without the use of contrast agents. Higher native T1 values are associated with excess water in edema and lower native T1 is related to the deposition of lipid or iron. The extracellular fraction (ECV) which is calculated from the values of native T1 and T1 after enhancement, reflects the enhancement based extracellular space [25]. Clinically, T1 mapping with ECV is particularly useful in the assessment of cardiac diseases with diffuse fibrosis. Furthermore, especially in cases with ambiguous LGE. Beyond differential diagnosis of cardiomyopathies, tissue characterization with T1 mapping can be useful in differentiating between pericardial fat *vs*. LGE, differentiating between epicardial fat *vs*. pericardial effusion [25].

Fig. (**3**) shows parametric mapping with CMR for a case with ischemia and diffuse fibrosis.

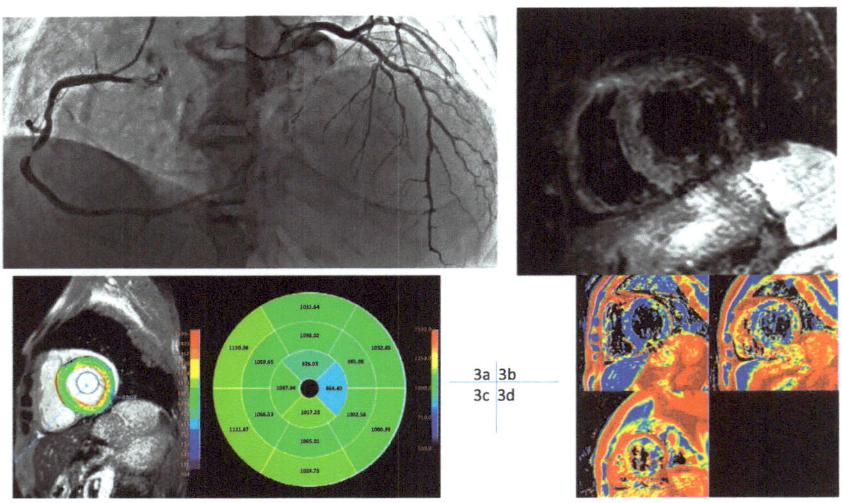

Fig. (3). A case of moderately reduced LV function without asynergy. (**3a**) CAG shows RCA stenosis; (**3b**) T2W image (SPIR) shows inferior high intensity in inferior; (**3c**) native T1 mapping shows diffuse longer value; (**3d**) T2 mapping shows apical inferior mild longer value.

CARDIAC COMPUTER TOMOGRAPHY (CCT)

Since approximately 10 years ago of the first introduction of 64-slice CT scanners, a CCT angiography (CCTA) has made substantial progress due to both imaging technology and clinical validation. However, the ability of CCTA for determination of the physiological significance of intermediate coronary stenosis remains shortcoming compared to other noninvasive methods such as SPECT, stress echocardiography, and stress CMR. New methods have been investigated recently such as CCT perfusion and fractional flow reserve (FFR) computed from

CCT (FFRct) [26, 27]. The diagnostic accuracy by combining the anatomical assessment of CCTA and a physiologic assessment *via* CT perfusion or FFRct reduces the need for invasive testing in the evaluation of ischemia. These results also reduced the excessed medical expense and the inappropriate risks associated with an invasive procedure. Consequently, it leads to improved patient outcomes. In addition to an anatomical imaging, CCTA additively produces plaque imaging of coronary arteries and also produced myocardial perfusion imaging (Fig. **4**) [35, 37].

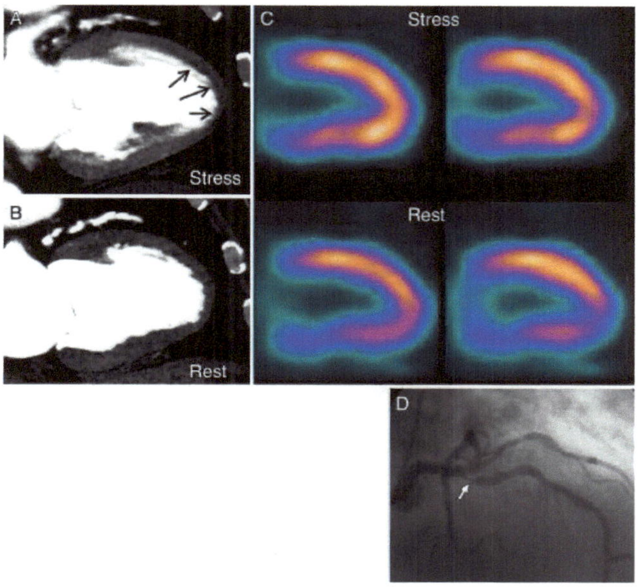

Fig. (4). Images of the man with chest pain. **A**, Myocardial CT perfusion image at stress demonstrates subendocardial perfusion defect in antero-apical and apical walls (arrows). **B**, Myocardial CT perfusion image at rest shows that defect is reversible. **C**, SPECT images demonstrate normal myocardial perfusion with subdiaphragmatic attenuation artifact. **D**, Image from invasive coronary angiography demonstrates 85% stenosis in proximal left anterior descending artery. FFRct and invasive FFR is good correlation. Cited [35].

In the emergency setting, use of a triple rule out (TRO) scan can provide a simultaneous evaluation of CAD, pulmonary embolism, and aortic disease, although its indiscriminate use is not warranted [36].

Standardized Reporting of CCTA

Clinically the decision support is a major focus of healthcare policies which aimed at improving guideline-directed care. From PROMISE study and CT coronary angiography in patients with suspected angina due to coronary heart disease (SCOT-HEART), CTCA clarifies the diagnosis, enables targeting of interventions, and might reduce the future risk of myocardial infarction in patients with suspected angina due to coronary heart disease [20, 28, 29]. Recently, Coronary Artery Disease - Reporting and Data System (CAD-RADS) was developed to standardize CCTA reporting includes clinical recommendations to facilitate patient management after examination of CCTA [30]. This reporting system clinically includes both stable chest pain and acute chest pain from CAD-RADS 0 (absence of atherosclerosis) to CAD-RADS 5 (presence of at least one total occlusion) the most relevant clinical patient findings. Typical imaging of CAD RAD 4a,4b,5, and Modified V are shown in Fig. (**5**). The CAD RADS 4 designation is divided into two categories: CAD RADS 4a describes a condition of a single vessel or two vessels demonstrating severe (70–99%) stenosis; while CAD RADS 4b identifies the presence of left main artery stenosis greater than 50% or three-vessel obstructive disease greater than 70%. CAD-RADS 5 is used to identify chronic total occlusion. The CAD-RADS system effectively identifies patients at risk for adverse events and its application is designed to both avoid unnecessary examination and perform evidence-based care.

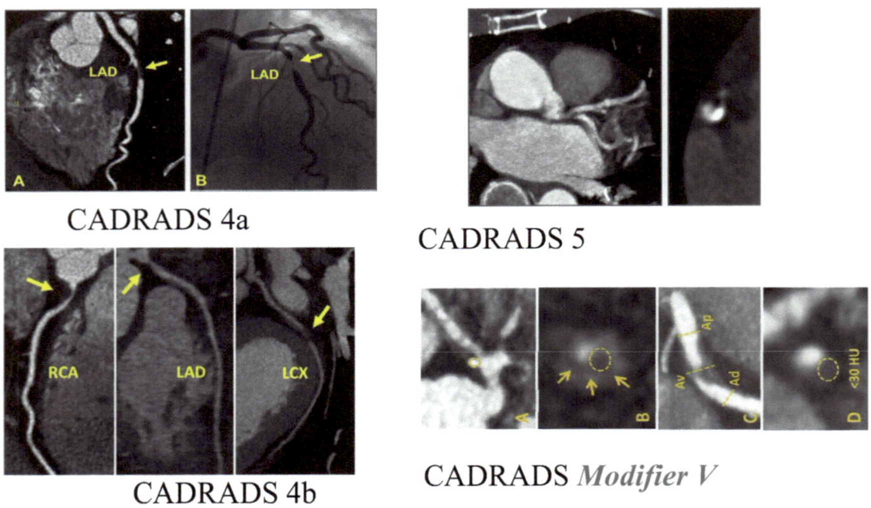

Fig. (5). CAD-RADS **4a**; Focal non-calcified plaque in the mid LAD with 70-99% diameter stenosis. Invasive coronary angiography confirming 70-99% stenosis in the mid LAD. CAD-RADS **4b**(left); Three-vessel obstructive disease (>70% stenosis), including in 70-99% stenosis of the proximal RCA, 70-99% stenosis of the proximal LAD and 70-99% stenosis of the mid LCX. CAD-RADS **4b**(right); Distal left main stenosis with circumferential calcified plaque resulting in > 50% stenosis. Oblique longitudinal plane of the left main coronary artery and crosssectional slice of the distal left main coronary artery also showed. Invasive coronary angiography confirming focal severe stenosis in the distal left main coronary artery. CAD-RADS **5**(Left): Focal, non-calcified occlusion of the proximal RCA. (Right): Total occlusion of the proximal LCX. High-Risk Plaque Features on coronary CTA. CAD-RADS the modifier "V" (vulnerability). These include (**A**) Spotty calcium, defined as punctate calcium within a plaque, "napkin ring sign", (**B**) defined as central low attenuation plaque with a peripheral rim of higher CT attenuation (arrows), (**C**) Positive remodeling, defined as the ratio of outer vessel diameter at the site of plaque divided by the average outer diameter of the proximal and distal vessel greater than 1.1mm (**D**) Low attenuation plaque, defined as non-calcified plaque with internal attenuation less than 30 HU (Cited [30]).

CAD-RADS 4b (left) ; Three-vessel obstructive disease (>70% stenosis), including in 70-99% stenosis of the proximal RCA, 70-99% stenosis of the proximal LAD and 70-99% stenosis of the mid LCX. CAD-RADS 4b (right); Distal left main stenosis with circumferential calcified plaque resulting in > 50% stenosis. Oblique longitudinal plane of the left main coronary artery and cross-sectional slice of the distal left main coronary artery also showed. Invasive coronary angiography confirming focal severe stenosis in the distal left main coronary artery. CAD-RADS 5. Left: Focal, non-calcified occlusion of the proximal RCA. Right: Total occlusion of the proximal LCX. High-Risk Plaque Features on coronary CTA.

CAD-RADS the modifier “V” (vulnerability).These include (A) Spotty calcium, defined as punctate calcium within a plaque, “napkin ring sign”, defined as central low attenuation plaque with a peripheral rim of higher CT attenuation (arrows), (C) Positive remodeling, defined as the ratio of outer vessel diameter at the site of plaque divided by the average outer diameter of the proximal and distal vessel greater than 1.1mm (D) Low attenuation plaque, defined as non-calcified plaque with internal attenuation less than 30 HU (Cited [30]).

Anatomical CCT Imaging and Other Functional Imaging

While coronary CTA may evaluate the location and extent of stenotic artery disease in addition to plaque morphology and characterization, stress MPI may depict the hemodynamic status of coronary stenosis (where stenosis > 50% is considered anatomically obstructive). When the detection of lesion-specific ischemia using FFR with invasive coronary angiography (ICA) is the gold standard, the diagnostic accuracy of CCTA was 69% and sensitivity, specificity, positive predictive value, and negative predictive values were 79%, 63%, 55%, and 83%, respectively [31]. In anatomical information, both CTA and ICA exhibited similar diagnostic performance for the detection and exclusion of lesion-specific CAD. The PROMISE trial reported that compared to functional testing, coronary CTA led to an increase in ICA and was less likely to demonstrate normal coronary arteries (4.3 *vs*. 3.4%; $p < 0.02$), and consequently, more likely to lead to coronary revascularization at 90 days (6.2 *vs*. 3.2%; $p < 0.001$). The risk of death or non-fatal MI was lower in the coronary CTA group (hazard ratio [HR]: 0.66; 95% CI: 0.44-1.00; $p < 0.049$), although this benefit did not persist throughout the study follow-up period [20]. In the SCOT-HEART trial, CCTA led to earlier decisions for performing ICA and subsequent invasive treatment for high-risk patients, while led to diminishing the use of unnecessary anti-anginal medication with clarifying and excluding the diagnosis of CHD [29]. This may have important implications for patients’ health-related quality of life.

Through identifying patients at moderate risk, CCTA provides better prognostic information than MPI functional testing in contemporary patients with stable chest pain. On the other hand, in the PROMISE study, it is noteworthy that adding the Framingham Risk Score to MPI functional test resulted significantly improved the prognostic value of functional testing [20, 28]. Coronary CTA is a Class IIa alternative to stress imaging techniques for ruling out coronary artery disease in patients with intermediate risk [32].

Functional Imaging with Coronary CTA

Despite that FFR with ICA is the gold standard and its feasibility and appropriate usefulness are clear, this method is more invasive than CCTA. Recent advances in computational fluid dynamics and image-based modeling have been permitted the determination of coronary flow and pressure from CCT scans, without additional acquisition protocols [27]. These techniques depict noninvasively compute fractional flow reserve (FFRct), which is the ratio of maximal coronary blood flow of a stenotic artery to the blood flow in the hypothetical normal value using CCTA imaging [27]. By using invasive FFR as the reference standard, the area under the ROC for FFRct was higher than ROC for anatomical coronary CTA at 0.90 (95% CI: 0.87–0.94) *versus* 0.81 (95% CI: 0.76–0.87) and $p < 0.0008$. In patients with intermediate stenosis (95% CI: 30–70), the diagnostic accuracy of FFRct remained high [33]. Compared to anatomical testing with CCTA, FFRct led to a marked increase in specificity for detecting ischemia. Patients with an FFRct value greater than 0.80 deferred from invasive coronary angiography have a favorable short-term prognosis [33]. Fig. (**6**) demonstrated a case which was noninvasively diagnosed as ischemic heart disease with using CTA.

CT Myocardial Perfusion Imaging

Recent technical advances in CCT have made the development of CT MPI feasible. CT MPI with rest and adenosine stress with 320-row CT is accurate in detecting obstructive atherosclerosis causing myocardial ischemia [34]. The sensitivity of CT perfusion imaging for single- and multivessel CAD was higher than that of SPECT MPI, with sensitivities for left main, three-vessel, two-vessel, and one-vessel disease of 92%, 92%, 89%, and 83%, respectively, for CT perfusion imaging, on the other hand 75%, 79%, 68%, and 41%, respectively, for SPECT. The area under the ROC (AUC) for combined coronary CTA and CT perfusion was similar (p = .36) to that for combined ICA and SPECT in the identification of major adverse cardiac event (MACE) at the two-year follow-up examination milestone [36]. Further, the radiation doses for the comprehensive CCT protocol (CT MPI and coronary CTA) and SPECT MPI were similar at 13.8 ± 2.9 mSv and 13.1 ± 1.7 mSv, respectively [35].

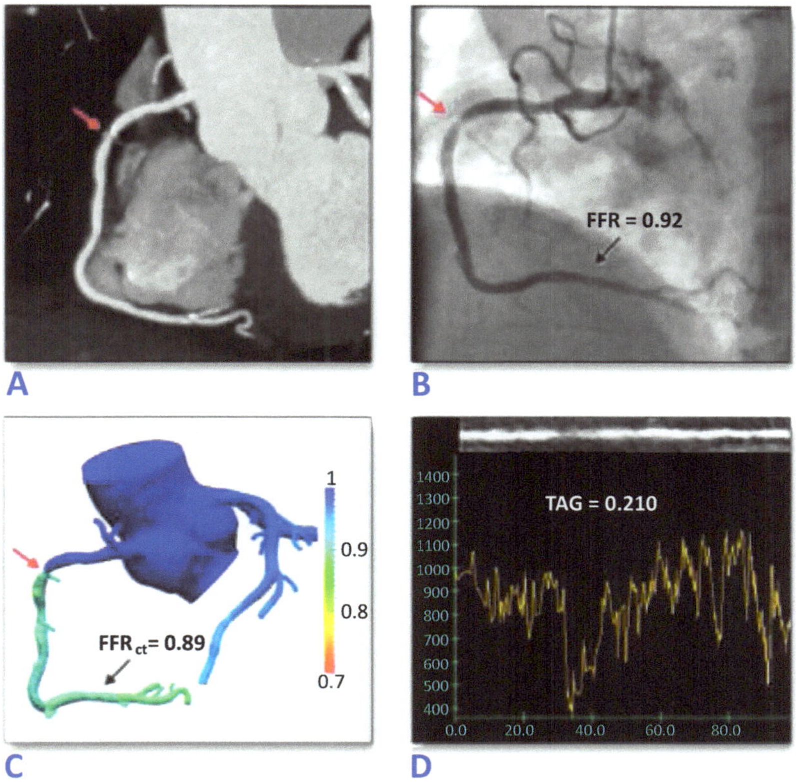

Fig. (6). (A) Coronary CTA detected obstructive (50%) stenosis (red arrow) in the proximal RCA. **(B)**Invasive coronary angiography also showed obstructive stenosis (red arrow) in the proximal RCA. FFR of 0.92 at the time of invasive coronary angiography demonstrates no ischemia of right coronary artery. **(C)** FFRct with a value of 0.89 and **(D)** transluminal attenuation gradient (TAG) of 0.210 demonstrate no ischemia in the RCA Cited [37].

Triple Rule Out with CT

In 8.9% of patients, the "triple rule out" with CT method could diagnose as a significant non-coronary artery disease in the of acute chest pain at the emergent department. Commonly detected diseases included pulmonary embolism (2.3%), aortic aneurysm (2.0%), and pneumonia (1.7%). On the other hand, 27.3% of pulmonary embolism and aortic pathologic findings would not have been detected with coronary CT angiography because of non-opaque filling of right-side circulation or limited z-axis coverage. The appropriate use of the triple rule out with CT method requires further investigation [36].

APPROPRIATE CRITERIA

The Asian Society of Cardiovascular Imaging (ASCI) published recommendations for CCT and CMR and revised their appropriate use criteria

(AUC) in 2016. The recommendations document lists the ratings of various noninvasive tests including exercise electrocardiogram, echocardiography, PET, SPECT, CMR, and CCTA in various clinical scenarios.

The recommendations classified appropriate use into four sections as follows: 1) detection of coronary artery disease, symptomatic or asymptomatic; 2) cardiac evaluation in various clinical scenarios; 3) use of imaging modality according to prior testing, and 4) evaluation of cardiac structure and function. The appropriateness of use criteria was defined with three ratings which include the following: appropriate (A), uncertain (U), and inappropriate (I). Each modality includes inherent risks such as radiation exposure, contrast enhancement hypersensitivity, and interpretation error, those are factors in interpreting the score. The assumption is made that each modality is only chosen after weighing the risks and benefits in the specific clinical scenario [38].

Table 1. Symptomatic: Non-Acute Chest Pain Suspected of Stable Coronary Artery Disease.

	ExerciseECG	**ECHO**	**SPECT**	**CMR**	**CCTA**	
ECG interpretable AND able to exercise						
Low pretest probability	A	I	I	I	U	
Intermediate pretest probability	A	A	A	A	A	
High pretest probability	A	A	A	A	A	
ECG uninterpretable or unable to exercise						
Low pretest probability	I	U	U	U	A	
Intermediate pretest probability	I	A	A	A	A	
High pretest probability	I	A	A	A	A	
1-2. Symptomatic: Acute Chest Pain Suspected of Acute Coronary Syndrome						
	Exercise ECG	ECHO	SPECT	CMR	CCTA	
Normal ECG AND cardiac biomarker						
Low global CAD risk	U	A	A	U	A	
Intermediate global CAD risk	U	A	A	U	A	
High global CAD risk	A	A	A	U	A	
Non-diagnostic ECG or equivocal cardiac biomarker						
Low global CAD risk	I	A	A	U	A	
Intermediate global CAD risk	I	A	A	U	A	
High global CAD risk	I	A	A	A	A	
Abnormal ECG (ischemic nature)	I	A	A	U	A	

(Table 1) cont.....

	ExerciseECG	**ECHO**	**SPECT**	**CMR**	**CCTA**	
Acute chest pain of uncertain cause in emergency department ("triple rule out")	I	A	I	U	A	
1-3. Asymptomatic (1)						
	Exercise ECG	ECHO	SPECT	CMR	CT calcification	CCTA
Framingham CHD risk						
Low	I	I	I	I	I	I
Intermediate	U	I	I	I	U	U
High	A	U	U	U	U	A
Abnormal or uncertain prior testing						
Abnormal rest ECG (potentially ischemic)	A	A	A	A	U	A
Abnormal prior exercise ECG test	U	A	A	A	A	A
Zero CAC > 5 years ago	I	I	I	I	I	I
Positive CAC > 2 years ago						
CAC < 100	I	I	I	I		U
CAC 100–400	U	I	U	I		A
CAC 401–1000	A	U	A	U		U
CAC > 1000	A	U	A	U		U
Abnormal prior stress SPECT	I	U	U	U		A
1-3. Asymptomatic (2): Post-Revascularization (PCI or CABG)						
	Exercise ECG	ECHO	SPECT	CMR	CCTA	
Post-revascularization (PCI or CABG)						
Incomplete revascularization (additional revascularization feasible)	U	U	A	A	A	
Prior left main coronary stent	U	U	U	U	A	
< 5 years after CABG	I	U	U	U	A	
≥ 5 years after CABG	U	U	U	U	A	
< 2 years after PCI	I	I	I	I	A	
≤ 2 years after PCI	U	U	U	U	A	
2-4. Coronary Revascularization						
	Exercise ECG	ECHO	SPECT	CMR	CCTA	
Before revascularization						
*Evaluation of complex lesions before PCI	I	U	U	U	A	
Myocardial viability	I	U	A	A	U	

(Table 1) cont.....

	ExerciseECG	ECHO	SPECT	CMR	CCTA	
Suspected post-PCI myocardial infarction	I	A	A	A	U	
Suspected ischemic chest pain after coronary revascularization	U	U	A	A	A	
* such as chronic total occlusions, bification						

CONSENT FOR PUBLICATION

Not applicable.

CONFLICT OF INTEREST

The authors declare no conflict of interest, financial or otherwise.

ACKNOWLEDGEMENTS

Declared none.

REFERENCES

[1] Salerno M, Kramer CM. Advances in parametric mapping with CMR imaging. JACC Cardiovasc Imaging 2013; 6(7): 806-22. [http://dx.doi.org/10.1016/j.jcmg.2013.05.005] [PMID: 23845576]

[2] Bustamante M, Petersson S, Eriksson J, *et al.* Atlas-based analysis of 4D flow CMR: automated vessel segmentation and flow quantification. J Cardiovasc Magn Reson 2015; 17(1): 87. [http://dx.doi.org/10.1186/s12968-015-0190-5] [PMID: 26438074]

[3] Mordini FE, Haddad T, Hsu LY, *et al.* Diagnostic accuracy of stress perfusion CMR in comparison with quantitative coronary angiography: Fully quantitative, semiquantitative, and qualitative assessment JACC Cardiovasc Imaging 2014; 7(1): 14-22.

[4] van Dijk R, van Assen M, Vliegenthart R, de Bock GH, van der Harst P, Oudkerk M. Diagnostic performance of semi-quantitative and quantitative stress CMR perfusion analysis: a meta-analysis. J Cardiovasc Magn Reson 2017; 19(1): 92-108. [http://dx.doi.org/10.1186/s12968-017-0393-z] [PMID: 29178905]

[5] Schwitter J, Wacker CM, Wilke N, *et al.* MR-IMPACT II: Magnetic Resonance Imaging for Myocardial Perfusion Assessment in Coronary artery disease Trial: perfusion-cardiac magnetic resonance *vs.* single-photon emission computed tomography for the detection of coronary artery disease: a comparative multicentre, multivendor trial. Eur Heart J 2013; 34(10): 775-81. [http://dx.doi.org/0.1093/eurheartj/ehs022] [PMID: 22390914]

[6] Greenwood JP, Maredia N, Radjenovic A, *et al.* Clinical evaluation of magnetic resonance imaging in coronary heart disease: the CE-MARC study. Trials 2009; 10(1): 62. [http://dx.doi.org/10.1186/1745-6215-10-62] [PMID: 19640271]

[7] Vincenti G, Masci PG, Monney P, *et al.* Stress perfusion CMR in patients with known and suspected CAD: prognostic value and optimal ischemic threshold for revascularization. JACC: Cardiovascular Imaging 2017; 10(5): 526-37. [http://dx.doi.org/10.1016/j.jcmg.2017.02.006]

[8] Jaarsma C, Leiner T, Bekkers SC, *et al.* Diagnostic performance of noninvasive myocardial perfusion imaging using single-photon emission computed tomography, cardiac magnetic resonance, and positron emission tomography imaging for the detection of obstructive coronary artery disease: a meta-analysis. J Am Coll Cardiol 2012; 59(19): 1719-28. [http://dx.doi.org/10.1016/j.jacc.2011.12.040] [PMID: 22554604]

[9] von Knobelsdorff-Brenkenhoff F, Schulz-Menger J. Role of cardiovascular magnetic resonance in the guidelines of the European Society of Cardiology. J Cardiovasc Magn Reson 2016; 18: 6. [http://dx.doi.org/10.1186/s12968-016-0225-6] [PMID: 26800662]

[10] Braunwald E. Myocardial reperfusion, limitation of infarct size, reduction of left ventricular dysfunction, and improved survival. Should the paradigm be expanded? Circulation 1989; 79(2): 441-4. [http://dx.doi.org/10.1161/01.CIR.79.2.441] [PMID: 2914356]

[11] Lipiecki J, Cachin F, Durel N, de Tauriac O, Ponsonnaille J, Maublant J. Influence of infarct-zone viability detected by rest Tc-99m sestamibi gated SPECT on left ventricular remodeling after acute myocardial infarction treated by percutaneous transluminal coronary angioplasty in the acute phase. J Nucl Cardiol 2004; 11(6): 673-81. [http://dx.doi.org/10.1016/j.nuclcard.2004.09.003] [PMID: 15592190]

[12] Hadamitzky M, Langhans B, Hausleiter J, *et al.* The assessment of area at risk and myocardial salvage after coronary revascularization in acute myocardial infarction: comparison between CMR and SPECT. JACC Cardiovasc Imaging 2013; 6(3): 358-69. [http://dx.doi.org/10.1016/j.jcmg.2012.10.018] [PMID: 23473113]

[13] Eitel I, Desch S, Fuernau G, *et al.* Prognostic significance and determinants of myocardial salvage assessed by cardiovascular magnetic resonance in acute reperfused myocardial infarction. J Am Coll Cardiol 2010; 55(22): 2470-9. [http://dx.doi.org/10.1016/j.jacc.2010.01.049] [PMID: 20510214]

[14] Robbers LF, Eerenberg ES, Teunissen PF, *et al.* Magnetic resonance imaging-defined areas of microvascular obstruction after acute myocardial infarction represent microvascular destruction and haemorrhage. Eur Heart J 2013; 34(30): 2346-53. [http://dx.doi.org/10.1093/eurheartj/eht100] [PMID: 23594591]

[15] Eitel I, Kubusch K, Strohm O, *et al.* Prognostic value and determinants of a hypointense infarct core in T2-weighted cardiac magnetic resonance in acute reperfused ST-elevation-myocardial infarction. Circ Cardiovasc Imaging 2011; 4(4): 354-62. [http://dx.doi.org/10.1161/CIRCIMAGING.110.960500] [PMID: 21518773]

[16] Hadamitzky M, Langhans B, Hausleiter J, *et al.* The assessment of area at risk and myocardial salvage after coronary revascularization in acute myocardial infarction: comparison between CMR and SPECT. JACC Cardiovasc Imaging 2013; 6(3): 358-69. [http://dx.doi.org/10.1016/j.jcmg.2012.10.018] [PMID: 23473113]

[17] von Knobelsdorff-Brenkenhoff F, Pilz G, Schulz-Menger J. Representation of cardiovascular magnetic resonance in the AHA / ACC guidelines. J Cardiovasc Magn Reson 2017; 19(1): 70. [http://dx.doi.org/10.1186/s12968-017-0385-z] [PMID: 28942735]

[18] Khan JN, McCann GP. Cardiovascular magnetic resonance imaging assessment of outcomes in acute myocardial infarction. World J Cardiol 2017; 9(2): 109-33. [http://dx.doi.org/10.4330/wjc.v9.i2.109] [PMID: 28289525]

[19] Choi KM, Kim RJ, Gubernikoff G, Vargas JD, Parker M, Judd RM. Transmural extent of acute myocardial infarction predicts long-term improvement in contractile function. Circulation 2001; 104(10): 1101-7. [http://dx.doi.org/10.1161/hc3501.096798] [PMID: 11535563]

[20] Hoffmann U, Ferencik M, Udelson JE, *et al.* Prognostic value of noninvasive cardiovascular testing in patients with stable chest pain: insights from the PROMISE Trial (Prospective Multicenter Imaging

Study for Evaluation of Chest Pain). Circulation 2017; 135(24): 2320-32.
[http://dx.doi.org/10.1161/CIRCULATIONAHA.116.024360] [PMID: 28389572]

[21] Bulluck H, Hausenloy DJ. Ischaemic conditioning: are we there yet? Heart 2015; 101(13): 1067-77.
[http://dx.doi.org/10.1136/heartjnl-2014-306531] [PMID: 25887783]

[22] Glaveckaite S, Valeviciene N, Palionis D, *et al.* Value of scar imaging and inotropic reserve combination for the prediction of segmental and global left ventricular functional recovery after revascularisation. J Cardiovasc Magn Reson 2011; 13(1): 35.
[http://dx.doi.org/10.1186/1532-429X-13-35] [PMID: 21787383]

[23] McCrohon JA, Moon JC, Prasad SK, *et al.* Differentiation of heart failure related to dilated cardiomyopathy and coronary artery disease using gadolinium-enhanced cardiovascular magnetic resonance. Circulation 2003; 108(1): 54-9.
[http://dx.doi.org/10.1161/01.CIR.0000078641.19365.4C] [PMID: 12821550]

[24] Mahrholdt H, Wagner A, Judd RM, Sechtem U, Kim RJ. Delayed enhancement cardiovascular magnetic resonance assessment of non-ischaemic cardiomyopathies. Eur Heart J 2005; 26(15): 1461-74.
[http://dx.doi.org/10.1093/eurheartj/ehi258] [PMID: 15831557]

[25] Haaf P, Garg P, Messroghli DR, Broadbent DA, Greenwood JP, Plein S. Cardiac T1 Mapping and Extracellular Volume (ECV) in clinical practice: a comprehensive review. J Cardiovasc Magn Reson 2016; 18(1): 89.
[http://dx.doi.org/10.1186/s12968-016-0308-4] [PMID: 27899132]

[26] Choi AD, Joly JM, Chen MY, Weigold WG. Physiologic evaluation of ischemia using cardiac CT: current status of CT myocardial perfusion and CT fractional flow reserve. J Cardiovasc Comput Tomogr 2014; 8(4): 272-81.
[http://dx.doi.org/10.1016/j.jcct.2014.06.006] [PMID: 25151919]

[27] Taylor CA, Fonte TA, Min JK. Computational fluid dynamics applied to cardiac computed tomography for noninvasive quantification of fractional flow reserve: scientific basis. J Am Coll Cardiol 2013; 61(22): 2233-41.
[http://dx.doi.org/10.1016/j.jacc.2012.11.083] [PMID: 23562923]

[28] Douglas PS, Hoffmann U, Patel MR, *et al.* Outcomes of anatomical *versus* functional testing for coronary artery disease. N Engl J Med 2015; 372(14): 1291-300.
[http://dx.doi.org/10.1056/NEJMoa1415516] [PMID: 25773919]

[29] Newby D. CT coronary angiography in patients with suspected angina due to coronary heart disease (SCOT-HEART): an open-label, parallel-group, multicentre trial. Lancet 2015; 385(9985): 2383-91.
[http://dx.doi.org/10.1016/S0140-6736(15)60291-4] [PMID: 25788230]

[30] Cury RC, Abbara S, Achenbach S, *et al.* Coronary Artery Disease - Reporting and Data System (CAD-RADS): An Expert Consensus Document of SCCT, ACR and NASCI: Endorsed by the ACC. JACC Cardiovasc Imaging 2016; 9(9): 1099-113.
[http://dx.doi.org/10.1016/j.jcmg.2016.05.005] [PMID: 27609151]

[31] Budoff MJ, Nakazato R, Mancini GBJ, *et al.* CT angiography for the prediction of hemodynamic significance in intermediate and severe lesions head-to-head comparison with quantitative coronary angiography using fractional flow reserve as the reference standard. JACC Cardiovasc Imaging 2016; 9(5): 559-64.
[http://dx.doi.org/10.1016/j.jcmg.2015.08.021] [PMID: 26897669]

[32] Montalescot G, Sechtem U, Achenbach S, *et al.* 2013 ESC guidelines on the management of stable coronary artery disease: the Task Force on the management of stable coronary artery disease of the European Society of Cardiology. Eur Heart J 2013; 34(38): 2949-3003.
[http://dx.doi.org/10.1093/eurheartj/eht296] [PMID: 23996286]

[33] Nørgaard BL, Hjort J, Gaur S, *et al.* Clinical use of coronary CTA-Derived FFR for decision-making in stable CAD. JACC Cardiovasc Imaging 2017; 10(5): 541-50.

[http://dx.doi.org/10.1016/j.jcmg.2015.11.025] [PMID: 27085447]

[34] George RT, Arbab-Zadeh A, Miller JM, *et al.* Computed tomography myocardial perfusion imaging with 320-row detector computed tomography accurately detects myocardial ischemia in patients with obstructive coronary artery disease. Circ Cardiovasc Imaging 2012; 5(3): 333-40. [http://dx.doi.org/10.1161/CIRCIMAGING.111.969303] [PMID: 22447807]

[35] George RT, Mehra VC, Chen MY, *et al.* Myocardial CT perfusion imaging and SPECT for the diagnosis of coronary artery disease: a head-to-head comparison from the CORE320 multicenter diagnostic performance study. Radiology 2014; 272(2): 407-16. [http://dx.doi.org/10.1148/radiol.14140806] [PMID: 24865312]

[36] Ayaram D, Bellolio MF, Murad MH, *et al.* Triple rule-out computed tomographic angiography for chest pain: a diagnostic systematic review and meta-analysis. Acad Emerg Med 2013; 20(9): 861-71. [http://dx.doi.org/10.1111/acem.12210] [PMID: 24050793]

[37] Yoon Y, Choi J, Kim J, *et al.* Noninvasive diagnosis of ischemia-causing coronary stenosis using CT angiography: Diagnostic value of transluminal attenuation gradient and fractional flow reserve computed from coronary CT angiography compared to invasively measured fractional flow reserve JACC: Cardiovascular Imaging 2012; 5(11): 1088-96. [http://dx.doi.org/10.1016/j.jcmg.2012.09.002]

[38] Beck KS, Kim JA, Choe YH, *et al.* 2017 Multimodality appropriate use criteria for noninvasive cardiac imaging: Expert consensus of the Asian Society of Cardiovascular Imaging. Korean J Radiol 2017; 18(6): 871-80. [http://dx.doi.org/10.3348/kjr.2017.18.6.871] [PMID: 29089819]

CHAPTER 7

Fatty Acid Imaging from Basic to Clinical

Iichiro Osawa[*,1], **Takashi Ushimi**[1], **Nanami Okano**[1], **Eito Kozawa**[1] and **Ichiro Matsunari**[2]

[1] *Department of Radiology, Saitama Medical University Hospital, Saitama, Japan*

[2] *Division of Nuclear Medicine, Department of Radiology, Saitama Medical University Hospital, Saitama, Japan*

Abstract: A number of radiolabeled fatty acids have been developed to assess myocardial fatty acid metabolism. Radioactive fatty acid analogues are classified into PET and SPECT tracers; carbon-11 is the most common isotope for PET, while iodine-123 is typically used in SPECT. The main approaches for the development in fatty acid tracers include shift from PET tracers to SPECT tracers, iodine stabilization, and prolonged retention of tracers in the myocardium. 15-(*p*-iodophenyl)-3-(R, S)-methyl pentadecanoic acid (BMIPP), an iodine-123 labeled branched-chain fatty acid analogue, has been widely available for routine clinical SPECT in Japan, and provides useful information on abnormal fatty acid metabolism in ischemic heart disease as well as nonischemic cardiomyopathy. This agent plays a crucial role in the diagnosis of these diseases, and the prediction of therapeutic effect and prognosis. Reduced BMIPP uptake than perfusion is often observed in ischemic heart disease such as myocardial infarction and angina pectoris. This mismatched uptake may reflect ischemic but viable myocardium, and is associated with stunned or hibernating myocardium. In addition, BMIPP can serve as a memory marker of transient myocardial ischemia because BMIPP abnormality may persist even after perfusion recovery following ischemia. On the other hand, heart-to-mediastinum (H/M) ratio is commonly used as an index of BMIPP uptake in nonischemic cardiomyopathy. This topic will overview basic principles and clinical applications of fatty acid metabolic imaging.

Keywords: BMIPP, Fatty Acid Metabolic Imaging, Ischemic Heart Disease, Nonischemic Cardiomyopathy, SPECT.

INTRODUCTION

Nuclear imaging has offered noninvasive technique to evaluate myocardial perfusion and metabolism. Normally, fatty acids are the principle substrates for generating energy in the myocardium. On the other hand, abnormalities of myocardial fatty acid metabolism are observed frequently under pathologic

* **Corresponding author Iichiro Osawa:** Department of Radiology, Saitama Medical University Hospital, Saitama, Japan; Tel: +8149 2761265; Fax: +81492958003; Email: oyabun@saitama-med.ac.jp

Shinro Matsuo (Ed.)

conditions such as ischemic heart disease and nonischemic cardiomyopathy. Thus, nuclear imaging for fatty acid metabolism has the potential to disclose the underlying etiology. Although a large number of tracers for myocardial fatty acid imaging have been introduced, 15-(*p*-iodophenyl)-3-(*R, S*)-methyl pentadecanoic acid (BMIPP) is the most widely used agent in clinical settings. This tracer can identify alterations of fatty acid metabolism caused by ischemia in patients with ischemic heart disease. Of these alterations, reduced BMIPP uptake may reflect metabolic shift from fatty acid to glucose within the myocardium. In addition, reduced BMIPP uptake than perfusion implies myocardial viability since such mismatched area may show improvement in wall motion. Moreover, the role of BMIPP scintigraphy has been extended to patients with nonischemic cardiomyopathy. This topic will review basic principles and clinical applications of fatty acid metabolic imaging. In the section of basic principles, we attempt to explain myocardial fatty acid metabolism, radiopharmaceuticals for positron emission tomography (PET) and single photon emission computed tomography (SPECT), and BMIPP. In the section of clinical applications, we will describe a role of BMIPP in ischemic heart disease and nonischemic cardiomyopathy.

BASIC PRINCIPLES

Myocardial Fatty Acid Metabolism

Myocardium requires a lot of energy to sustain cardiac function, and utilizes various substrates including free fatty acids, glucose, lactose, pyruvate, keton bodies, and amino acids to produce energy. Among them, free fatty acids and glucose represent primary sources of energy in the adult heart. Under fasting and aerobic conditions, oxidation of fatty acids covers 60% to 90% of the myocardial energy requirements [1]. The remainder is mostly derived from glucose oxidation. Of circulating free fatty acids, palmitate is most abundant and is a rich source of adenosine triphosphate (ATP), although the need for more oxygen compared with carboxylate catabolism makes fatty acid oxidation less desirable during ischemia. Both fatty acids and glucose are metabolized to acetyl coenzyme A (acetyl-CoA) through β oxidation and glycolysis, and the metabolite is oxidized to the tricarboxylic acid (TCA) cycle, also known as the Krebs or citric acid cycle. However, the dependency of fatty acid metabolism on oxygen makes this process vulnerable to ischemia. During anaerobic conditions such as ischemia and hypoxia, lack of oxygen causes shift from aerobic to anaerobic metabolism because fatty acid oxidation needs large amounts of oxygen. There is a switch of substrate from fatty acid to glucose which is utilized by anaerobic glycolysis with decreased oxygen consumption.

Fig. (**1**) shows schematically fatty acid metabolism in normal myocardial cell. Because of their hydrophobicity, fatty acids are transported to the myocardium bound to plasma proteins or albumin, or covalently bound in the triacylglycerol core of lipoproteins. After dissociation of the albumin-fatty acid complex or hydrolysis of the triacylglycerols, fatty acids are transported from capillary lumen to the myocardium through the capillary endothelium and interstitial compartment. Fatty acids cross the myocardial membrane via passive diffusion or protein-mediated transport mechanism involving a number of fatty acid transporters. CD38, also known as fatty acid translocase (FAT), is one of the fatty acid transporters, which plays a pivotal role in both facilitating and regulating myocardial fatty acid uptake. After uptake into the cytosol, fatty acids are activated by acyl-CoA synthetase into acyl-CoA. Subsequently, fatty acids are carried into the mitochondria via a carnitine carrier system and metabolized by β oxidation into two-carbon intermediate, acetyl-CoA. Acetyl-CoA then enters the TCA cycle to be oxidized for energy production. A part of acyl-CoA is not oxidized and is incorporated into intracellular lipid pool as triglycerides or phospholipids.

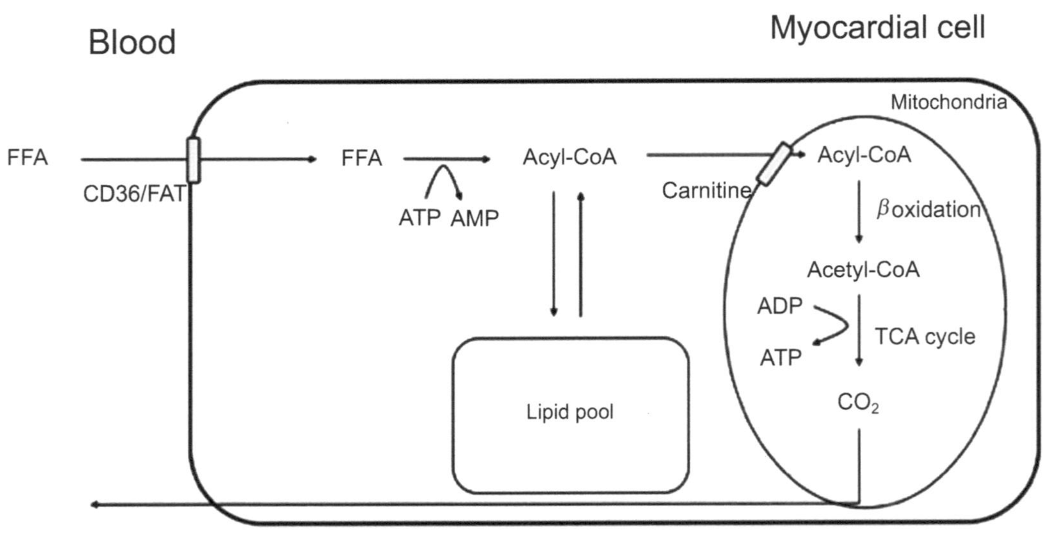

Fig. (1). Fatty acid metabolism in normal myocardium. *FFA* free fatty acid, *FAT* fatty acid translocase, *ATP* adenosine triphosphate, *AMP* adenosine monophosphate, *CoA* coenzyme A, *ADP* adenosine diphosphate.

On the other hand, the fetal heart utilizes glucose and lactate as major sources of energy [2] since the fetal heart develops in a relatively hypoxic environment and receives a supply of nutrients rich in carbohydrates. After birth, the newborn receives milk rich in fatty acids. As the newborn heart matures, fatty acids become the preferred oxidative substrates for the heart.

Myocardial metabolism and kinetics of fatty acid change dynamically in response to ischemia-reperfusion injury. As this process is complicated, the exact mechanism remains unclear. Ischemic stress causes catecholamine discharge, resulting in elevation of plasma catecholamine levels. Catecholamines stimulate adipose tissue lipolysis which leads to elevation of plasma fatty acid levels and increased delivery of fatty acid to the myocyte. The increased fatty acid delivery to the myocardium can affect myocardial metabolism and kinetics of fatty acid during ischemia and reperfusion. Excess fatty acid can have toxic effect, including fatal arrhythmias [3] and depressed contractility [4]. To avoid the toxic effect, the lipid pool expands and stores excess fatty acid. A canine study demonstrated that the lipid pool increased the size in the ischemic regions than that in the nonischemic regions [5].

Several reports indicated serial changes in metabolism and kinetics of fatty acid from the acute to the subacute and chronic phase of ischemia, using BMIPP scintigraphy in animal [6] and human studies [7]. Ito *et al.* studied 10 patients with stunned myocardium to evaluate dynamic changes in BMIPP uptake and washout [7]. The authors showed nondecreasing uptake and reduced washout of BMIPP during the acute phase of ischemia. They suggested that this phenomenon may be explained by expanded lipid pool to incorporate excess fatty acid, and suppressed washout from the lipid pool into the bloodstream. By contrast, BMIPP demonstrated decreased accumulation and increased washout during the subacute phase of ischemia. The decreased accumulation of BMIPP may be explained by shrunk lipid pool, and decreased fatty acid metabolism with increased glucose metabolism, whereas the increased washout of BMIPP may reflect accelerated washout from the lipid pool into the bloodstream.

Radiopharmaceuticals for PET and SPECT

There have been a number of radiolabeled fatty acid analogues since Evans *et al.* initially reported iodine-131 oleic acid [8]. Fig. (**2**) and Table **1** show well-known fatty acid tracers. According to the type of nuclear imaging procedures, radiolabeled fatty acid analogues are classified into two categories: PET tracer and SPECT tracer. Another classification includes two groups based on the type of carbon chain: straight-chain and branched-chain. While straight-chain fatty acids are metabolized by β oxidation, branched-chain with a β-methyl group theoretically cannot. Three directions of development in fatty acid tracers are as follows: 1) shift from PET tracers to SPECT tracers 2) iodine stabilization 3) prolonged retention of tracers in the myocardium. First, PET tracers require a cyclotron and a special camera, both of which are expensive. By contrast, SPECT tracers do not require a cyclotron, and SPECT cameras are more readily available and less expensive. The introduction of radioactive iodine to the terminal position of fatty acids has made the shift to SPECT tracers possible.

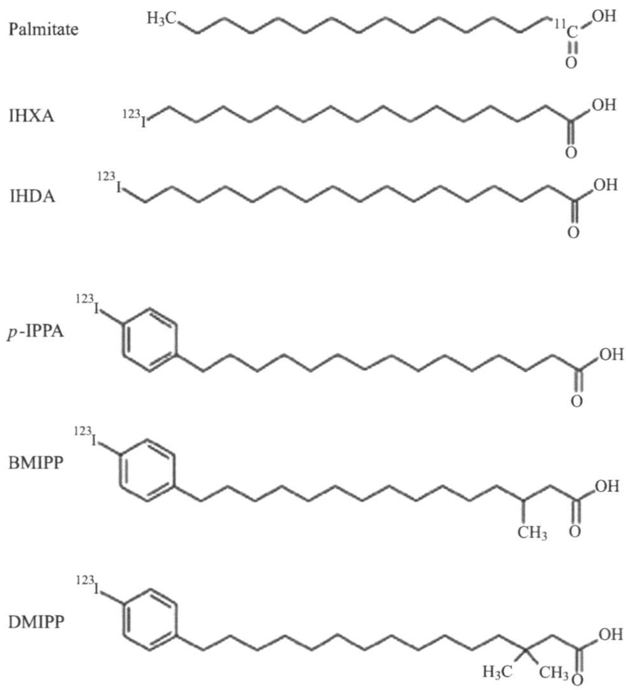

Fig. (2). Structural formula of radiolabeled fatty acids. *IPPA* iodophenyl pentadecanoic acid, *IHXA* 16-iodohexadecanoic acid, *IHDA* 17-iodoheptadecanoic acid, *BMIPP* β-methyl-iodophenyl pentadecanoic acid, *DMIPP* dimethyl iodophenyl pentadecanoic acid.

Second, deiodination is an essential issue for iodinated alkyl fatty acids among straight-chain fatty acids. This phenomenon may result in degeneration of image quality. Iodinated phenyl fatty acids, in which iodide is attached to the phenyl ring of straight-chain fatty acids, can prevent the deiodination.

Table 1. Straight-chain and branched-chain fatty acids for PET and SPECT. *IPPA* iodophenyl pentadecanoic acid, *IHXA* 16-iodohexadecanoic acid, *IHDA* 17-iodoheptadecanoic acid, *BMIPP* β-methyl-iodophenyl pentadecanoic acid, *DMIPP* dimethyl iodophenyl pentadecanoic acid.

Isotope	Straight-chain fatty acids	Branched-chain fatty acids
PET tracers 11C	Palmitate	
SPECT tracers 123I	IHXA IHDA IPPA	BMIPP DMIPP

Third, iodinated straight-chain phenyl fatty acids have relatively rapid washout from the myocardium, which may make clinical applications difficult. Branched-chain fatty acids with a β-methyl group have been introduced to overcome the problem. β-methyl group can prevent β oxidation and prolong retention of fatty acids within the myocardium.

This topic will provide a brief history on the development of fatty acid tracers, concentrating on 11C-palmitate, 16-iodohexadacanoic acid (IHXA), 17-iodoheptadecanoic acid (IHDA), 15-(*p*-iodophenyl)-pentadecanoic acid (IPPA), 15-(*p*-iodophenyl)-3, 3-dimethyl pentadecanoic acid (DMIPP) and BMIPP.

PET Tracer

As a PET tracer, carbon-11 is a widely used isotope of carbon which radiolabels fatty acid analogues such as 11C-palmitate. 11C-palmitate is a radiolabeled straight-chain fatty acid, and most commonly used among PET tracers to evaluate myocardial fatty acid metabolism. Its kinetics including uptake and clearance are biologically identical to those of unlabeled palmitate. 11C-palmitate uptake into the myocardium depends on several factors as follows: regional blood flow, passive diffusion and protein mediated transport via the sarcolemmal membrane, and acceptance in the cytosol by binding to acyl-CoA. 11C-palmitate clearance follows a biexponential kinetic model, where an early component reflects β oxidation and a late slower washout reflects incorporation of the tracer into lipid pools [9]. β oxidation reduces the carbon-chain by two carbons to produce acetyl-CoA. This 11C-acetyl-CoA enters the TCA cycle in the mitochondrial matrix, and is oxidized to CO_2 which finally is released from the myocardium. Under ischemic conditions, the uptake and clearance are decreased, consistent with reduction of oxidative metabolism. Unfortunately, the tracer has several drawbacks including short imaging time because of rapid catabolism, complicated analysis due to differential tissue distribution with variable turnover rate, need for an onsite cyclotron, which allow only basic practice. Investigations focused on developing new radiotracers to overcome the problems.

SPECT Tracer

Iodinated Straight-Chain Fatty Acids

Alkyl Fatty Acids

An initial effort was made to develop radiolabeled straight-chain fatty acids. Iodine-123 is a most commonly used isotope of straight-chain fatty acids. Poe *et al.* reported that iodine-123 hexadacanoic acid (IHXA) and iodine-123 hepta-decanoic acid (IHDA) as potential myocardial perfusion tracers [10, 11]. After rapid first extraction, the two tracers show biexponential clearance similar to that of 11C-palmitate. Generally, the rapid clearance fraction reflects β oxidation, whereas the slow clearance fraction corresponds to storage of fatty acids in lipid pools.

However, the ability to evaluate myocardial metabolism remains doubtful. Some animal and clinical studies showed rapid release of free radioiodine and deterioration of image quality [12, 13]. Visser *et al.* examined a canine model to evaluate metabolic fate of IHDA [12]. The authors demonstrated that washout rate of radioactivity was reflective of the back diffusion of free radioiodine, not β oxidation. Moreover, Freundlieb *et al.* studied patients with prior myocardial infarction to evaluate IHDA [13]. IHDA showed rapid deterioration of image quality because of a low myocardium-to-background ratio. Degradation of images caused by deiodination encouraged further investigation to create new fatty acids with iodine stabilization.

Phenyl Fatty Acids

To stabilize the radioiodine attached to fatty acid, 15-(*p*-iodophenyl)-pentadecanoic acid (IPPA) was introduced by Machulla *et al.* [14]. *p*-IPPA is a straight-chain phenyl fatty acid with iodine-123 attached to the para position of phenyl ring. This agent has been examined in animal [15 - 17] and human [18 - 20] studies, under physiological and pathological conditions. As compared with the alkyl fatty acids, IPPA has the characteristics of iodine stabilization, and rapid uptake and clearance. In murine model, Reske *et al.* demonstrated rapid accumulation of the agent in the myocardium, with fast clearance from the heart following a biexponential function characteristic of 14C-palmitate [15]. Therefore, β oxidation can be directly evaluated by the clearance of IPPA. In canine study, Caldwell *et al.* showed IPPA uptake during exercise increased in proportion to myocardial perfusion [16]. In rat study, Ercan *et al.* revealed that IPPA was metabolized *via* β oxidation into iodobenzoic acid and iodohippurate [17]. These metabolites were rapidly extracted from kidneys with iodine stabilization, which led to high-quality images.

The ability of IPPA to evaluate patients with ischemic heart disease [18, 19] or nonischemic cardiomyopathy [20] has been studied. Under ischemic conditions, IPPA usually shows reduced uptake and slow washout. Using IPPA imaging, patients with ischemic heart disease were studied to assess myocardial viability and functional recovery, compared with or without perfusion scan [18, 19]. Patients with nonischemic cardiomyopathy also have been evaluated by IPPA scan. In patients with dilated cardiomyopathy, IPPA showed heterogeneous uptake and rapid washout compared with those in healthy volunteers [20].

Although IPPA enhanced image quality compared with the alkyl fatty acids, a conventional SPECT camera was not sufficient to assess relatively rapid metabolism of IPPA. Investigators moved onto the next stage of development to create radiolabeled fatty acids with slowed metabolism.

Iodinated Branched-Chain Fatty Acids

To slow metabolism and prolong cardiac retention of fatty acids, branched-chain fatty acid analogues were developed. Knapp *et al.* initially introduced BMIPP and 15-(*p*-iodophenly)-3,3-dimethyl-pentadecanoic acid (DMIPP) [21]. BMIPP and DMIPP are modified fatty acid analogues of IPPA in which a methyl group or dimethyl group is introduced into β-3 positon of the fatty acid chain, respectively. β-methyl group inhibits mitochondrial β oxidation and allows prolonged myocardial retention of BMIPP.

Animal studies revealed that both BMIPP and DMIPP had prolonged myocardial retention compared with IPPA [22]. In addition, DMIPP showed greater retention in the myocardium than BMIPP [21]. Sloof *et al.* studied patients with coronary artery disease to compare DMIPP and BMIPP, indicating that BMIPP appeared to be superior to DMIPP because lower uptake of the liver improved image quality [23]. Up to now, BMIPP has been extensively studied in Japan and Europe, and more recently in the USA.

BMIPP

Kinetics

Fig. (**3**) shows schematically myocardial metabolism of BMIPP. BMIPP uptakes from the plasma to myocytes *via* the CD38/FAT transporter protein on the sarcolemmal membrane. After uptake into the myocardial cytosol, BMIPP can take two pathways: nonmetabolic and metabolic. Nonmetabolized BMIPP is released immediately into the plasma by back diffusion (early back diffusion).

On the other hand, metabolic pathway includes storage in the lipid pool and oxidation to create energy. First, BMIPP is activated ATP-dependently by the enzyme acetyl-CoA synthetase to BMIPP-CoA. Thus, BMIPP uptake may indirectly reflect ATP concentrations [24]. Subsequently, a large amount of activated BMIPP is esterified and retained in the lipid pool, whereas a small amount of BMIPP is metabolized through α oxidation as the first step, followed by β oxidation to 123I-*p*-iodophenyl acetic acid (PIPA) as the final metabolite [22, 25]. BMIPP in the lipid pool is released into the bloodstream (late back diffusion), whereas α and β oxidation metabolites leave the myocyte. Fujibayashi *et al.* used an open-chest dog model to evaluate the metabolism and kinetics of

BMIPP [25]. BMIPP showed quick extraction into the myocardium (74% of infused BMIPP) followed by retention (65.3%). The retained radioactivity was washed out slowly, most of which consisted of α and β oxidation metabolites.

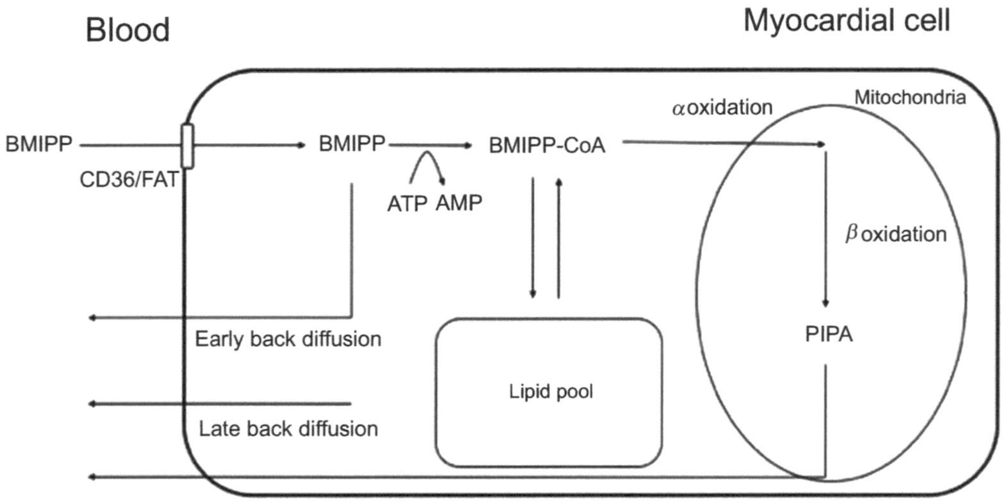

Fig. (3). BMIPP metabolism in normal myocardium. *BMIPP* β-methyl-iodophenyl pentadecanoic acid, *FAT* fatty acid translocase, *ATP* adenosine triphosphate, *AMP* adenosine monophosphate, *PIPA* *p*-iodophenyl acetic acid.

Imaging Protocols

Researchers have designed experiments with the use of BMIPP under various conditions such as subjects (animals or human), diseases (ischemic heart disease or nonischemic cardiomyopathy), comparison with perfusion/metabolic radionuclide imaging or non-nuclear techniques (echocardiography, magnetic resonance imaging, or contrast ventriculography), and evaluation contents (diagnostic accuracy, viability, area at risk, therapeutic efficacy, functional recovery, risk stratification, or prognostic value). One of the most important factors to the success of BMIPP scan is an imaging protocol. Imaging protocols consist of static/dynamic and rest/(exercise) stress procedures. Static images are acquired 15 to 30 minutes or 3 to 4 hours after intravenous injection of BMIPP. Dynamic images are usually obtained with 2 minute-intervals. BMIPP is usually imaged with SPECT, although heart-to-mediastinum (H/M) ratio is derived from conventional planar images.

Typically, BMIPP is administered under fasting conditions in non-emergency settings, and static imaging starts 15 to 30 minutes later. Some researchers have obtained static images 3 to 4 hours after tracer administration, combined with or without dynamic images [26, 27]. Fujiwara *et al.* reported that oral glucose loading increased sensitivity for identification of severe coronary stenosis compared with preloading in the fasting state [28].

It is desirable to compare BMIPP imaging with perfusion imaging for perfusion assessment because such combination is required to identify viable myocardium. Although BMIPP scintigraphy usually uses a single-isotope protocol, a dual-isotope protocol is utilized when images from both of BMIPP and a perfusion tracer are acquired simultaneously. Perfusion tracers consist of thallium and technetium-labeled tracers (sestamibi/MIBI and tetrofosmin). Injection protocols for intravenous administration of a perfusion tracer include as follows: one-injection and two-injection. On both of injection protocols, BMIPP imaging is usually compared with rest perfusion imaging, whereas Hatano *et al.* showed that BMIPP uptake less than stress thallium perfusion may assist better identification of patients with cardiovascular disease [29]. On a two-injection protocol, thallium is injected after stress redistribution imaging, which improves the identification of myocardial viability [30]. A single BMIPP scan can be applied in emergency unit to diagnose acute coronary syndrome [31, 32]. Although some investigators used exercise stress imaging [27, 33], this is not currently performed because of poor image quality.

Normal subjects show a homogenous distribution of BMIPP uptake throughout the left ventricular myocardium [34]. Also, higher BMIPP uptake than thallium perfusion may be normally seen in septal and inferior regions, probably due to the greater photon attenuation of thallium.

Qualitative, semiquantitative and quantitative analysis have been used to assess BMIPP uptake and washout. Typically, BMIPP uptake is semiquantitatively assessed on the basis of a segmental scoring system. Recently, some researchers have provided automated quantitative methods to improve the reproducibility and objectivity [35 - 38].

Various parameters such as extent, degree, H/M ratio or washout rate of BMIPP uptake can be extracted from these images. The relationship between BMIPP and a perfusion tracer is theoretically classified into two categories: match and non-matched patterns. Match pattern includes BMIPP uptake equal to perfusion tracer uptake normally or concordant defects in BMIPP uptake and perfusion tracer uptake, while non-matched patterns consist of lower BMIPP uptake than perfusion tracer uptake (mismatch or discordance) or higher BMIPP uptake than perfusion tracer uptake (reverse mismatch). Concordant defects are indicative of scar tissue.

Mismatch BMIPP uptake has been often reported in patients with both ischemic heart disease and nonischemic cardiomyopathy. In patients with acute myocardial infarction following reperfusion therapy, such mismatch uptake is frequently seen in the subacute phase of ischemic attack. However, reverse mismatch is occasionally observed in various conditions including acute and chronic ischemic heart disease, and nonischemic heart disease, specifically in the acute phase of acute myocardial infarction [7, 39 - 41]. Although several factors may determine such reverse mismatch, this phenomenon could be explained partially by the timing of image acquisition. In other words, serial changes of tracers are crucial to interpret underlying pathophysiology accurately.

Serial Changes of BMIPP Imaging

The imaging characteristics of BMIPP can vary dependent on the timing of acquisition. These time-dependent changes include short-term serial alterations after injection of BMIPP and long-term serial alterations after onset of ischemia. Short-term alterations after injection are usually analyzed using dynamic and static (early and delayed) imaging in the clinical settings [26, 27]. Kobayashi *et al.* revealed that the combined analysis of early dynamic acquisition (2 to 5 minutes) and late gated acquisition of BMIPP SPECT has the potential to evaluate myocardial perfusion, fatty acid metabolism, and left ventricular function simultaneously with a single injection of BMIPP [26].

Mastunari *et al.* studied 26 patients with prior myocardial infarction using rest BMIPP (dynamic and static) and exercise stress BMIPP (static) imaging, compared with exercise stress thallium (static) imaging [27]. Dynamic SPECT imaging revealed that the washout of BMIPP was observed in the early phase (2 to 6 minutes after injection) in the segments with reversible thallium defects, but not in the segments with normal uptake and fixed defects of thallium, suggestive of contribution of back diffusion to the early washout of BMIPP.

These evidences are supported by animal studies [42, 43]. Hosokawa *et al.* assessed the effects of mild and severe ischemia on the back diffusion and metabolism of BMIPP with an open-chest canine model [42]. Severe ischemia (30 minutes of coronary occlusion followed by 20 minutes of reperfusion) significantly increased early back diffusion of nonmetabolized BMIPP. In mild ischemia (10 minutes of coronary occlusion), back diffusion of BMIPP was closely correlated with lactate production. Hosokawa *et al.* also studied the effects of Etomoxir, a carnitine palmitoyltransferase I inhibitor, on the kinetics of BMIPP using an open-chest dog model [43]. Etomoxir inhibits the transport of fatty acids into the mitochondria resulting in reduction of β oxidation. These investigators suggested that the early washout of radioactivity was increased until 8 minutes after injection due to back diffusion of BMIPP.

By contrast, long-term alterations represent temporal continuum of ischemia from onset to acute, subacute and chronic phases. As mentioned before, Ito *et al.* found serial changes in BMIPP uptake and washout in 10 patients experiencing a first episode of angina without myocardial infarction but with regional wall motion abnormalities [7]. Significant BMIPP abnormalities were not seen during the acute phase (< 27 hours from the first episode) despite severe wall motion and perfusion abnormalities. On the other hand, a significant decrease in BMIPP uptake with increased washout from the myocardium was seen during the subacute phase (5 to 12 days from the first episode). In contrast, perfusion and systolic function showed only moderate improvement. These preliminary results suggest serial significant changes in BMIPP kinetics during the recovery phase of ischemic episodes. Such dynamic changes may be associated with changes in the lipid pool size and back diffusion of BMIPP from the fatty acid pool.

Some of animal studies can support the clinical findings [6, 44, 45]. Higuchi *et al.* used an occlusion-reperfusion rat model to assess the time course of BMIPP and thallium uptake [45]. BMIPP uptake in area at risk showed transient increase in the acute phase (20 minutes and 1 day), subsequent decrease in the subacute phase (3 and 7 days), followed by recovery in the chronic phase (30 days). On the other hand, thallium uptake changed minimally from the acute to chronic phase. Therefore, reverse mismatch of BMIPP uptake was observed in the acute phase, whereas mismatch was seen in the subacute phase. These results encourage careful interpretation of BMIPP uptake after ischemia.

CLINICAL APPLICATIONS

Ischemic Heart Disease

Myocardial Infarction

Many investigators have reported reduced BMIPP uptake as well as BMIPP-perfusion mismatch in patients with acute myocardial infarction especially after reperfusion therapy [46, 47]. Fig. (**4**) shows an example of BMIPP-tetrofosmin mismatch in acute myocardial infarction on the subacute phase after revascularization. Tamaki *et al.* studied 28 patients with prior myocardial infarction to compare rest BMIPP uptake with rest thallium perfusion and with wall motion assessed by contrast ventriculography [46]. Greater reduction of BMIPP uptake than thallium perfusion was more frequently observed in acute (< 4 weeks after onset) than in chronic (> 4 weeks after onset) myocardial infarction, and in revascularized than in nonrevascularized coronary arteries. In addition, regional wall motion was more severely impaired in mismatched area.

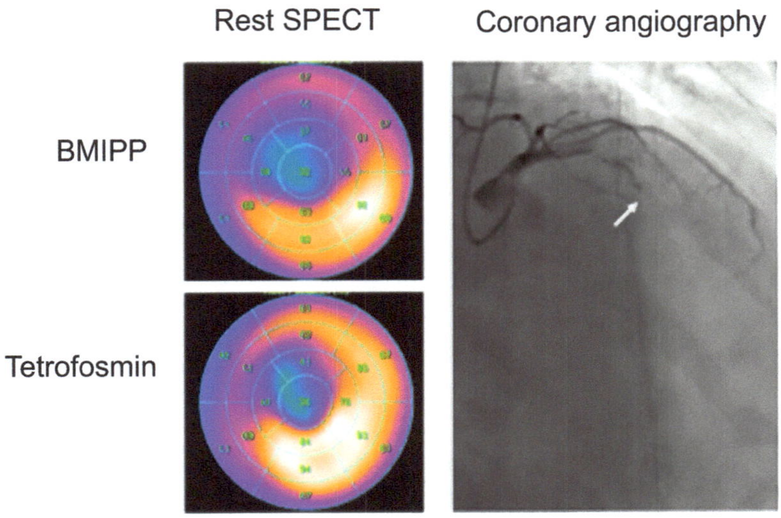

Fig. (4). BMIPP-tetrofosmin mismatch from a 55-year old man with acute myocardial infarction 16 days after reperfusion therapy. Polar maps demonstrate reduced BMIPP less than tetrofosmin perfusion in the anteroseptal segment. The apical segment shows matched uptake, indicating nonviable myocardium. Coronary angiography shows the infarct-related occlusion in the left anterior descending artery (arrow).

Franken *et al.* studied 22 patients with acute myocardial infarction 4 to 10 days after coronary thrombolysis to compare rest BMIPP SPECT with rest sestamibi perfusion and with wall motion assessed by low-dose dobutamine echocardiography [47]. SPECT studies identified three segmental patterns: normal uptake of both tracers, mismatched defects with more reduced BMIPP uptake, and matched defects. All segments with normal uptake of both tracers showed normal wall motion. Most segments with mismatched defects demonstrated normal wall motion at rest or showed inotropic reserve during low-dose dobutamine stimulation. By contrast, segments with matched defects always demonstrated abnormal wall motion and did not demonstrate inotropic reserve.

The two reports did not evaluate long-term serial alterations of either tracer uptake (BMIPP or perfusion tracer) or wall motion, both of which are necessary to assess myocardial metabolism or perfusion more accurately, and to evaluate functional recovery.

Estimation of Area at Risk

Area at risk is defined as the myocardial tissue within the perfusion territory of occluded coronary artery. After coronary occlusion, the infarct progresses as wavefront from the subendocardium to the subepicardium [48]. This area is the most important determinant of the ultimate infarct size [49]. Early reperfusion therapy can salvage myocardium at risk from ischemic injury. Myocardial salvage is defined as the difference between the initial area at risk and final area of infarction. Area at risk can be measured in several ways such as perfusion SPECT with a technetium-based tracer.

Perfusion SPECT imaging usually requires intravenous injection of a tracer before reperfusion therapy and image acquisition relatively soon after perfusion therapy. This logistic difficulty makes clinical application of this method limited. By contrast, BMIPP imaging has the potential of estimating area at risk in patients with acute myocardial infarction because reduced BMIPP uptake after reperfusion may reflect delayed metabolic recovery from ischemic injury even after perfusion is improved. This phenomenon is termed metabolic stunning where BMIPP can memorize the antecedent ischemic event. "Ischemic memory" represents biochemical or functional abnormalities which persist even after the recovery of myocardial perfusion to indicate the footprint of the prior ischemia.

Hasegawa *et al.* used a rat model of left coronary occlusion and reperfusion to evaluate whether BMIPP scan can identify the area at risk defined by histological examination [50]. BMIPP was injected at the acute or subacute stage after reperfusion. During both stages, the risk area showed lower uptake of BMIPP than the remote area did. Moreover, the area with reduced BMIPP uptake correlated with the area at risk. These investigators indicated that BMIPP can evaluate the area at risk at the acute and subacute stages.

Furutani *et al.* performed phantom and clinical study for quantification of area at risk in acute myocardial infarction using BMIPP SPECT [35]. Phantom study revealed that a simple threshold technique can quantify the defect size from BMIPP SPECT. Clinical study indicated that BMIPP SPECT in the subacute phase permits determination of the amount of myocardium at risk after acute myocardial infarction.

Kawai *et al.* investigated 65 patients with acute myocardial infarction after revascularization to assess whether BMIPP SPECT can estimate areas at risk. BMIPP SPECT was performed at rest 1 week after revascularization, compared with tetrofosmin perfusion imaging before and after revascularization [51]. Among a total of 1300 segments, the BMIPP defect score was identical to the tetrofosmin score before revascularization in 1156 segments (88.9%). These authors concluded that BMIPP imaging at 1 week after revascularization can identify areas at risk in patients with acute myocardial infarction similarly to tetrofosmin perfusion imaging before revascularization.

Katsunuma *et al.* studied 36 patients with acute myocardial infarction after reperfusion therapy to evaluate myocardial viability, contractile reserve and coronary stenotic progression, using BMIPP, thallium, and pyrophosphate scintigraphy [52]. Left ventricular angiography and coronary angiography were performed in the emergency setting, and were followed up 6 months later to evaluate functional recovery, coronary stenotic progression, and contractile reserve. Contractile reserve was estimated by the response to postextrasystolic potentiation testing. Thallium/pyrophosphate dual-isotope SPECT and BMIPP SPECT were performed 3 to 6 days, 10 to 14 days after the onset, respectively. BMIPP and stress thallium SPECT were repeated 6 months later. The size of reduced BMIPP uptake was more extensive than that of pyrophosphate accumulation, which suggested that reduced BMIPP uptake was indicative of risk area. BMIPP-thallium mismatch may be useful for evaluating myocardial viability and contractile reserve. Moreover, most patients with improved BMIPP had no coronary stenotic progression. This result suggested serial alterations of BMIPP had the ability to predict the progression of coronary stenosis.

Tanaka *et al.* studied 17 patients with acute myocardial infarction to serially evaluate tetrofosmin perfusion SPECT before and after reperfusion (1, 4, 7, and 20 days) [53]. Perfusion images after reperfusion were obtained 30 minutes (early) and 6 hours (delayed) after injection of tetrofosmin. Rest BMIPP SPECT was also performed after reperfusion (7 ± 1.8 days). The authors propose 7 days as the interval between reperfusion and tetrofosmin SPECT to assess the salvage effect. Moreover, they suggest that delayed perfusion and BMIPP images provide useful information on estimation of area at risk.

Mochizuki *et al.* examined 14 patients with acute myocardial infarction after reperfusion to compare BMIPP scintigraphy with pyrophosphate/thallium dual-isotope SPECT [54]. Dual-isotope SPECT was performed within 1 week of the onset, whereas BMIPP SPECT was undertaken 1 week after the dual-isotope SPECT. Positive uptake of pyrophosphate was concordant with defect in BMIPP in 13 out of 14 patients, indicating that BMIPP scan can commonly memorize the area at risk even after reperfusion.

Assessment of Myocardial Viability and Prediction of Functional Recovery

Viable myocardium is dysfunctional but non-scarred myocardium which has the potential for functional recovery with time either spontaneously or following revascularization. Both stunned and hibernating myocardium are dysfunctional but viable myocardium from ischemic injury. Stunned myocardium is characterized by a transient acute ischemia with maintained or nearly maintained perfusion, whereas hibernating myocardium is characterized by ongoing ischemia with chronic poor perfusion [55].

Clinically, stunned myocardium is typically encountered in patients with acute myocardial infarction after reperfusion. Many researchers have showed that less BMIPP uptake than perfusion in the acute or subacute phase of myocardial infarction after reperfusion is associated with improvement of wall motion abnormalities on the chronic phase. Such mismatched area is suggestive of stunned myocardium. Therefore, BMIPP imaging can provide useful information on predicting whether reperfused myocardium is viable or infarct.

Kawamoto *et al.* examined 22 patients with acute myocardial infarction to assess combined BMIPP and thallium SPECT, compared with stress redistribution thallium scintigraphy (n = 20) and 18F-fluorodeoxyglucose (FDG) PET (n = 10) [56]. Rest BMIPP and rest thallium SPECT were performed 2 weeks to 1 year after the last onset of infarction. Most segments of mismatch BMIPP uptake showed thallium redistribution, and increased FDG uptake, whereas fewer segments of matched BMIPP uptake did. These researchers indicated that BMIPP-thallium mismatch was indicative of viable myocardium.

Tamaki *et al.* evaluated BMIPP-thallium mismatch in 16 patients with coronary artery disease to compare relative FDG uptake assessed by FDG PET and clearance rate constant assessed by 11C-acetate PET [57]. Coronary artery disease consisted of acute myocardial infarction at least 1 month previously and unstable angina. Mismatch BMIPP uptake showed that both of relative FDG uptake and clearance rate constant were higher than matched BMIPP uptake. These authors confirmed that BMIPP and thallium imaging may have the potential to detect viable myocardium.

Ito *et al.* studied 37 patients with first acute myocardial infarction to assess functional recovery, compared with BMIPP and thallium SPECT after reperfusion [58]. Rest BMIPP and rest thallium SPECT were performed 3.2 ± 1.6 days, 6.2 ± 1.6 days after the onset, respectively. The extent of BMIPP-thallium mismatch correlated with the extent of functional recovery, indicating that such mismatch is an early predictor of myocardial viability at risk area.

Franken *et al.* assessed functional outcome in 18 patients with acute myocardial infarction using rest BMIPP and rest sestamibi scintigraphy, compared with dobutamine echocardiography [59]. All of the imaging procedures were performed 4 to 10 days after infarction. Dobutamine echocardiography assessed contractile reserve as an indicator of myocardial viability. Echocardiography was repeated 6 months later to evaluate functional outcome. Functional recovery was observed in most segments with BMIPP-sestamibi mismatch, whereas not observed in most segments with matched BMIPP uptake. For prediction of functional outcome, the accuracy of combined BMIPP and sestamibi SPECT was higher (85%) than that of sestamibi SPECT alone (77%), and that of dobutamine echocardiography (69%). These investigators concluded that BMIPP-sestamibi mismatch indicated myocardial viability and predicted functional recovery in patients with acute myocardial infarction.

Hashimoto *et al.* examined 56 patients with acute myocardial infarction to evaluate serial alterations in BMIPP and thallium uptake, compared with functional recovery after primary percutaneous transluminal coronary angioplasty (n = 32, group A) or conservational treatment (n = 24, group B) [60]. Group A showed that abnormal BMIPP uptake and BMIPP-thallium mismatch at the acute stage decreased significantly during follow-up, whereas group B did not. Recovery of BMIPP uptake was correlated with functional recovery. Group A showed that the mismatch at the acute stage was associated with functional recovery.

Nishimura *et al.* studied rest BMIPP and rest thallium SPECT in the subacute phase of acute myocardial infarction to predict functional recovery and cardiac events [61]. A total of 167 patients with first acute myocardial infarction were studied. BMIPP imaging at rest and thallium imaging were repeated in the chronic phase. For all patients, the investigators evaluated cardiac events including serious cardiac events and recurrent ischemia for at least 90 days after onset. All patients were divided into three groups: Subgroup A, B, and C. In Subgroup A, the association between recurrent ischemia and changes in radionuclide parameters was evaluated. They also assessed functional recovery by left ventriculography to calculate ejection fraction at discharge (Subgroup B) and 90 days or more after the onset of acute myocardial infarction (Subgroup C). Cox multivariate regression analysis revealed a high probability of serious cardiac events in patients with a high BMIPP defect score. Subgroup A had a tendency to show high probability of recurrent ischemia in patients with a large BMIPP-thallium mismatch during the subacute to chronic phase. Ejection fraction at discharge, and ejection fraction 90 days or more after the onset correlated more highly with defect score and extent score of BMIPP, and were predicted better by BMIPP defect parameters. These authors concluded that rest BMIPP and thallium SPECT during the subacute phase of acute myocardial infarction were valuable in predicting prognosis and ventricular function.

Naruse *et al.* studied 41 patients with acute myocardial infarction to evaluate the ability of BMIPP and thallium imaging for identifying stunned myocardium after revascularization [62]. Rest BMIPP imaging, and initial and delayed thallium imaging at rest were performed during the subacute phase (2 to 3 weeks after the onset and revascularization). Wall motion was assessed by echocardiography during the acute stage (immediately after revascularization). BMIPP uptake highly correlated with wall motion during the acute phase than other imaging procedures did. Improvement of wall motion showed a good correlation with BMIPP-delayed thallium mismatch.

Tani *et al.* studied 30 patients with acute myocardial infarction to assess viable myocardium and functional recovery, using five imaging techniques as follows: FDG PET, rest redistribution thallium SPECT, exercise reinjection thallium SPECT, BMIPP SPECT, and dobutamine stress echocardiography [63]. All of the techniques were performed at 10 ± 3 days after the onset, except for exercise reinjection thallium SPECT which was undergone at 14 ± 2 days. Echocardiography was followed up 5 ± 3 months after interventional therapy, which assessed functional recovery. All of the imaging procedures could identify viable myocardium and predict functional recovery, although there were some differences among these methods in the ability of predicting functional recovery.

Seki *et al.* compared the combination of three nuclear imaging techniques (FDG PET, BMIPP SPECT and tetrofosmin SPECT) to predict functional recovery in 10 patients with large acute myocardial infarction after revascularization [64]. The combination consisted of BMIPP-tetrofosmin, FDG-BMIPP, and FDG-tetrofosmin. Sensitivity, specificity and accuracy in prediction of functional recovery were calculated in each of these combinations. The authors concluded that BMIPP-tetrofosmin SPECT was practical for predicting the functional recovery in large acute myocardial infarction, compared favorably with FDG-BMIPP or FDG-tetrofosmin scan.

Biswas *et al.* studied 40 patients with acute myocardial infarction to compare BMIPP-tetrofosmin mismatch with recovery of systolic and diastolic parameters obtained from echocardiography [65]. BMIPP and tetrofosmin SPECT, and echocardiography were performed on 7 ± 3 days of admission. Follow up echocardiography was performed 3 months later. These authors concluded that the degree of mismatch correlated with the recovery of both systolic and diastolic function. Biswas *et al.* also confirmed that BMIPP-tetrofosmin mismatch correlated with the improvement of not only systolic and diastolic but also global left ventricular dysfunction after revascularization in patients with acute myocardial infarction [66].

Biswas *et al.* assessed the washout rate of BMIPP in 20 patients successfully reperfused with percutaneous coronary intervention after presenting with ST elevation myocardial infarction [67]. BMIPP imaging was performed at 7 ± 3 days after admission. Echocardiography was undertaken within 24 hours of admission and at 3 months. These authors proved that the washout of BMIPP is a promising indicator of improvement of left ventricular wall motion following ST elevation myocardial infarction and successful reperfusion.

Risk Stratification and Prognostic Value

Risk stratification and prognostication are crucial after acute myocardial infarction, since high-risk patients can benefit from earlier and customized treatments, whereas low-risk patients can avoid unnecessary interventions. Nakata *et al.* studied 101 patients with acute myocardial infarction to evaluate the prognostic value of BMIPP scan during a mean follow-up of 28 months [68]. Multivariate analysis revealed that reduced BMIPP uptake and greater BMIPP-thallium mismatch were prognostic predictors for cardiac events.

Nanasato *et al.* examined 159 patients with acute myocardial infarction to assess additional predictive value of BMIPP scintigraphy compared to variables from catheterization alone during a mean follow-up of 34.5 months [69]. BMIPP defects and BMIPP-thallium mismatch indicated a high probability of cardiac events, and increased predictive value above variables from catheterization.

Fukushima *et al.* evaluated relationship among non ST elevation myocardial infarction, BMIPP and thallium SPECT, and myocardial enzymes [70]. BMIPP/thallium dual-isotope SPECT was performed approximately 8 days after the onset. A total of 86 patients with acute myocardial infarction were studied. Patients were divided into two groups: 53 patients with increased cardiac troponin T and with creatine kinase-MB (Group A), and 33 patients with increased troponin T and without increased creatine kinase-MB (Group B). Most patients in group A showed ST elevation, whereas no patients in group B had ST elevation. Furthermore, group B was subdivided into two groups: with severe BMIPP defects (Group B(S)) and with mild BMIPP defects (Group B(M)). The authors assessed defect scores of the two tracers and the sensitivity for detecting the culprit coronary lesions, and compared the prognosis between the three groups over a period of 2 years. Group A showed higher scores of total BMIPP and thallium defects than group B. For detecting the culprit lesions, group B demonstrated the higher sensitivity of BMIPP imaging than that of thallium imaging, whereas group A showed no difference between the two sensitivities. Follow-up study revealed that group B(S) and group A had higher incidence of hard cardiac events than group B(M). These researchers conclude that BMIPP scan provides a useful method to identify the culprit lesions and predicts the prognosis in patients with acute myocardial infarction exhibiting neither ST elevation nor creatine kinase-MB but increased troponin T.

Inaba and Bergmann conducted a meta-analysis of six studies including 607 patients with acute myocardial infarction to evaluate the prognostic value of BMIPP [71]. They confirmed that large BMIPP defect was related to cardiac death and hard events.

Angina Pectoris and Acute Coronary Syndrome

Unstable Angina

In patients with unstable angina, reduced BMIPP uptake as well as discordant BMIPP uptake less than perfusion have also been observed frequently. Tateno *et al.* evaluated BMIPP scan in patients with ischemic heart disease and no prior infarction, compared with rest/stress thallium SPECT, coronary arteriography and left ventriculography [72]. Nineteen patients with unstable angina and 12 patients with stable angina were studied. They revealed that mismatched BMIPP uptake was observed more often in patients with unstable angina than in patients with stable angina, and was related to ventricular dysfunction.

Identification of Ischemia and Culprit Artery, and Decision-Making for Treatment

The identification of myocardial ischemia is crucial to diagnose unstable angina, because the presence of ischemic myocardium can encourage appropriate treatment. On the other hand, the detection of culprit artery is important, since multivessel disease makes it hard to determine which stenotic arteries are responsible for ischemic attack. Although a 12 lead electrocardiography is the first choice of method for suspected unstable angina, a nondiagnostic electrocardiogram may make decision-making with these patients difficult. Moreover, the 12 lead electrocardiography alone cannot evaluate the location and severity of myocardial ischemia.

Another noninvasive method is a radionuclear imaging technique including perfusion imaging and BMIPP imaging. Sestamibi SPECT performed during angina attack has higher sensitivity in detection of ischemia than electrocardiography. However, false negative results are often seen in perfusion imaging performed during a symptom-free period. By contrast, BMIPP has the potential to overcome the problems.

Takeishi *et al.* assessed patients with unstable angina using rest BMIPP imaging and rest sestamibi imaging during a symptom-free period [73]. Sensitivity for BMIPP and sestamibi in detection of ischemia was 77% and 45%, respectively. The authors indicated that BMIPP scintigraphy identified myocardial ischemia more sensitively than sestamibi imaging.

Saitoh *et al.* studied 54 patients with unstable angina to evaluate the ability of 12 lead electrocardiogram and BMIPP-thallium mismatch to identify coronary artery disease [74]. Electrocardiographic alterations during the attack showed high sensitivity and low specificity, whereas mismatched BMIPP uptake demonstrated the inverse results. Mismatched BMIPP uptake showed that both of sensitivity and specificity were high in patients with ST depression during the attack. These investigators concluded that both of electrocardiogram and BMIPP-perfusion mismatch are valuable methods for identifying coronary artery disease in patients with unstable angina.

Inaba and Bergmann performed a meta-analysis of seven studies to confirm the diagnostic accuracy of rest BMIPP scintigraphy for identification of cardiovascular disease [75]. Sensitivity and specificity were 78% and 84%, respectively, in patients with a high prevalence of cardiovascular disease. These results compared favorably with the diagnostic performance of stress perfusion SPECT. The investigators concluded that rest BMIPP imaging may offer great value for patients with acute chest pain and patients who should avoid stress perfusion imaging.

Morimoto *et al.* used rest BMIPP scan to assess the ability for predicting culprit lesions in 100 patients with unstable angina [76]. BMIPP and thallium imaging, and left ventricular cineangiography were performed 1 week after the last episode of angina. As severity scores of BMIPP became worse, the number of stenotic coronary arteries and the severity of individual arterial stenosis increased. In addition, severity scores of BMIPP recovered 1 month after revascularization, and correlated with left ventricular dysfunction. Sensitivity of BMIPP and thallium scan in detection of significant coronary stenosis was 74% and 31%, respectively, and specificity was 86% and 91%, respectively. These researchers concluded that rest BMIPP scintigraphy is effective for predicting coronary lesions of patients with unstable angina without provocation.

BMIPP scan may assist therapeutic decision-making in patients with unstable angina. Takeishi *et al.* evaluated BMIPP scintigraphy in 20 patients with unstable angina, compared with angiography [75]. Eleven out of 20 patients showed BMIPP abnormalities. These patients had more severe coronary stenosis and collateral circulation, and underwent revascularization more frequently than 9 patients with normal images. These authors concluded that BMIPP imaging is helpful for interventional strategy.

Prognostic Value

BMIPP may be a useful prognostic indicator in patients with unstable angina. Matsuki *et al.* assessed prognostic value of BMIPP imaging in 167 patients with angina pectoris and no prior infarction [77]. Patients underwent rest BMIPP and stress thallium imaging, and were followed up for hard and soft cardiac events during a period of 48 months. Multivariate Cox analysis revealed independent predictors as follows: BMIPP defect score, stress thallium score, diabetes, and ejection fraction. Patients with normal BMIPP uptake showed no hard event, while 2 patients with abnormal BMIPP uptake and nearly normal stress perfusion demonstrated hard cardiac events. These authors reported that normal BMIPP uptake provides excellent prognostic value independent of stress perfusion imaging in patients with angina without prior myocardial infarction.

Inaba and Bergmann conducted a meta-analysis of three studies to assess prognostic value of patients with suspected acute coronary syndrome after exclusion of acute myocardial infarction [71]. Abnormal BMIPP imaging was significantly associated with hard events. Over a 3.5-year follow-up, the negative predictive value of normal BMIPP imaging for hard and soft events was 98.9% and 92.3%, respectively.

Acute Coronary Syndrome

Acute coronary syndrome is the umbrella term for any kind of clinical signs and symptoms compatible with acute myocardial ischemia. The spectrum of clinical conditions ranges from unstable angina to myocardial infarction with or without ST elevation. Patients with acute coronary syndrome may present to emergency department exhibiting acute chest pain. However, because a large number of chest pain episodes are due to noncardiac causes, accurate diagnosis is crucial in the emergency department. The diagnosis of acute coronary syndrome is challenging in patients with nondiagnostic electrocardiography and normal cardiac biomarkers. Rest myocardial perfusion imaging has been proven to be useful, especially in such situation with a lower probability of an ischemic attack. Technetium-99m based perfusion radiotracers are more suitable for use in the emergency department than thallium-201. A rest-only perfusion SPECT has a high negative predictive value for acute coronary syndrome during active chest pain, although stress SPECT is more sensitive than rest SPECT after pain relief. However, stress perfusion study may not be safe in unstable patients. BMIPP imaging is another method to identify patients with acute coronary syndrome who visit emergency department due to acute chest pain. This method has the ability to assess these patients at rest and during the pain-free period. Because BMIPP imaging usually does not require a provocation test, this imaging is suitable for patients with unstable acute coronary syndrome or severe coronary disease.

Kawai *et al.* used rest BMIPP SPECT in 111 patients with acute chest pain and no infarction, compared with rest tetrofosmin SPECT and coronary angiography [31]. These patients included 66 patients with organic stenosis, 21 patients with spasm, and 24 patients without stenosis or spasm. BMIPP and tetrofosmin SPECT were performed at rest within 48 hours and 24 hours of the last chest pain, respectively. BMIPP abnormalities were associated with coronary stenosis and spasm. Sensitivity in identifying significant coronary stenosis of BMIPP and tetrofosmin was 74% and 38%, respectively, whereas specificity was 92% and 96%, respectively. These investigators indicated that BMIPP SPECT may detect prior myocardial ischemia after improvement of chest pain.

Dilsizian *et al.* studied 32 patients with exercise-induced ischemia on thallium SPECT to evaluate whether rest BMIPP imaging can detect the ischemia within 30 hours after the induction of ischemia [78]. SPECT images were obtained both 10 minutes (early) and 30 minutes (delayed) after injection of BMIPP. For ischemic abnormalities, there was 91% agreement between early BMIPP and stress thallium data, and 94% agreement between delayed BMIPP and stress thallium data. The authors concluded that BMIPP imaging identifies recent ischemia induced by exercise stress.

Kantos *et al.* performed a multicenter study of 507 patients with chest pain who presented to emergency department to assess diagnostic ability of BMIPP imaging for acute coronary syndrome [32]. BMIPP scan was performed within 30 hours of symptom resolution. BMIPP imaging alone had higher sensitivity in the diagnosis of acute coronary syndrome (73%) than initial clinical diagnosis alone (43%). Adding BMIPP imaging to the initial clinical diagnosis increased sensitivity form 43% to 81%. The specificity of BMIPP imaging alone was similar to that of the initial clinical diagnosis (63% *vs* 61%). These investigators concluded that the addition of BMIPP scintigraphy to the initial clinical diagnosis provides incremental value for the early diagnosis of acute coronary syndrome.

Vasospastic Angina

Vasospastic angina is characterized by transient spasm of coronary arteries, resulting in myocardial ischemia and wall motion abnormality. Provocative testing is a well-established method of vasospastic angina, directly identifying coronary spasm with intracoronary administration of ergonovine or acetylcholine. Because more invasive, this technique has encouraged the development of other methods to less invasively diagnose vasospastic angina.

Rest or stress perfusion imaging is a noninvasive technique to detect myocardial ischemia, although these methods have several disadvantages in diagnosis of vasospastic angina. Rest perfusion imaging identifies myocardial ischemia less sensitively on pain-free conditions, whereas stress perfusion scintigraphy insufficiently induces ischemia in patients with vasospastic angina.

Conversely, BMIPP scan can detect ischemic myocardium by vasospasm, because repetitive ischemic episodes may result in changes of fatty acid metabolism. Since altered fatty acid metabolism may persist even after perfusion recovery, BMIPP scan, unlike perfusion imaging, can identify ischemia during symptom-free period after disappearance of spasm. Moreover, BMIPP scan is performed at rest without the need of stress testing. In fact, decreased BMIPP uptake is often observed in patients with vasospastic angina [79 - 83].

Nakajima *et al.* examined 32 patients with vasospastic angina to compare rest BMIPP SPECT with stress perfusion SPECT using thallium or MIBI [79]. Reduced BMIPP uptake was seen in these patients more frequently (78%) than reduced perfusion (31%) was. Twenty-three patients were followed up for a mean period of 206 days to evaluate response to therapy, and these researchers revealed that improved BMIPP showed improved symptom more often than nonimproved BMIPP did.

Watanabe *et al.* compared BMIPP uptake in 53 patients with vasospastic angina with coronary vasospastic regions induced by ergonovine and ventricular wall motion assessed by left ventriculography [80]. Patients with vasospastic angina showed reduced BMIPP uptake (89%) and regional wall motion (36%). Reduced BMIPP uptake was seen in the coronary vasospastic regions and abnormality of wall motion. The sensitivity and specificity of BMIPP in identifying spasm-induced arteries were 71% and 88%, respectively. Patients with spasm-reinduced arteries after treatment had lower improvement of reduced BMIPP uptake than patients without spasm-reinduced arteries. The authors concluded that BMIPP scintigraphy can accurately detect ischemia induced by vasospasm based on alterations of fatty acid metabolism.

Watanabe *et al.* also examined 50 patients with vasospastic angina to assess BMIPP and 123I-metaiodobenzylguanidine (MIBG) scintigraphy [81]. They showed that BMIPP scan had higher specificity and MIBG had higher sensitivity, both of which may indicate myocardial injury more accurately than thallium or left ventriculography.

Yamabe *et al.* conducted a multicenter study of patients with chest pain to evaluate rest BMIPP imaging for the diagnosis of coronary artery disease and the prediction of therapeutic outcome [82]. A total of 104 patients had angina pectoris (stable, unstable and vasospastic) or noncoronary artery disease. BMIPP scintigraphy was performed under pain-free conditions. Reduced BMIPP uptake was observed more often in stable angina and unstable angina with organic stenosis (54%) than in vasospastic angina without organic stenosis (22%), and was correlated highly with subsequent intervention than normal BMIPP uptake. These investigators suggested that BMIPP imaging was valuable for the diagnosis of angina pectoris and decision-making in interventional therapy.

Kawai *et al.* studied patients with acute chest pain to compare rest BMIPP SPECT with rest stress tetrofosmin SPECT and coronary angiography [83]. A total of 150 patients with acute chest pain were divided into three groups: 46 patients with organic stenosis, 27 patients with spasm induced by provocation testing, and 77 patients without coronary stenosis or spasm. All imaging techniques were performed within 6 days after the last episode of chest pain. Rest BMIPP imaging had higher sensitivity in identifying organic stenosis (54%) than rest tetrofosmin imaging (33%), but lower sensitivity than stress tetrofosmin imaging (76%). On the other hand, rest BMIPP scintigraphy showed higher sensitivity in detecting spasm (63%) than both rest (15%) and stress (19%) tetrofosmin imaging. These researchers concluded that rest BMIPP scan was alternative to stress perfusion imaging for identifying organic stenosis and spasm in patients with acute chest pain.

Chronic Coronary Aartery Disease

Stable Angina and Old Myocardial Infarction

Reduced uptake of BMIPP and BMIPP-perfusion mismatch are observed often in patients with chronic coronary artery disease including stable angina and old myocardial infarction. Some investigators reported the diagnostic value of BMIPP scan for the disease and stenotic vessels [82, 84]. In addition, BMIPP abnormalities are associated with various parameters including abnormalities of electrocardiography, ischemia, coronary artery, myocardial flow reserve, and wall motion.

Tateno *et al.* studied 31 patients with ischemic heart disease without myocardial infarction, using rest BMIPP SPECT, rest/stress thallium SPECT, coronary arteriography and left ventriculography [72]. These patients consisted of 19 with unstable angina and 12 with stable angina. They reported that BMIPP abnormalities were related to severe ischemia, severe coronary stenosis, and wall motion abnormalities.

Yamabe *et al.* studied patients with effort angina pectoris to assess the diagnostic value of rest BMIPP scintigraphy, compared with coronary angiography [82]. These patients were divided into three subsets: stable type, new onset type, and worsening type. Worsening type showed a higher detection rate of both disease and stenotic vessels than the other two types. These authors concluded that rest BMIPP scan provided diagnostic value specifically in patients with worsening type.

Takeishi *et al.* examined 46 patients with stable effort angina pectoris to evaluate rest BMIPP scintigraphy, compared with rest and exercise MIBI imaging [84]. BMIPP abnormalities were associated with exercise-induced ST depression, severe coronary stenosis, collateral vessels, and severe wall motion abnormalities.

BMIPP scan also could identify coronary artery stenosis and exercise-induced ischemia with moderate sensitivity.

Kageyama *et al.* evaluated relation of BMIPP to myocardial flow reserve in 21 patients with chronic stable angina [85]. Myocardial flow reserve was assessed with 15O-water PET. They reported that reduction of BMIPP uptake implies reduction of myocardial flow reserve.

Akashi *et al.* used BMIPP planar imaging to assess the H/M ratio and washout rate in patients with heart disease (20 with chronic heart failure and 30 with stable angina), compared with control subjects [86]. BMIPP planar imaging was performed 30 minutes (early) and 4 hours (delayed) after intravenous administration of a tracer. Delayed H/M ratio showed greater reduction in patients with chronic heart disease than patients with stable angina and controls, and correlated with ejection fraction and brain natriuretic peptide (BNP) in all subjects. Washout rate was higher in patients with heart disease than in controls, and related to BNP. The authors suggest that delayed H/M ratio and washout rate of BMIPP enhance assessment of impaired fatty acid metabolism in patients with heart disease.

Assessment of Myocardial Viability and Prediction of Functional Recovery

Identification of viable myocardium is crucial for patients with chronic coronary artery disease, because reperfusion has effects only if affected area is viable. Many investigators have indicated that discordant BMIPP uptake in patients with chronic coronary artery disease may represent viable myocardium, also known as hibernating myocardium. Thus, BMIPP imaging has the potential to predict functional recovery in these patients. Multiple noninvasive methods have been developed to assess myocardial viability, including nuclear imaging, dobutamine stress echocardiography, and magnetic resonance imaging. Of nuclear imaging techniques, FDG PET is considered as the gold standard to evaluate viability, while perfusion SPECT is a well-established modality and more practical than PET because of low cost and wide availability. Dobutamine stress echocardiography evaluates myocardial contractile reserve which is increased in dysfunctional but viable tissue after administration of low-dose dobutamine. Mismatch BMIPP uptake has accumulated evidence to support myocardial viability by comparing such noninvasive techniques [40, 56, 87, 88] and pathological study [89]. Moreover, assessment of left ventricular function is necessary to determine whether discordant BMIPP reflects myocardial viability [90, 91]. In particular, several studies have been performed in terms of association between the degree of mismatch and the degree of ventricular dysfunction, and serial alterations of mismatch and function before and after reperfusion.

Taki *et al.* studied 45 patients with chronic coronary artery disease using rest BMIPP scan compared with exercise reinjection thallium imaging and wall motion [87]. Discordant BMIPP less than reinjection thallium was seen frequently in stress-induced ischemia, whereas BMIPP and reinjection thallium decreased concordantly in a majority of fixed perfusion defects. The more severely BMIPP uptake reduced than reinjection thallium perfusion, the more extensively wall motion decreased. The authors concluded that such discordant BMIPP uptake may reflect alterations of myocardial metabolism and wall motion independent of perfusion abnormalities.

Matsunari *et al.* examined 55 patients with coronary artery disease and fixed defects on exercise redistribution thallium scan [88]. Rest BMIPP and exercise redistribution reinjection thallium imaging were performed. Discordant BMIPP uptake (less than reinjection thallium) was observed in most of myocardial segments with fill-in, while such discordant BMIPP uptake was seen in only 19% of segments with no fill-in. The researchers concluded fatty acid uptake was impaired especially in ischemic myocardium identified by thallium reinjection.

Kawamoto *et al.* studied 22 patients with myocardial infarction using combined BMIPP and thallium imaging at rest, compared with stress redistribution thallium SPECT and FDG PET [56]. The segments with discordant BMIPP uptake (less than thallium uptake) showed thallium redistribution and increased FDG uptake, more often than those with concordant BMIPP uptake. Therefore, the area with discordant BMIPP uptake represented ischemic but viable myocardium. The investigators concluded that BMIPP-thallium mismatch is useful for evaluation of tissue viability in patients with coronary artery disease.

Hambÿe *et al.* examined 25 patients with chronic and severe left ventricular dysfunction after infarction to evaluate whether combined BMIPP and sestamibi SPECT can identify viable myocardium, compared with dobutamine stress echocardiography [40]. They concluded that the combined analysis correlates well with contractile response to dobutamine and detects viable myocardium more sensitively than sestamibi alone.

Kudoh *et al.* studied 15 patients with non-acute myocardial infarction and angina pectoris to compare BMIPP and thallium SPECT with myocardial fibrosis by histologic analysis at cardiac surgery [89]. As fibrosis progressed, each of BMIPP and thallium uptake decreased in a different manner. Unlike thallium uptake, BMIPP uptake seemed to exhibit a biphasic pattern with a steep decline in mild fibrosis, followed by a gradual decline in moderate to severe fibrosis. Moreover, BMIPP-thallium mismatch was observed only in patients with mild fibrosis.

Taki *et al.* studied 34 patients with chronic coronary artery disease to serially evaluate rest BMIPP and stress reinjection thallium imaging, and left ventricular function before and after revascularization [90]. The recovery of function after revascularization correlated with the recovery of BMIPP uptake. In addition, the area of discordant BMIPP uptake (less than reinjection thallium) before revascularization was a good predictor of ejection fraction improvement after revascularization.

Hambye *et al.* evaluated BMIPP-sestamibi mismatch to predict functional recovery in 20 patients with chronic left ventricular dysfunction after myocardial infarction [91]. These patients underwent radionuclide angiography, echocardiography, BMIPP scan and gated sestamibi scintigraphy before and > 6 months after treatment (revascularization and conservative therapy). On a patient basis, mismatch BMIPP uptake was observed in 15 out of 20 patients before treatment, and could predict functional recovery with 75% accuracy. On a segmental basis, adding BMIPP to sestamibi data improved the accuracy from 63% to 80%. The authors concluded that in patients with chronic dysfunction after infarction, BMIPP-sestamibi mismatch detects viable myocardium and predicts functional recovery with an accuracy similar to that previously reported in the acute and subacute phases of the infarction.

Risk Stratification and Prognostic Value

BMIPP scintigraphy has been shown to yield important information regarding risk stratification and prognostic value in patients with chronic coronary artery disease. Chikamori *et al.* used rest BMIPP scan to assess the prognostic value for hard and significant events in 270 patients with known or suspected coronary artery disease during a median follow-up of 3.9 years [92]. Kaplan-Meier survival estimates revealed that event-free survival rates for both hard and significant events were higher in patients with a BMIPP defect score < 5 than with a BMIPP defect score ≥ 5. These authors indicate that rest BMIPP imaging has the prognostic value and may hold potential for risk stratification of patients with known or suspected coronary artery disease.

Tamaki *et al.* studied 50 patients with chronic myocardial infarction to evaluate prognostic value of BMIPP scintigraphy in a median follow-up of 23 months [93]. Cox regression analysis revealed that among clinical, angiographic, and radionuclide variables, discordant BMIPP was the best predictor of future cardiac events, followed by coronary stenosis.

Fukuzawa *et al.* studied 76 patients with chronic coronary artery disease and left ventricular dysfunction to evaluate the prognostic value of BMIPP-thallium mismatch [94]. Patients underwent revascularization and were followed up for cardiac function and events. The larger BMIPP-thallium mismatch was, the better recovery of ejection fraction was. Functional recovery with a large BMIPP-thallium mismatch was associated with a low rate of cardiac events and better event free survival. These investigators revealed that BMIPP-thallium mismatch can predict the prognosis in revascularized patients with chronic coronary artery disease and cardiac dysfunction.

Inaba and Bergmann performed a meta-analysis of two studies with stable coronary artery disease to evaluate the prognostic value of BMIPP-perfusion mismatch [71]. A total of 166 patients underwent revascularization. The results obtained from these two studies were contrast, depending whether BMIPP scintigraphy was performed before or after revascularization; BMIPP mismatch before revascularization was related to fewer events after successful revascularization, while such mismatch resulting after revascularization was associated with more events.

Nonischemic Cardiomyopathy

Hypertrophic Cardiomyopathy

BMIPP Imaging

Hypertrophic cardiomyopathy is a genetic disease characterized by abnormal thickness of the heart muscle. Alterations of fatty acid metabolism, which are often observed in patients with this entity, have been extensively assessed using BMIPP scintigraphy in Japan. This condition often has shown reduced BMIPP uptake, which is usually distributed heterogeneously and frequently seen in the ventricular septum and apex.

Ohtsuki *et al.* studied 30 patients with asymmetric septal hypertrophy to evaluate regional BMIPP accumulation [95]. They concluded that in some patients with asymmetric septal hypertrophy, BMIPP defects are seen most markedly and frequently in the anterior and posterior junctions between the ventricular septum and the left and right ventricular free walls.

Kuribayashi *et al.* revealed that myocardial disarray most frequently seen at the junction of ventricular free walls in patients with hypertrophic cardiomyopathy [96]. These results suggest the presence of association between impaired fatty acid metabolism and myocardial disarray.

BMIPP Imaging Compared with Perfusion Imaging and other Metabolic Imaging Techniques

Several investigators have studied patients with hypertrophic cardiomyopathy to compare BMIPP imaging with rest or stress perfusion scan. Abnormalities of fatty acid metabolism assessed with BMIPP may precede perfusion defects. BMIPP mismatch less than perfusion is often observed especially in hypertrophic segments [97 - 99], whereas Nishimura *et al.* reported that such mismatch was seen even in nonhypertrophic myocardium [100]. Stress thallium SPECT often demonstrates reversible thallium defect in patients with hypertrophic cardiomyopathy [101].

Taki *et al.* studied 17 patients with hypertrophic cardiomyopathy using rest BMIPP scintigraphy (20 minutes and 3 hours after injection of a tracer), compared with exercise stress redistribution thallium SPECT (10 minutes and 3 hours after injection) [102]. BMIPP uptake (20 minutes) in the hypertrophic areas was lower than thallium uptake (3 hours). Some patients showed that BMIPP-thallium mismatch was associated with thallium redistribution.

Tadamura *et al.* studied 28 patients with hypertrophic cardiomyopathy to compare BMIPP scintigraphy with 11C-acetate and 18F-FDG PET imaging [103]. These authors concluded abnormalities of fatty acid metabolism assessed with BMIPP preceded oxygen metabolism assessed with acetate and glucose metabolism with FDG.

BMIPP Imaging for Evaluation of Cardiac Dysfunction and Prognosis

BMIPP scintigraphy has the potential to evaluate cardiac function and predict prognosis in patients with hypertrophic cardiomyopathy. Shimonagata *et al.* studied 12 patients with asymmetric septal hypertrophy and 5 normal subjects to assess discordant BMIPP uptake less than thallium perfusion and left ventricular function [104]. Patients with hypertrophic cardiomyopathy showed discordant BMIPP uptake, while normal subjects demonstrated homogenous uptake without discrepancy between the two traces. BMIPP score correlated significantly with left ventricular ejection fraction, whereas thallium score did not. The authors suggested BMIPP is useful in the assessment of left ventricular function in hypertrophic cardiomyopathy.

Nishimura *et al.* used BMIPP and thallium perfusion SPECT to study 25 patients with myocardial infarction (group A) and 16 patients with hypertrophic cardiomyopathy (group B) [99]. Group A showed BMIPP-perfusion mismatch more frequently seen in patients with successful reperfusion than in patients without reperfusion and patients with reinfarction. By contrast, group B demonstrated such mismatch observed in hypertrophic myocardium. In addition, nonhypertrophic myocardium also showed reduced BMIPP uptake. In both groups, BMIPP severity scores were related to left ventricular function compared with thallium severity scores. These results indicate that BMIPP is suitable for the assessment of functional integrity.

Narita *et al.* examined 18 patients with asymptomatic hypertrophic cardiomyopathy using BMIPP and stress perfusion imaging [105]. These two imaging procedures were performed (first scan), and were repeated 4.0 ± 0.8 years after the first scan (second scan). The second scan showed that total defect score of BMIPP increased and %uptake of BMIPP decreased compared with the first scan, whereas no deficiencies in perfusion were observed between the two scans. Some of patients who presented with exertional dyspnea showed the greatest reduction of %uptake during the follow-up, and deterioration of %fractional shortening and volume in left ventricle on the second scan. These authors concluded that BMIPP abnormalities, which were seen frequently with asymptomatic hypertrophic cardiomyopathy, showed progression over time. Moreover, the greatest reduction of %uptake reflected the deterioration of left ventricular function.

Nishimura *et al.* studied 65 patients with hypertrophic cardiomyopathy to evaluate the usefulness of BMIPP SPECT in predicting the prognosis [100]. Patients were followed up for cardiac events during a mean period of 3.0 ± 0.6 years. The BMIPP severity score was high in patients with fatal heart failure, and correlated negatively with left ventricular function. The mortality over 3 years increased together with the increase in extent of the BMIPP severity score. These researchers concluded that BMIPP imaging provided a useful method in evaluating the disease severity and predicting the outcome in patients with hypertrophic cardiomyopathy.

Dilated Cardiomyopathy

BMIPP Imaging Compared with Perfusion Imaging

Nuclear imaging techniques have shown abnormality of myocardial fatty acid metabolism in patients with dilated cardiomyopathy [20, 106]. Of these imaging techniques, BMIPP scan is extensively used in the clinical settings. Compared with ischemic cardiomyopathy, dilated cardiomyopathy demonstrates less reduced uptake of BMIPP and lower frequency of mismatched BMIPP uptake [107], and is more often assessed with heart-to-mediastinum (H/M) ratio of BMIPP than with BMIPP-perfusion mismatch. BMIPP as well as thallium may distribute heterogeneously in patients with dilated cardiomyopathy. BMIPP abnormality correlates with left ventricular function, whereas thallium abnormality does not [41].

BMIPP Imaging for Therapy Monitoring

BMIPP may have the ability to monitor therapeutic effects of medications and cardiac resynchronization therapy in patients with dilated cardiomyopathy. Medications used to treat with this entity include β-blocker, angiotensin-converting enzyme inhibitor (ACE-I), and coenzyme Q10. Yoshinaga *et al.* revealed that H/M ratio of BMIPP uptake can predict the response to β-blocker in patients with dilated cardiomyopathy [108]. Ito *et al.* also showed that %BM uptake (percentage of cardiac uptake of BMIPP to total injected dose) may predict functional recovery induced by β-blocker therapy [109].

Yamauchi *et al.* studied 25 patients with congestive heart failure to evaluate whether ACE-I improved myocardial fatty acid metabolism [110]. Causative diseases included idiopathic dilated cardiomyopathy (n = 20), ischemic cardiomyopathy (n = 2), valvular heart disease (n = 2), and hypertensive heart disease (n = 1). The authors showed that ACE-I improved the delayed H/M ratio and washout rate of BMIPP.

Kim *et al.* confirmed that BMIPP SPECT can evaluate the therapeutic effects of coenzyme Q10 in patients with idiopathic dilated cardiomyopathy [111]. Moreover, the authors suggested that BMIPP imaging is a more sensitive indicator of the effects compared with functional parameters.

Zavadovsky *et al.* used BMIPP and MIBI SPECT to predict therapeutic effect of cardiac resynchronization therapy in patients with dilated cardiomyopathy [112]. BMIPP and MIBI imaging were performed before cardiac resynchronization therapy, whereas echocardiography was undertaken to evaluate cardiac hemodynamics before and 6 months after the therapy. Patients were divided into two groups based on the response to therapy: responders and non-responders. Preoperatively, responders had greater defect size of both BMIPP and thallium than non-responders. Receiver operating characteristic (ROC) curve analysis revealed BMIPP defect predicted the indication of cardiac resynchronization therapy with greater efficacy than thallium defect.

BMIPP Imaging for Prognostic Prediction

Identification of abnormal BMIPP uptake can provide useful information on prognostic prediction in patients with dilated cardiomyopathy. Inoue *et al.* suggested that the extent score of BMIPP could be a valuable predictor of cardiac events in dilated cardiomyopathy [113].

Nakae *et al.* studied 32 patients with congestive heart failure compared with 18 normal control subjects [114]. They evaluated the initial and delayed H/M ratio and washout rate using BMIPP scintigraphy, and association with left ventricular ejection fraction and BNP. Causative diseases varied including idiopathic dilated cardiomyopathy as the most frequent condition. Patients with congestive heart failure had lower H/M ratio on initial and delayed images than control subjects. Both of the initial and delayed H/M ratio correlated with left ventricular ejection fraction. On the other hand, patients with congestive heart failure demonstrated higher washout rate than control subjects, and the washout rate correlated with BNP. Kaplan-Meier analysis showed that cardiac events occurred more frequently in a lower initial H/M ratio than in a higher initial H/M ratio. The investigators concluded that BMIPP abnormality was associated with the severity of congestive heart failure and may be a useful predictor of cardiac events.

Sasaki *et al.* studied patients with left ventricular dysfunction and chronic heart failure to evaluate whether BMIPP can predict cardiac death [115]. Causative diseases included ischemic heart disease, dilated cardiomyopathy, hypertrophic cardiomyopathy followed by other myocardial diseases in order of decreasing frequency. The multivariate analysis revealed that value of H/M ratio of BMIPP divided by H/M ratio of thallium was an independent prognostic factor in patients with nonischemic heart disease.

Takotsubo Cardiomyopathy

Takotsubo cardiomyopathy is characterized by a reversible left ventricular dysfunction without coronary artery stenosis, with clinical features such as symptoms or electrocardiographic alterations similar to acute myocardial infarction. Left ventriculography typically shows hypokinesis or akinesis in the mid and apical segments, and hyperkinesis in the basal segments. The shape of systolic apical ballooning in the left ventricle resembles “takotsubo”, the term taken from Japanese octopus pot by Sato *et al.* in 1990 [116]. There are several publications about nuclear imaging to evaluate myocardial metabolism or perfusion in patients with Takotsubo cardiomyopathy. Some reports show abnormal BMIPP uptake in this entity [117 - 120].

Kurisu *et al.* studied patients with Takotsubo cardiomyopathy to serially assess rest BMIPP imaging compared with rest thallium perfusion imaging and left ventricular function [117]. Reduced BMIPP uptake was observed in parallel with an apical akinetic region during the acute phase (5 ± 3 days after onset). Abnormal BMIPP uptake usually persisted even after recovery of left ventricular dysfunction. Mismatched BMIPP was also seen during the acute phase. The mismatched uptake improved gradually from the subacute phase (15 ± 3 days after onset) to follow-up (29 ± 6 days after onset).

Owa *et al.* examined 4 patients with Takotsubo cardiomyopathy to chronologically evaluate three tracers (MIBG, BMIPP, and thallium) using SPECT imaging [118]. SPECT imaging was assessed at 2 to 3 days (acute phase), 2 to 3 weeks, 3 months, and 12 months after the initial admission. In the acute phase, MIBG and BMIPP imaging demonstrated higher uptake defects than thallium uptake. BMIPP and thallium uptake recovered 2 weeks later, whereas uptake defects of MIBG persisted for several months.

Ito *et al.* studied 7 patients with Takotsubo cardiomyopathy compared with 7 patients with acute myocardial infarction to chronologically assess four tracers (BMIPP, tetrofosmin, pyrophosphate, and MIBG) by SPECT imaging and wall motion by echocardiography [119]. SPECT imaging and echocardiography were performed on admission (acute phase), and 2 to 14 days (subacute phase), 1 month (chronic phase) and 3 months (chronic II phase) after the attack. Patients with Takotsubo cardiomyopathy demonstrated the serial alterations of BMIPP and MIBG which resembled those of acute myocardial infarction despite different recovery time. These results suggested an affected myocardial tissue of this entity might be a type of stunned myocardium.

Matsuo *et al.* also examined 16 patients with Takotsubo cardiomyopathy compared with 12 patients with acute myocardial infarction in the left anterior descending artery [120]. Rest BMIPP and rest perfusion (sestamibi or tetrofosmin) imaging were performed at 11.1 ± 2.1 days and 14.6 ± 2.5 days after admission, respectively. Unlike patients with acute myocardial infarction, patients with Takotsubo cardiomyopathy showed both defect score and BMIPP-perfusion mismatch extensively in the apical area. The investigators suggested utility of BMIPP scan in differentiation between the two diseases.

CONSENT FOR PUBLICATION

Not applicable.

CONFLICT OF INTEREST

The authors declare no conflict of interest, financial or otherwise.

ACKNOWLEDGEMENTS

Declared none.

REFERENCES

[1] Stanley WC, Lopaschuk GD, Hall JL, McCormack JG. Regulation of myocardial carbohydrate metabolism under normal and ischaemic conditions. Potential for pharmacological interventions. Cardiovasc Res 1997; 33(2): 243-57.

[http://dx.doi.org/10.1016/S0008-6363(96)00245-3] [PMID: 9074687]

[2] Lopaschuk GD, Collins-Nakai RL, Itoi T. Developmental changes in energy substrate use by the heart. Cardiovasc Res 1992; 26(12): 1172-80.
[http://dx.doi.org/10.1093/cvr/26.12.1172] [PMID: 1288863]

[3] Oliver MF, Kurien VA, Greenwood TW. Relation between serum-free-fatty acids and arrhythmias and death after acute myocardial infarction. Lancet 1968; 1(7545): 710-4.
[http://dx.doi.org/10.1016/S0140-6736(68)92163-6] [PMID: 4170959]

[4] Katz AM, Messineo FC. Lipid-membrane interactions and the pathogenesis of ischemic damage in the myocardium. Circ Res 1981; 48(1): 1-16.
[http://dx.doi.org/10.1161/01.RES.48.1.1] [PMID: 7438341]

[5] Straeter-Knowlen IM, Evanochko WT, den Hollander JA, *et al.* 1H NMR spectroscopic imaging of myocardial triglycerides in excised dog hearts subjected to 24 hours of coronary occlusion. Circulation 1996; 93(7): 1464-70.
[http://dx.doi.org/10.1161/01.CIR.93.7.1464] [PMID: 8641037]

[6] Noriyasu K, Mabuchi M, Kuge Y, *et al.* Serial changes in BMIPP uptake in relation to thallium uptake in the rat myocardium after ischaemia. Eur J Nucl Med Mol Imaging 2003; 30(12): 1644-50.
[http://dx.doi.org/10.1007/s00259-003-1305-z] [PMID: 12955484]

[7] Ito K, Sugihara H, Kawasaki T, Katoh S, Azuma A, Nakagawa M. Dynamic changes in cardiac fatty acid metabolism in the stunned human myocardium. Ann Nucl Med 2001; 15(4): 343-50.
[http://dx.doi.org/10.1007/BF02988241] [PMID: 11577759]

[8] Evans JR, Gunton RW, Baker RG, Beanlands DS, Spears JC. Use of radioiodinated fatty acid for photoscans of the heart. Circ Res 1965; 16(1): 1-10.
[http://dx.doi.org/10.1161/01.RES.16.1.1] [PMID: 14252152]

[9] Schön HR, Schelbert HR, Najafi A, *et al.* C- 11 labeled palmitic acid for the noninvasive evaluation of regional myocardial fatty acid metabolism with positron-computed tomography. II. Kinetics of C- 11 palmitic acid in acutely ischemic myocardium. Am Heart J 1982; 103(4 Pt 1): 548-61.
[http://dx.doi.org/10.1016/0002-8703(82)90342-8] [PMID: 6801945]

[10] Poe ND, Robinson GD Jr, Graham LS, MacDonald NS. Experimental basis of myocardial imaging with 123I-labeled hexadecenoic acid. J Nucl Med 1976; 17(12): 1077-82.
[PMID: 993841]

[11] Poe ND, Robinson GD Jr, Zielinski FW, Cabeen WR Jr, Smith JW, Gomes AS. Myocardial imaging with 123I-hexadecenoic acid. Radiology 1977; 124(2): 419-24.
[http://dx.doi.org/10.1148/124.2.419] [PMID: 141683]

[12] Visser FC, van Eenige MJ, Westera G, *et al.* Metabolic fate of radioiodinated heptadecanoic acid in the normal canine heart. Circulation 1985; 72(3): 565-71.
[http://dx.doi.org/10.1161/01.CIR.72.3.565] [PMID: 4017208]

[13] Freundlieb C, Höck A, Vyska K, Feinendegen LE, Machulla HJ, Stöcklin G. Myocardial imaging and metabolic studies with [17-123I]iodoheptadecanoic acid. J Nucl Med 1980; 21(11): 1043-50.
[PMID: 7431103]

[14] Machulla HJ, Marsmann M, Dutschka K. Biochemical concept and synthesis of a radioiodinated phenylfatty acid for *in vivo* metabolic studies of the myocardium. Eur J Nucl Med 1980; 5(2): 171-3.
[http://dx.doi.org/10.1007/BF00252480] [PMID: 7379820]

[15] Reske SN, Sauer W, Machulla HJ, Winkler C. 15(p-[123I]Iodophenyl)pentadecanoic acid as tracer of lipid metabolism: comparison with [1-14C]palmitic acid in murine tissues. J Nucl Med 1984; 25(12): 1335-42.
[PMID: 6334144]

[16] Caldwell JH, Martin GV, Link JM, Krohn KA, Bassingthwaighte JB. Iodophenylpentadecanoic acid-myocardial blood flow relationship during maximal exercise with coronary occlusion. J Nucl Med

1990; 31(1): 99-105.
[PMID: 2295946]

[17] Ercan M, Senekowitsch R, Bauer R, Reidel G, Kriegel H, Pabst HW. *In vivo* and *in vitro* studies with ω-[rho-123I-phenyl]-pentadecanoic acid in rats. Int J Appl Radiat Isot 1983; 34(11): 1519-24.
[http://dx.doi.org/10.1016/0020-708X(83)90286-7] [PMID: 6642711]

[18] Hansen CL, Heo J, Oliner C, Van Decker W, Iskandrian AS. Prediction of improvement in left ventricular function with iodine-123-IPPA after coronary revascularization. J Nucl Med 1995; 36(11): 1987-93.
[PMID: 7472586]

[19] Iskandrian AS, Powers J, Cave V, Wasserleben V, Cassell D, Heo J. Assessment of myocardial viability by dynamic tomographic iodine 123 iodophenylpentadecanoic acid imaging: comparison with rest-redistribution thallium 201 imaging. J Nucl Cardiol 1995; 2(2 Pt 1): 101-9.
[PMID: 9420774]

[20] Ugolini V, Hansen CL, Kulkarni PV, Jansen DE, Akers MS, Corbett JR. Abnormal myocardial fatty acid metabolism in dilated cardiomyopathy detected by iodine-123 phenylpentadecanoic acid and tomographic imaging. Am J Cardiol 1988; 62(13): 923-8.
[http://dx.doi.org/10.1016/0002-9149(88)90894-6] [PMID: 3263035]

[21] Knapp FF Jr, Goodman MM, Callahan AP, Kirsch G. Radioiodinated 15-(p-iodophenyl)-- ,3-dimethylpentadecanoic acid: a useful new agent to evaluate myocardial fatty acid uptake. J Nucl Med 1986; 27(4): 521-31.
[PMID: 3712065]

[22] Ambrose KR, Owen BA, Goodman MM, Knapp FF Jr. Evaluation of the metabolism in rat hearts of two new radioiodinated 3-methyl-branched fatty acid myocardial imaging agents. Eur J Nucl Med 1987; 12(10): 486-91.
[http://dx.doi.org/10.1007/BF00620471] [PMID: 3569336]

[23] Sloof GW, Visser FC, van Lingen A, *et al.* Evaluation of heart-to-organ ratios of 123I-BMIPP and the dimethyl-substituted 123I-DMIPP fatty acid analogue in humans. Nucl Med Commun 1997; 18(11): 1065-70.
[http://dx.doi.org/10.1097/00006231-199711000-00010] [PMID: 9423207]

[24] Nohara R, Okuda K, Ogino M, *et al.* Evaluation of myocardial viability with iodine-123-BMIPP in a canine model. J Nucl Med 1996; 37(8): 1403-7.
[PMID: 8708784]

[25] Fujibayashi Y, Nohara R, Hosokawa R, *et al.* Metabolism and kinetics of iodine-123-BMIPP in canine myocardium. J Nucl Med 1996; 37(5): 757-61.
[PMID: 8965141]

[26] Kobayashi H, Kusakabe K, Momose M, *et al.* Evaluation of myocardial perfusion and fatty acid uptake using a single injection of iodine-123-BMIPP in patients with acute coronary syndromes. J Nucl Med 1998; 39(7): 1117-22.
[PMID: 9669379]

[27] Matsunari I, Saga T, Taki J, *et al.* Kinetics of iodine-123-BMIPP in patients with prior myocardial infarction: assessment with dynamic rest and stress images compared with stress thallium-201 SPECT. J Nucl Med 1994; 35(8): 1279-85.
[PMID: 8046479]

[28] Fujiwara S, Takeishi Y, Atsumi H, Takahashi K, Tomoike H. Fatty acid metabolic imaging with iodine-123-BMIPP for the diagnosis of coronary artery disease. J Nucl Med 1997; 38(2): 175-80.
[PMID: 9025730]

[29] Hatano T, Chikamori T, Usui Y, Morishima T, Hida S, Yamashina A. Diagnostic significance of positive I-123 BMIPP despite negative stress Tl-201 myocardial imaging in patients with suspected coronary artery disease. Circ J 2006; 70(2): 184-9.

[http://dx.doi.org/10.1253/circj.70.184] [PMID: 16434813]

[30] Tamaki N, Ohtani H, Yonekura Y, *et al.* Significance of fill-in after thallium-201 reinjection following delayed imaging: comparison with regional wall motion and angiographic findings. J Nucl Med 1990; 31(10): 1617-23.
[PMID: 2213182]

[31] Kawai Y, Tsukamoto E, Nozaki Y, Morita K, Sakurai M, Tamaki N. Significance of reduced uptake of iodinated fatty acid analogue for the evaluation of patients with acute chest pain. J Am Coll Cardiol 2001; 38(7): 1888-94.
[http://dx.doi.org/10.1016/S0735-1097(01)01634-5] [PMID: 11738290]

[32] Kontos MC, Dilsizian V, Weiland F, *et al.* Iodofiltic acid I 123 (BMIPP) fatty acid imaging improves initial diagnosis in emergency department patients with suspected acute coronary syndromes: a multicenter trial. J Am Coll Cardiol 2010; 56(4): 290-9.
[http://dx.doi.org/10.1016/j.jacc.2010.03.045] [PMID: 20633821]

[33] Mori T, Hayakawa M, Hattori K, *et al.* Exercise beta-methyl iodophenyl acid (BMIPP) and resting thalium delayed single photon emission computed tomography (SPECT) in the assessment of ischemia and viability. Jpn Circ J 1996; 60(1): 17-26.
[http://dx.doi.org/10.1253/jcj.60.17] [PMID: 8648880]

[34] Matsuo S, Nakajima K, Yamashina S, *et al.* Characterization of Japanese standards for myocardial sympathetic and metabolic imaging in comparison with perfusion imaging. Ann Nucl Med 2009; 23(6): 517-22.
[http://dx.doi.org/10.1007/s12149-009-0269-x] [PMID: 19521747]

[35] Furutani Y, Shiigi T, Nakamura Y, *et al.* Quantification of area at risk in acute myocardial infarction by tomographic imaging. J Nucl Med 1997; 38(12): 1875-82.
[PMID: 9430461]

[36] Hambÿe AS, Vervaet A, Dobbeleir A, Dendale P, Franken P. Prediction of functional outcome by quantification of sestamibi and BMIPP after acute myocardial infarction. Eur J Nucl Med 2000; 27(10): 1494-500.
[http://dx.doi.org/10.1007/s002590000332] [PMID: 11083538]

[37] Yoshinaga K, Matsuki T, Hashimoto A, Tsukamoto K, Nakata T, Tamaki N. Validation of automated quantitation of myocardial perfusion and fatty acid metabolism abnormalities on SPECT images. Circ J 2011; 75(9): 2187-95.
[http://dx.doi.org/10.1253/circj.CJ-10-1272] [PMID: 21747199]

[38] Nakata T, Hashimoto A, Matsuki T, Yoshinaga K, Tsukamoto K, Tamaki N. Prognostic value of automated SPECT scoring system for coronary artery disease in stress myocardial perfusion and fatty acid metabolism imaging. Int J Cardiovasc Imaging 2013; 29(1): 253-62.
[http://dx.doi.org/10.1007/s10554-012-0069-6] [PMID: 22782310]

[39] Sloof GW, Visser FC, Bax JJ, *et al.* Increased uptake of iodine-123-BMIPP in chronic ischemic heart disease: comparison with fluorine-18-FDG SPECT. J Nucl Med 1998; 39(2): 255-60.
[PMID: 9476931]

[40] Hambÿe AS, Vaerenberg MM, Dobbeleir AA, Van den Heuvel PA, Franken PR. Abnormal BMIPP uptake in chronically dysfunctional myocardial segments: correlation with contractile response to low-dose dobutamine. J Nucl Med 1998; 39(11): 1845-50.
[PMID: 9829568]

[41] Hashimoto Y, Yamabe H, Yokoyama M. Myocardial defect detected by 123I-BMIPP scintigraphy and left ventricular dysfunction in patients with idiopathic dilated cardiomyopathy. Ann Nucl Med 1996; 10(2): 225-30.
[http://dx.doi.org/10.1007/BF03165396] [PMID: 8800452]

[42] Hosokawa R, Nohara R, Fujibayashi Y, *et al.* Myocardial kinetics of iodine-123-BMIPP in canine myocardium after regional ischemia and reperfusion: implications for clinical SPECT. J Nucl Med

1997; 38(12): 1857-63.
[PMID: 9430458]

[43] Hosokawa R, Nohara R, Fujibayashi Y, *et al.* Metabolic fate of iodine-123-BMIPP in canine myocardium after administration of etomoxir. J Nucl Med 1996; 37(11): 1836-40.
[PMID: 8917188]

[44] Hosokawa R, Nohara R, Fujibayashi Y, *et al.* Myocardial metabolism of 123I-BMIPP in a canine model with ischemia: implications of perfusion-metabolism mismatch on SPECT images in patients with ischemic heart disease. J Nucl Med 1999; 40(3): 471-8.
[PMID: 10086713]

[45] Higuchi T, Taki J, Nakajima K, Kinuya S, Namura M, Tonami N. Time course of discordant BMIPP and thallium uptake after ischemia and reperfusion in a rat model. J Nucl Med 2005; 46(1): 172-5.
[PMID: 15632049]

[46] Tamaki N, Kawamoto M, Yonekura Y, *et al.* Regional metabolic abnormality in relation to perfusion and wall motion in patients with myocardial infarction: assessment with emission tomography using an iodinated branched fatty acid analog. J Nucl Med 1992; 33(5): 659-67.
[PMID: 1569474]

[47] Franken PR, De Geeter F, Dendale P, Demoor D, Block P, Bossuyt A. Abnormal free fatty acid uptake in subacute myocardial infarction after coronary thrombolysis: correlation with wall motion and inotropic reserve. J Nucl Med 1994; 35(11): 1758-65.
[PMID: 7965152]

[48] Reimer KA, Jennings RB. The "wavefront phenomenon" of myocardial ischemic cell death. II. Transmural progression of necrosis within the framework of ischemic bed size (myocardium at risk) and collateral flow. Lab Invest 1979; 40(6): 633-44.
[PMID: 449273]

[49] Califf RM, Phillips HR III, Hindman MC, *et al.* Prognostic value of a coronary artery jeopardy score. J Am Coll Cardiol 1985; 5(5): 1055-63.
[http://dx.doi.org/10.1016/S0735-1097(85)80005-X] [PMID: 3989116]

[50] Hasegawa S, Kusuoka H, Fukuchi K, Hori M, Nishimura T. Estimation of the area at risk in myocardial infarction of rats by means of I-123 beta-methyliodophenyl pentadecanoic acid imaging. Ann Nucl Med 2000; 14(5): 347-52.
[http://dx.doi.org/10.1007/BF02988694] [PMID: 11108163]

[51] Kawai Y, Tsukamoto E, Nozaki Y, Kishino K, Kohya T, Tamaki N. Use of 123I-BMIPP single-photon emission tomography to estimate areas at risk following successful revascularization in patients with acute myocardial infarction. Eur J Nucl Med 1998; 25(10): 1390-5.
[http://dx.doi.org/10.1007/s002590050313] [PMID: 9818278]

[52] Katsunuma E, Kurokawa S, Takahashi M, Fukuda N, Kurosawa T, Izumi T. Usefulness of BMIPP SPECT to evaluate myocardial viability, contractile reserve and coronary stenotic progression after reperfusion in acute myocardial infarction. Jpn Heart J 2001; 42(4): 435-49.
[http://dx.doi.org/10.1536/jhj.42.435] [PMID: 11693280]

[53] Tanaka R, Nakamura T. Time course evaluation of myocardial perfusion after reperfusion therapy by 99mTc-tetrofosmin SPECT in patients with acute myocardial infarction. J Nucl Med 2001; 42(9): 1351-8.
[PMID: 11535724]

[54] Mochizuki T, Murase K, Higashino H, *et al.* Ischemic "memory image" in acute myocardial infarction of 123I-BMIPP after reperfusion therapy: a comparison with 99mTc-pyrophosphate and 201Tl dual-isotope SPECT. Ann Nucl Med 2002; 16(8): 563-8.
[http://dx.doi.org/10.1007/BF02988634] [PMID: 12593422]

[55] Schulz R, Heusch G. Characterization of hibernating and stunned myocardium Eur Heart J 1995; 16 (J): 19-25.

[http://dx.doi.org/10.1093/eurheartj/16.suppl_J.19]

[56] Kawamoto M, Tamaki N, Yonekura Y, *et al.* Combined study with I-123 fatty acid and thallium-201 to assess ischemic myocardium: comparison with thallium redistribution and glucose metabolism. Ann Nucl Med 1994; 8(1): 47-54.
[http://dx.doi.org/10.1007/BF03164986] [PMID: 8204397]

[57] Tamaki N, Tadamura E, Kawamoto M, *et al.* Decreased uptake of iodinated branched fatty acid analog indicates metabolic alterations in ischemic myocardium. J Nucl Med 1995; 36(11): 1974-80.
[PMID: 7472584]

[58] Ito T, Tanouchi J, Kato J, *et al.* Recovery of impaired left ventricular function in patients with acute myocardial infarction is predicted by the discordance in defect size on 123I-BMIPP and 201Tl SPET images. Eur J Nucl Med 1996; 23(8): 917-23.
[http://dx.doi.org/10.1007/BF01084365] [PMID: 8753680]

[59] Franken PR, Dendale P, De Geeter F, Demoor D, Bossuyt A, Block P. Prediction of functional outcome after myocardial infarction using BMIPP and sestamibi scintigraphy. J Nucl Med 1996; 37(5): 718-22.
[PMID: 8965133]

[60] Hashimoto A, Nakata T, Tsuchihashi K, Tanaka S, Fujimori K, Iimura O. Postischemic functional recovery and BMIPP uptake after primary percutaneous transluminal coronary angioplasty in acute myocardial infarction. Am J Cardiol 1996; 77(1): 25-30.
[http://dx.doi.org/10.1016/S0002-9149(97)89129-1] [PMID: 8540452]

[61] Nishimura T, Nishimura S, Kajiya T, *et al.* Prediction of functional recovery and prognosis in patients with acute myocardial infarction by 123I-BMIPP and 201Tl myocardial single photon emission computed tomography: a multicenter trial. Ann Nucl Med 1998; 12(5): 237-48.
[http://dx.doi.org/10.1007/BF03164908] [PMID: 9839484]

[62] Naruse H, Arii T, Kondo T, *et al.* Clinical usefulness of iodine 123-labeled fatty acid imaging in patients with acute myocardial infarction. J Nucl Cardiol 1998; 5(3): 275-84.
[http://dx.doi.org/10.1016/S1071-3581(98)90129-5] [PMID: 9669582]

[63] Tani T, Teragaki M, Watanabe H, *et al.* Detecting viable myocardium and predicting functional improvement: comparisons of positron emission tomography, rest-redistribution thallium-201 single-photon emission computed tomography (SPECT), exercise thallium-201 reinjection SPECT, I-123 BMIPP SPECT and dobutamine stress echocardiography. Circ J 2004; 68(10): 950-7.
[http://dx.doi.org/10.1253/circj.68.950] [PMID: 15459470]

[64] Seki H, Toyama T, Higuchi K, *et al.* Prediction of functional improvement of ischemic myocardium with (123I-BMIPP SPECT and 99mTc-tetrofosmin SPECT imaging: a study of patients with large acute myocardial infarction and receiving revascularization therapy. Circ J 2005; 69(3): 311-9.
[http://dx.doi.org/10.1253/circj.69.311] [PMID: 15731537]

[65] Biswas SK, Sarai M, Toyama H, *et al.* (123)I-BMIPP and (99m)Tc-TF discordance on myocardial scintigraphy and it's correlation with functional recovery following acute myocardial infarction: role of conventional echocardiography. Int J Cardiovasc Imaging 2009; 25(8): 765-75.
[http://dx.doi.org/10.1007/s10554-009-9497-3] [PMID: 19768573]

[66] Biswas SK, Sarai M, Yamada A, *et al.* Fatty acid metabolism and myocardial perfusion imaging for the evaluation of global left ventricular dysfunction following acute myocardial infarction: comparisons with echocardiography. Int J Cardiol 2010; 138(3): 290-9.
[http://dx.doi.org/10.1016/j.ijcard.2008.11.170] [PMID: 19157585]

[67] Biswas SK, Sarai M, Yamada A, *et al.* The washout rate of (123)I-BMIPP and the evolution of left ventricular function in patients with successfully reperfused ST-segment elevation myocardial infarction: comparisons with the echocardiography. Int J Cardiovasc Imaging 2010; 26 (Suppl. 1): 155-64.
[http://dx.doi.org/10.1007/s10554-009-9575-6] [PMID: 20058081]

[68] Nakata T, Kobayashi T, Tamaki N, *et al.* Prognostic value of impaired myocardial fatty acid uptake in patients with acute myocardial infarction. Nucl Med Commun 2000; 21(10): 897-906. [http://dx.doi.org/10.1097/00006231-200010000-00003] [PMID: 11130330]

[69] Nanasato M, Hirayama H, Ando A, *et al.* Incremental predictive value of myocardial scintigraphy with 123I-BMIPP in patients with acute myocardial infarction treated with primary percutaneous coronary intervention. Eur J Nucl Med Mol Imaging 2004; 31(11): 1512-21. [http://dx.doi.org/10.1007/s00259-004-1556-3] [PMID: 15232655]

[70] Fukushima Y, Toba M, Ishihara K, *et al.* Usefulness of 201TlCl/ 123I-BMIPP dual-myocardial SPECT for patients with non-ST segment elevation myocardial infarction. Ann Nucl Med 2008; 22(5): 363-9. [http://dx.doi.org/10.1007/s12149-007-0126-8] [PMID: 18600413]

[71] Inaba Y, Bergmann SR. Prognostic value of myocardial metabolic imaging with BMIPP in the spectrum of coronary artery disease: a systematic review. J Nucl Cardiol 2010; 17(1): 61-70. [http://dx.doi.org/10.1007/s12350-009-9157-y] [PMID: 19851821]

[72] Tateno M, Tamaki N, Yukihiro M, *et al.* Assessment of fatty acid uptake in ischemic heart disease without myocardial infarction. J Nucl Med 1996; 37(12): 1981-5. [PMID: 8970518]

[73] Takeishi Y, Sukekawa H, Saito H, *et al.* Impaired myocardial fatty acid metabolism detected by 123I-BMIPP in patients with unstable angina pectoris: comparison with perfusion imaging by 99mTc-sestamibi. Ann Nucl Med 1995; 9(3): 125-30. [http://dx.doi.org/10.1007/BF03165038] [PMID: 8534584]

[74] Saitoh M, Hasegawa K, Hasegawa K, Kondoh T, Yanagawa T. Detection of coronary artery disease using 12-lead electrocardiogram and simultaneous dual myocardial imaging with iodine-123-be-a-methyl iodophenyl-pentadecanoic acid (BMIPP) and thallium-201 in patients with unstable angina. Intern Med 1995; 34(11): 1064-70. [http://dx.doi.org/10.2169/internalmedicine.34.1064] [PMID: 8774965]

[75] Inaba Y, Bergmann SR. Diagnostic accuracy of β-methyl-p-[123I]-iodophenyl-pentadecanoic acid (BMIPP) imaging: a meta-analysis. J Nucl Cardiol 2008; 15(3): 345-52. [http://dx.doi.org/10.1016/j.nuclcard.2008.02.019] [PMID: 18513641]

[76] Morimoto K, Tomoda H, Yoshitake M, Aoki N, Handa S, Suzuki Y. Prediction of coronary artery lesions in unstable angina by iodine 123 beta-methyl iodophenyl pentadecanoic acid (BMIPP), a fatty acid analogue, single photon emission computed tomography at rest. Angiology 1999; 50(8): 639-48. [http://dx.doi.org/10.1177/000331979905000804] [PMID: 10451231]

[77] Matsuki T, Tamaki N, Nakata T, *et al.* Prognostic value of fatty acid imaging in patients with angina pectoris without prior myocardial infarction: comparison with stress thallium imaging. Eur J Nucl Med Mol Imaging 2004; 31(12): 1585-91. [http://dx.doi.org/10.1007/s00259-004-1551-8] [PMID: 15583913]

[78] Dilsizian V, Bateman TM, Bergmann SR, *et al.* Metabolic imaging with beta-methyl-p-[(123-I]-iodophenyl-pentadecanoic acid identifies ischemic memory after demand ischemia. Circulation 2005; 112(14): 2169-74. [http://dx.doi.org/10.1161/CIRCULATIONAHA.104.530428] [PMID: 16186423]

[79] Nakajima K, Shimizu K, Taki J, *et al.* Utility of iodine-123-BMIPP in the diagnosis and follow-up of vasospastic angina. J Nucl Med 1995; 36(11): 1934-40. [PMID: 7472578]

[80] Watanabe K, Ohta Y, Toba K, *et al.* Abnormal fatty acid metabolism in patients with coronary vasospasm. Ann Nucl Med 1999; 13(1): 33-41. [http://dx.doi.org/10.1007/BF03165425] [PMID: 10202946]

[81] Watanabe K, Takahashi T, Miyajima S, *et al.* Myocardial sympathetic denervation, fatty acid

metabolism, and left ventricular wall motion in vasospastic angina. J Nucl Med 2002; 43(11): 1476-81.
[PMID: 12411551]

[82] Yamabe H, Fujiwara S, Rin K, *et al.* Resting 123I-BMIPP scintigraphy for detection of organic coronary stenosis and therapeutic outcome in patients with chest pain. Ann Nucl Med 2000; 14(3): 187-92.
[http://dx.doi.org/10.1007/BF02987858] [PMID: 10921483]

[83] Kawai Y, Morita K, Nozaki Y, Ohkusa T, Sakurai M, Tamaki N. Diagnostic value of 123I-betamethyl-p-iodophenyl-pentadecanoic acid (BMIPP) single photon emission computed tomography (SPECT) in patients with chest pain. Comparison with rest-stress 99mTc-tetrofosmin SPECT and coronary angiography. Circ J 2004; 68(6): 547-52.
[http://dx.doi.org/10.1253/circj.68.547] [PMID: 15170090]

[84] Takeishi Y, Sukekawa H, Saito H, *et al.* Clinical significance of decreased myocardial uptake of 123I-BMIPP in patients with stable effort angina pectoris. Nucl Med Commun 1995; 16(12): 1002-8.
[http://dx.doi.org/10.1097/00006231-199512000-00003] [PMID: 8719980]

[85] Kageyama H, Morita K, Katoh C, *et al.* Reduced 123I-BMIPP uptake implies decreased myocardial flow reserve in patients with chronic stable angina. Eur J Nucl Med Mol Imaging 2006; 33(1): 6-12.
[http://dx.doi.org/10.1007/s00259-005-1863-3] [PMID: 16041617]

[86] Akashi YJ, Kida K, Suzuki K, *et al.* The significance of 123I-BMIPP delayed scintigraphic imaging in cardiac patients. Int J Cardiol 2007; 117(2): 145-51.
[http://dx.doi.org/10.1016/j.ijcard.2006.04.056] [PMID: 16843549]

[87] Taki J, Nakajima K, Matsunari I, Bunko H, Takada S, Tonami N. Impairment of regional fatty acid uptake in relation to wall motion and thallium-201 uptake in ischaemic but viable myocardium: assessment with iodine-123-labelled beta-methyl-branched fatty acid. Eur J Nucl Med 1995; 22(12): 1385-92.
[http://dx.doi.org/10.1007/BF01791146] [PMID: 8586083]

[88] Matsunari I, Fujino S, Taki J, *et al.* Impaired fatty acid uptake in ischemic but viable myocardium identified by thallium-201 reinjection. Am Heart J 1996; 131(3): 458-65.
[http://dx.doi.org/10.1016/S0002-8703(96)90523-2] [PMID: 8604624]

[89] Kudoh T, Tadamura E, Tamaki N, *et al.* Iodinated free fatty acid and 201Tl uptake in chronically hypoperfused myocardium: histologic correlation study. J Nucl Med 2000; 41(2): 293-6.
[PMID: 10688114]

[90] Taki J, Nakajima K, Matsunari I, *et al.* Assessment of improvement of myocardial fatty acid uptake and function after revascularization using iodine-123-BMIPP. J Nucl Med 1997; 38(10): 1503-10.
[PMID: 9379183]

[91] Hambye AS, Dobbeleir AA, Vervaet AM, Van den Heuvel PA, Franken PR. BMIPP imaging to improve the value of sestamibi scintigraphy for predicting functional outcome in severe chronic ischemic left ventricular dysfunction. J Nucl Med 1999; 40(9): 1468-76.
[PMID: 10492367]

[92] Chikamori T, Fujita H, Nanasato M, Toba M, Nishimura T. Prognostic value of I-123 15-(--iodophenyl)-3-(R,S) methylpentadecanoic acid myocardial imaging in patients with known or suspected coronary artery disease. J Nucl Cardiol 2005; 12(2): 172-8.
[http://dx.doi.org/10.1016/j.nuclcard.2004.12.293] [PMID: 15812371]

[93] Tamaki N, Tadamura E, Kudoh T, *et al.* Prognostic value of iodine-123 labelled BMIPP fatty acid analogue imaging in patients with myocardial infarction. Eur J Nucl Med 1996; 23(3): 272-9.
[http://dx.doi.org/10.1007/BF00837625] [PMID: 8599958]

[94] Fukuzawa S, Ozawa S, Shimada K, Sugioka J, Inagaki M. Prognostic values of perfusion-metabolic mismatch in Tl-201 and BMIPP scintigraphic imaging in patients with chronic coronary artery disease and left ventricular dysfunction undergoing revascularization. Ann Nucl Med 2002; 16(2): 109-15.

[http://dx.doi.org/10.1007/BF02993713] [PMID: 12043904]

[95] Ohtsuki K, Sugihara H, Kuribayashi T, Nakagawa M. Impairment of BMIPP accumulation at junction of ventricular septum and left and right ventricular free walls in hypertrophic cardiomyopathy. J Nucl Med 1999; 40(12): 2007-13.
[PMID: 10616878]

[96] Kuribayashi T, Roberts WC. Myocardial disarray at junction of ventricular septum and left and right ventricular free walls in hypertrophic cardiomyopathy. Am J Cardiol 1992; 70(15): 1333-40.
[http://dx.doi.org/10.1016/0002-9149(92)90771-P] [PMID: 1442587]

[97] Takeishi Y, Chiba J, Abe S, Tonooka I, Komatani A, Tomoike H. Heterogeneous myocardial distribution of iodine-123 15-(p-iodophenyl)-3-R,S-methylpentadecanoic acid (BMIPP) in patients with hypertrophic cardiomyopathy. Eur J Nucl Med 1992; 19(9): 775-82.
[http://dx.doi.org/10.1007/BF00182819] [PMID: 1396872]

[98] Kurata C, Tawarahara K, Taguchi T, *et al.* Myocardial emission computed tomography with iodine-123-labeled beta-methyl-branched fatty acid in patients with hypertrophic cardiomyopathy. J Nucl Med 1992; 33(1): 6-13.
[PMID: 1530969]

[99] Nishimura T, Uehara T, Shimonagata T, Nagata S, Haze K. Clinical results with beta-methyl-p-(123I)iodophenylpentadecanoic acid, single-photon emission computed tomography in cardiac disease. J Nucl Cardiol 1994; 1(2 Pt 2): S65-71.
[http://dx.doi.org/10.1007/BF02940071] [PMID: 9420700]

[100] Nishimura T, Nagata S, Uehara T, *et al.* Prognosis of hypertrophic cardiomyopathy: assessment by 123I-BMIPP (beta-methyl-p-(123I)iodophenyl pentadecanoic acid) myocardial single photon emission computed tomography. Ann Nucl Med 1996; 10(1): 71-8.
[http://dx.doi.org/10.1007/BF03165056] [PMID: 8814730]

[101] Cannon RO III, Dilsizian V, O'Gara PT, *et al.* Myocardial metabolic, hemodynamic, and electrocardiographic significance of reversible thallium-201 abnormalities in hypertrophic cardiomyopathy. Circulation 1991; 83(5): 1660-7.
[http://dx.doi.org/10.1161/01.CIR.83.5.1660] [PMID: 2022023]

[102] Taki J, Nakajima K, Bunko H, Shimizu M, Taniguchi M, Hisada K. 123I-labelled BMIPP fatty acid myocardial scintigraphy in patients with hypertropic cardiomyopathy: SPECT comparison with stress 201Tl. Nucl Med Commun 1993; 14(3): 181-8.
[http://dx.doi.org/10.1097/00006231-199303000-00006] [PMID: 8455908]

[103] Tadamura E, Kudoh T, Hattori N, *et al.* Impairment of BMIPP uptake precedes abnormalities in oxygen and glucose metabolism in hypertrophic cardiomyopathy. J Nucl Med 1998; 39(3): 390-6.
[PMID: 9529280]

[104] Shimonagata T, Nishimura T, Uehara T, *et al.* Discrepancies between myocardial perfusion and free fatty acid metabolism in patients with hypertrophic cardiomyopathy. Nucl Med Commun 1993; 14(11): 1005-13.
[http://dx.doi.org/10.1097/00006231-199311000-00012] [PMID: 8290156]

[105] Narita M, Kurihara T. Is I-123-beta-methyl-p-iodophenyl-methylpentadecanoic acid imaging useful to evaluate asymptomatic patients with hypertrophic cardiomyopathy? I-123 BMIPP imaging to evaluate asymptomatic hypertrophic cardiomyopathy. Int J Cardiovasc Imaging 2003; 19(6): 499-510.
[http://dx.doi.org/10.1023/B:CAIM.0000004262.48898.5d] [PMID: 14690189]

[106] Höck A, Freundlieb C, Vyska K, Lösse B, Erbel R, Feinendegen LE. Myocardial imaging and metabolic studies with [17-123I]iodoheptadecanoic acid in patients with idiopathic congestive cardiomyopathy. J Nucl Med 1983; 24(1): 22-8.
[PMID: 6848699]

[107] Ishida Y, Yasumura Y, Nagaya N, *et al.* Myocardial imaging with 123I-BMIPP in patients with congestive heart failure. Int J Card Imaging 1999; 15(1): 71-7.

[http://dx.doi.org/10.1023/A:1006152804670] [PMID: 10453405]

[108] Yoshinaga K, Tahara M, Torii H, Kihara K. Predicting the effects on patients with dilated cardiomyopathy of beta-blocker therapy, by using iodine-123 15-(p-iodophenyl)-3- R,S-methylpentadecanoic acid (BMIPP) myocardial scintigraphy. Ann Nucl Med 1998; 12(6): 341-7. [http://dx.doi.org/10.1007/BF03164923] [PMID: 9972371]

[109] Ito T, Hoshida S, Nishino M, *et al.* Relationship between evaluation by quantitative fatty acid myocardial scintigraphy and response to beta-blockade therapy in patients with dilated cardiomyopathy. Eur J Nucl Med 2001; 28(12): 1811-6. [http://dx.doi.org/10.1007/s00259-001-0668-2] [PMID: 11734920]

[110] Yamauchi S, Takeishi Y, Minamihaba O, *et al.* Angiotensin-converting enzyme inhibition improves cardiac fatty acid metabolism in patients with congestive heart failure. Nucl Med Commun 2003; 24(8): 901-6. [http://dx.doi.org/10.1097/01.mnm.0000084579.51410.69] [PMID: 12869823]

[111] Kim Y, Sawada Y, Fujiwara G, Chiba H, Nishimura T. Therapeutic effect of co-enzyme Q10 on idiopathic dilated cardiomyopathy: assessment by iodine-123 labelled 15-(p-iodophenyl)-3(R-S)-methylpentadecanoic acid myocardial single-photon emission tomography. Eur J Nucl Med 1997; 24(6): 629-34. [http://dx.doi.org/10.1007/BF00841400] [PMID: 9169569]

[112] Zavadovsky KV, Gulya MO, Lishmanov YB, Lebedev DI. Perfusion and metabolic scintigraphy with (123)I-BMIPP in prognosis of cardiac resynchronization therapy in patients with dilated cardiomyopathy. Ann Nucl Med 2016; 30(5): 325-33. [http://dx.doi.org/10.1007/s12149-016-1064-0] [PMID: 26872805]

[113] Inoue A, Fujimoto S, Yamashina S, Yamazaki J. Prediction of cardiac events in patients with dilated cardiomyopathy using 123I-BMIPP and 201Tl myocardial scintigraphy. Ann Nucl Med 2007; 21(7): 399-404. [http://dx.doi.org/10.1007/s12149-007-0045-8] [PMID: 17876553]

[114] Nakae I, Matsuo S, Koh T, Mitsunami K, Horie M. Iodine-123 BMIPP scintigraphy in the evaluation of patients with heart failure. Acta Radiol 2006; 47(8): 810-6. [http://dx.doi.org/10.1080/02841850600855354] [PMID: 17050361]

[115] Sasaki R, Mitani I, Usui T, *et al.* Clinical value of iodine-123 beta-methyliodophenyl pentadecanoic acid (BMIPP) myocardial single photon emission computed tomography for predicting cardiac death among patients with chronic heart failure. Circ J 2003; 67(11): 918-24. [http://dx.doi.org/10.1253/circj.67.918] [PMID: 14578597]

[116] Sato H, Tateishi H, Uchida T. Takotsubo-type cardiomyopathy due to multivessel spasm.Clinical aspect of myocardial injury: from ischemia to heart failure. Kagakuhyouronsha 1990; pp. 56-64.

[117] Kurisu S, Inoue I, Kawagoe T, *et al.* Myocardial perfusion and fatty acid metabolism in patients with tako-tsubo-like left ventricular dysfunction. J Am Coll Cardiol 2003; 41(5): 743-8. [http://dx.doi.org/10.1016/S0735-1097(02)02924-8] [PMID: 12628716]

[118] Owa M, Aizawa K, Urasawa N, *et al.* Emotional stress-induced 'ampulla cardiomyopathy': discrepancy between the metabolic and sympathetic innervation imaging performed during the recovery course. Jpn Circ J 2001; 65(4): 349-52. [http://dx.doi.org/10.1253/jcj.65.349] [PMID: 11316138]

[119] Ito K, Sugihara H, Kawasaki T, *et al.* Assessment of ampulla (Takotsubo) cardiomyopathy with coronary angiography, two-dimensional echocardiography and 99mTc-tetrofosmin myocardial single photon emission computed tomography. Ann Nucl Med 2001; 15(4): 351-5. [http://dx.doi.org/10.1007/BF02988242] [PMID: 11577760]

[120] Matsuo S, Nakajima K, Kinuya S, Yamagishi M. Diagnostic utility of 123I-BMIPP imaging in patients with Takotsubo cardiomyopathy. J Cardiol 2014; 64(1): 49-56. [http://dx.doi.org/10.1016/j.jjcc.2013.10.019] [PMID: 24331764]

CHAPTER 8

Recent Advances in BMIPP Imaging

Takashi Kudo*, Altay Myssayev and **Reiko Ideguchi**

Department of Radioisotope Medicine, Atomic Bomb Disease Institute, Nagasaki University, Nagasaki, Japan

Abstract: Impairments in the myocardial metabolism of fatty acids occurs not only as a result of ischemic insults, but also with any type of myocardial damage, such as radiation injuries and genetic alterations. Changes in myocardial metabolism persist after these events. BMIPP (I-123-labeled beta-methyl-p-iode-phenyl-pentadecanoic acid) is a unique radiopharmaceutical with the ability to image changes in myocardial fatty acid metabolism. Therefore, BMIPP has been widely used in the diagnosis and risk stratification of ischemic heart diseases, cardiomyopathies, and other disease conditions in Japan since its introduction to the commercial market in 1993. The main clinical target is the detection of severe ischemia and a damaged myocardium due to acute and chronic coronary artery diseases without a stress test. A recent study on BMIPP in a population of hemodialysis patients revealed that it also has potential as an important tool for managing and triaging patients with a poor prognosis in this specific population group. Furthermore, it is useful for differential diagnoses and prognostic assessments of cardiomyopathies, such as hypertrophic, dilated, and Takotsubo cardiomyopathies. The clinical utility of BMIPP has recently expanded to radiation injuries, chronic thromboembolism pulmonary hypertension (CTEPH), triglyceride deposit cardiomyovasculopathy (TGCV), and mitochondrial cardiomyopathy. The proper use of BMIPP provides important information that cannot be obtained using myocardial perfusion imaging (MPI). BMIPP; more than meets the MPI.

Keywords: BMIPP, Cardiac Sarcoidosis, Cardiomyopathy, Chronic Thromboembolism Pulmonary Hypertension, Dilated Cardiomyopathy, Fatty Acid Metabolism, Hemodialysis, Heart Failure, Hypertrophic Cardiomyopathy, Ischemia, Mitochondrial Cardiomyopathy, Prognosis, Radiation, Risk Assessment, Solid State Detector, Takotsubo Cardiomyopathy, Triglyceride Deposit Cardiomyovasculopathy.

BMIPP: MECHANISM OF UPTAKE AND THEORY FOR DIAGNOSIS

BMIPP (I-123 labeled beta-methyl-*p*-iodo-phenyl-pentadecanoic acid) is a branched long chain fatty acid tracer that images the myocardial uptake and

* **Corresponding author Takashi Kudo:** Department of Radioisotope Medicine, Atomic Bomb Disease Institute, Nagasaki University, Nagasaki, Japan; Tel: +81958197101; Fax: +81958197104; E-mail: tkudo123@nagasaki-u.ac.jp

Shinro Matsuo (Ed.)

metabolism of free fatty acids (FFA). The energy source of the myocardium is mainly FFA. When the myocardium is damaged not only due to ischemic heart disease, but also under other conditions, such as hypertrophy and cardiomyopathy, the main source of energy switches from FFA to glucose because glucose provides ATP even in the presence of a low oxygen supply. Thus, the hypothesis of "if it is possible to image the metabolism of fatty acids, myocardial damage may also be imaged" was proposed. This was the main concept for the development of BMIPP. The following properties of tracers are required to image myocardial fatty acid metabolism. The tracer needs to enter the myocardium according to fatty acid transfer and remain for a sufficient period of time for the acquisition of SPECT images. To fulfil this requirement, several tracers labeled with I-123 have been developed, such as radio-iodinated branched long chain fatty acids (BMIPP [1], I-123 labeled 15-(p-iodophenyl)-9-R,S-methyl pentadecanoic acid (9MPA) [2]), radio-iodinated straight long chain fatty acids (I-123 labeled phenylpentadecanoic acid (IPPA) [3], and I-123 labeled 17-iodine-heptadecanoic acid (HDA) [4]). BMIPP was developed according to the above concept and is still widely used in clinical settings even 20 years after its development. Myocardial perfusion imaging (MPI) using Tc-99m-labeled tracers (or Tl-201) images perfusion distribution to the myocardium, namely, energy supply to the myocardium. BMIPP images myocardial metabolic changes, and, thus, myocardial damage itself. Based on this concept, it is possible to extract more important information from BMIPP than from MPI.

Recent Findings on the Uptake/Metabolism Mechanism CD36

BMIPP is considered to be trapped in the myocardium through the same process as physiological fatty acids. Thus, under normal conditions, BMIPP is expected to accumulate homogenously in the myocardium. However, previous studies reported some groups of patients in which myocardial BMIPP uptake was not detected [5, 6]. This phenomenon is known to be related to a deficiency in CD36 [6, 7], which plays a key role in fatty acid uptake in various tissues. Previous human studies showed increased FDG uptake in these patients [5, 6]. This accelerated FDG uptake was recently proven in a mouse model with the knockout of CD36 [8]. They also demonstrated that the myocardial concentration of ATP was preserved in CD36 knockout mice by compensation *via* glucose and ketone metabolism. CD36 is expressed not only in the heart, but also in skeletal muscle, the endothelium, macrophages, platelets, and adipose tissue. A recent study reported that CD36 is indispensable for thermogenesis in brown adipose tissue (BAT) [9]. The uptake of FDG and BMIPP in BAT was severely impaired in CD36-deficient rats. These findings indicate that a relationship exists between FDG, BMIPP, and heat production mechanisms in humans.

Single Ischemic Insult

The accelerated myocardial uptake of BMIPP was reported in several animal studies, which is discordant with findings obtained in clinical patients consistently showing the decreased uptake of BMIPP [10, 11]. A recent study by Fukushima *et al.* proved this phenomenon in an isolated rat heart model with a tracer kinetic analysis [12]. They demonstrated that K_1 (rate of uptake to the myocardium) was decreased with MIBI, but increased with BMIPP in a 15-30 min no-flow ischemia model. This phenomenon was partly suggested by previous studies. Hosokawa *et al.* investigated the kinetics of BMIPP in detail in a dog ischemia model and revealed that tracer retention was not reduced, whereas the back diffusion of non-metabolized BMIPP was accelerated in a single ischemic event [13, 14]. These discrepancies between the findings obtained from animal models and clinical patients suggest the difficulty of introducing data from experiments to clinical disease conditions. In humans, ischemia occurs in the atherosclerotic coronary artery. In the background of one symptomatic ischemic event, there are frequent subclinical ischemic events. Pure single ischemic events, such as those observed in animal models, are unlikely to occur in human patients with coronary artery disease. Based on the memory effect of BMIPP, the finding of BMIPP in human subjects is the sum of not only a visible ischemic event, but all symptomatic and asymptomatic events.

ISCHEMIC HEART DISEASE

When damage occurs in the myocardium without necrosis/apoptosis, the damaged but viable myocardium shows the reduced uptake of BMIPP. This phenomenon remains even after recovery from low perfusion. Therefore, the reduced uptake of BMIPP shows a memory (persistence?) of myocardial damage. This is a very unique characteristic from other perfusion tracers that provide real-time information on the myocardium only. The unique advantages of BMIPP are as follows.

1. Showing a memory of acute myocardial damage, such as acute coronary syndrome (ACS) after an acute event.
2. Visualizing the memory of severe ischemic damage in patients who are not suitable for real-time stress/resting MPI.
3. Evaluating ischemic damage that repeatedly occurs.
4. Evaluating myocardial damage other than ischemic insults.

A large number of studies have evaluated the diagnostic value of BMIPP for coronary artery diseases (CAD) [15], including vasospastic angina [16], worsening (progressive?) angina [17], unstable angina [18], ACS [19], and hemodialysis (HD) patients with CAD [20]. Inaba *et al.* performed a meta-analysis [21] to define the diagnostic accuracy of BMIPP for CAD. They concluded that BMIPP has moderate sensitivity and high specificity.

Acute Conditions: Unstable Angina and ACS

The condition of patients with ACS, including unstable angina, changes rapidly, and, thus, it is important but is very hard to evaluate the condition of the myocardium during very early stage of ACS in real-time.

Using BMIPP, the condition of the myocardial damage can be evaluated even after the actual ACS events. In an early study on unstable angina, Takeishi *et al.* revealed very abnormal BMIPP images associated with severe CAD, which led to proper management with coronary interventions, such as PCI and CABG. A total of 82% of patients with severely abnormal BMIPP findings underwent interventions, in contrast to only 22% of those with normal BMIPP findings [18]. Saito *et al.* suggested the use of electrocardiogram (ECG) findings with BMIPP to overcome the low sensitivity of BMIPP image findings alone for patients with unstable angina [22]. A recent study that performed BMIPP imaging one day after the cessation of acute chest pain showed that BMIPP imaging can distinguish the patients with significant coronary disease (including vasospastic angina) from those without stenosis or spasm in coronary artery [19]. The findings of this study showed that patients with acute chest pain, but no coronary disease had almost normal BMIPP uptake, suggesting that BMIPP imaging is very helpful for triaging patients with acute chest pain with equivocal evidence of ACS in daily clinical practice.

Subacute Conditions and After Interventions

In patients with acute myocardial infarction (AMI), it is very important to evaluate the condition of the myocardium in order to select proper therapeutic interventions. Decreased BMIPP uptake indicates a damaged (=damaged but viable + non-viable) myocardium. A perfusion defect theoretically indicates scar tissue. Thus, differences between BMIPP and perfusion defects (a so-called mismatch) indicate the extent and severity of a damaged but viable myocardium, which is crucial for the selection of proper therapeutic procedures. This information on a viable myocardium may theoretically be obtained with an FDG/perfusion mismatch. However, due to inflammatory cell activity in an infarcted myocardium, the image interpretation of FDG PET just after AMI is difficult. Additionally, recent studies indicated that under AMI conditions, some patients showed larger FDG defects than perfusion (a reverse flow-glucose metabolism mismatch), which resulted in successful PCI [23] and preserved oxygen metabolism [24]. These conflicting findings indicate that FDG PET is not appropriate for use in AMI patients.

The mismatch between BMIPP and perfusion (the defect of BMIPP being larger than that of perfusion) after AMI indicates that the area is still viable, but was previously damaged. This finding is available even after successful PCI procedures because BMIPP can memorize myocardial damage. This area is called a "risked area". The myocardium in this area is on the brink of survival and death, and may receive great benefits from proper management, but is also expected to deteriorate to a poor condition when management is not properly performed. Previous studies indicated that patients with a BMIPP/perfusion mismatch showed good wall motion recovery after coronary interventions, such as PCI and CABG [25 - 29]. These studies generally included patients with large AMI, and patients showing a large mismatch received greater benefits from interventions than those without. A previous study that measured the BMIPP washout rate indicated that it was useful for predicting ventricular functional recovery after successful interventions [30].

However, this is not the case for patient prognoses. A previous study reported that patients with a BMIPP/perfusion mismatch showed a high probability of future cardiac events [31]. Nanasato *et al.* [32] also demonstrated that a large BMIPP/perfusion mismatch was an independent predictor of major cardiac adverse events. A study that performed serial BMIPP/perfusion scans within 30 days and after 11 months of the onset of AMI revealed that the first, but not the second BMIPP scan is a strong predictor of future cardiac events [33]. Those finding indicates that BMIPP can provide useful prognostic information even after PCI procedure and it is not required to BMIPP image before PCI. Fukushima *et al.* selectively examined patients with non-ST segment elevation myocardial infarction (NSTEMI) [34]. The findings obtained showed that patients with a large BMIPP defect (Total defect score: TDS>7) without serum CK-MB elevations had a worse prognosis than those with a small BMIPP defect (TDS≤7), which is similar to the prognosis of patients with serum CK-MB elevations. To summarize, most data suggest that large BMIPP defects and a BMIPP/perfusion mismatch after an AMI event predict a poor outcome regardless of the intervention performed.

However, when a stunned myocardium was selected, data appeared to be different. Ueda *et al.* examined patients with a stunned myocardium only [35]. The findings obtained showed that patients with a mismatch showed clearly better wall motion recovery 6 months after the cardiac event than those without a mismatch. It is important to note that cardiac troponin T levels were not measured in that study, and detailed scoring of the magnitude of the mismatch was not reported.

These discrepancies between the outcomes of wall motion recovery and patient prognosis may be related to the difficulties associated with the viability assessment itself. In the STICH trial [36], myocardial viability measured using nuclear cardiology imaging (and dobutamine echo) failed to show the benefits of coronary surgery over optimal medical therapy alone. The gap between optimal medical therapy and invasive interventions has been decreasing with advances in medical therapy. Furthermore, many factors, such as restenosis, microvascular damage, and remodeling, modify the effects of interventions. This complexity may result in discrepant findings between the outcomes of wall motion recovery and prognosis. A recent systematic review [37] reported that the relationship between BMIPP findings and risk was closely influenced by the timing of BMIPP imaging relative to revascularization. BMIPP abnormalities found before revascularization was associated with lower risk of future cardiac events, whereas those detected after revascularization were associated with higher risk. In the same study, they showed that negative BMIPP findings provided a very strong assurance that the patient will not experience hard events (98.9% free over 3.5 years). Fujita *et al.* performed serial BMIPP scans before and 3 weeks after CABG and found that the recovery of BMIPP uptake 3 weeks after CABG was a strong predictor of wall motion recovery [38]. Therefore, BMIPP findings need to be interpreted with detailed clinical information. In combination with detailed data, such as timing after an event and the history of interventions, BMIPP will provide important information for precise and personalized patient management.

Chronic Ischemia

BMIPP has the potential to diagnose chronic ischemic heart disease. In an early study by Takeishi *et al.* [39], resting BMIPP imaging detected 43% of patients with significant coronary stenosis, and 59% with exercise-induced ischemia. They also noted that the severity of ischemic findings (such as the early termination of stress and ST depression) was related to the severity of BMIPP findings. Yamabe *et al.* [17] examined different types of angina pectoris, including the stable, new onset, and worsening types. The detection rates of patients with CAD were 48.1, 47.6, and 77.1% for each type, respectively. Overall sensitivity was 62.6% and specificity was 95.2%, which indicates that BMIPP is a specific, but not sensitive method for detecting angina pectoris. A study by Fujiwara *et al.* showed similar sensitivity and specificity (55 and 78%, respectively) for the detection of significant coronary stenosis [15]. They also performed BMIPP under oral glucose loading and reported that this technique increased sensitivity to 75% without sacrificing specificity. Nakamura *et al.* scored rest Thallium and BMIPP image using 17 segment/4 grade scoring method according to the American Heart Association criteria. Then, they calculated difference between total BMIPP score and Thallium score as mismatch score and assessed the threshold to detect a mismatch with a receiver-operator-characteristic (ROC) analysis [40]. They identified a mismatch score of 4 as the threshold. Using this threshold value, they achieved 80% sensitivity and 63% specificity; sensitivity was low due to the high incidence of false positive cases because of non-ischemic heart diseases, such as sarcoidosis and DCM. These findings generally indicate that BMIPP imaging is relatively specific, but not sensitive for detecting chronic ischemic heart disease. Therefore, the application of BMIPP to detect chronic ischemic heart disease in routine clinical practice needs to be limited to specific patient groups, such as patients who are unsuitable for stress testing (such as very old patients and those with severe disabilities) or the requirement to triage severely ischemic subjects from a specific group with a large population, such as HD patients.

BMIPP is useful in prognostic assessments of chronic ischemic heart disease and ACS. In an early study by Tamaki *et al.*, 50 patients with stable myocardial infarction were examined using BMIPP imaging and stress Thallium (Tl) imaging. A stepwise regression model analysis revealed that a Tl/BMIPP mismatch, not Tl stress imaging was a strong predictor of future cardiac events [41]. Matsuki *et al.* studied a group of patients without a previous history of myocardial infarction [42] and also found that reduced BMIPP uptake was the second strongest predictor of all cardiac events. In that study, the strongest predictor was LVEF followed by BMIPP. Summed difference scores for stress MPI (performed with Tl) was the fourth predictor after diabetes mellitus (DM). A multicenter study that including four hospitals and 274 patients with a BMIPP defect score of less than 5 was performed, and showed a very good survival rate of 92% in a 3-year follow-up [43]. When patients with a BMIPP defect score of 5 or greater also had DM, the event rate increased to 41%.

These studies were all performed using visual interpretation and scoring. Recent advances in nuclear cardiology have provided many types of automated analysis software. Nakata *et al.* attempted to use one type of software and performed an analysis on patient prognosis [44]. In their study, BMIPP defect scores were identified as a significant predictor of cardiac events in a univariate analysis, but not in a multivariate analysis, which is discordant with previous studies. Therefore, the use of an automatic analysis for BMIPP warrants further development.

Vasospasm

The non-invasive diagnosis of vasospastic angina is challenging. Stress testing, even with exercise, does not necessarily induce vasospasm at the moment of maximum stress, resulting in relatively low sensitivity and specificity. Based on the capability of BMIPP to memorize ischemic insults in the myocardium, BMIPP is expected to be useful for detecting vasospastic angina without stress testing.

Nakajima *et al.* studied 32 patients with known VSA [45]. BMIPP abnormalities were observed in 78% of patients, while perfusion abnormalities measured using Thallium were only detected in 31% of patients, indicating the clear superiority of BMIPP for detecting VSA. Watanabe *et al.* included a group of patients who were initially suspected of having vasospasms, although this was denied by ergonovine provocation as a control to calculate sensitivity and specificity. Their findings showed very high sensitivity and specificity (89 and 81%, respectively).

Yoneyama *et al.* compared BMIPP findings with TIMI (thrombolysis in myocardial infarction) flow grades during acetylcholine (ACH) provocation [46]. They found no significant differences in BMIPP defect scores between the TIMI0-2 and TIMI3 groups. They performed a BMIPP imaging study 14 days after the ACH provocation. Thus, the BMIPP defects measured in their study were not only related to the ACH provocation, but also to all ischemic insults during daily life. The magnitudes of BMIPP defects should relates to the extent and severity of ischemia in addition to its frequency.

SPECIFIC DISEASE GROUPS

CKD/HD

Due to its relatively high specificity and low sensitivity for diagnosing ischemic heart disease, BMIPP cannot replace stress MPI. However, BMIPP is advantageous in specific groups of patients. One of these patient populations that have been extensively studied is chronic kidney disease (CKD), particularly patients receiving HD.

Fig. (**1**) shows incidentally found myocardial damage detected by Tl/BMIPP dual isotope SPECT imaging. Low perfusion on the inferolateral wall was noted with more severe reductions in BMIPP in the same area, which indicated severe myocardial damage caused by ischemic insults. The very high prevalence of cardiovascular disease in patients with end-stage kidney disease resulted in a high rate of cardiac events and the poor survival of HD patients [47, 48]. A nationwide survey performed in 2007 in Japan showed that cardiovascular death accounted for more than one fourth of all-cause mortality [49]. Although the prevalence of CAD appears to be declining due to improvements in medical management [50], it is still a major issue in HD patients. Thus, the evaluation of cardiac disease contributes to the management of these patients and helps to prolong their survival. However, due to the large number of CKD/HD patients, it is unrealistic to evaluate all of these patients with stress MPI. BMIPP has relatively low sensitivity to detect all types of ischemic heart diseases [21]. However, BMIPP findings are related to the severity of myocardial damage [39]. BMIPP also has the potential to identify patients with a poor prognosis [37]. Based on these findings and its easy imaging procedure, BMIPP has potential as an alternative to stress MPI for CKD/HD patients. Nishimura *et al.* extensively examined a HD patient population and demonstrated that BMIPP was useful for the detection of CAD in these patients [20]. The sensitivity, specificity, and accuracy of detecting CAD with BMIPP were 98.0, 65.6, and 90%, respectively, which were markedly better than those of Tl SPECT acquired at rest [20]. This high accuracy of the diagnosis of CAD in HD subjects was kept equally high regardless of the concurrence of DM [51].

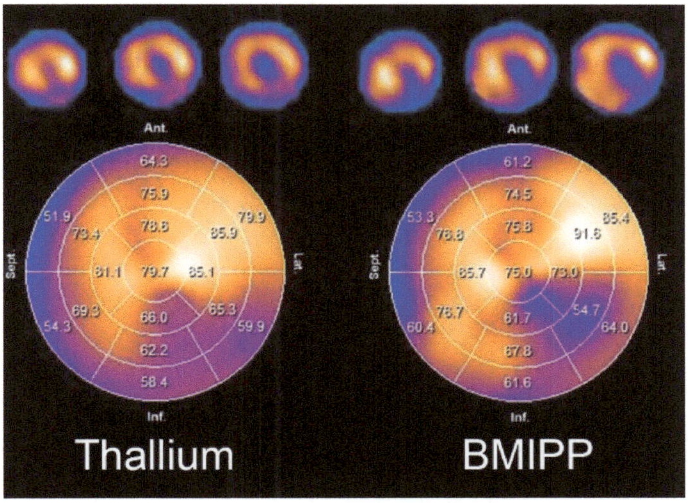

Fig. (1). Ischemic cardiac damage in HD patients on Thallium/BMIPP dual isotope images. Note the infero-lateral wall showing marked reductions in BMIPP uptake.

The reduced myocardial uptake of BMIPP also indicates a significant hard event rate in CKD patients [52]. Even in a group of HD patients without symptoms, a similar poor prognosis was noted in patients with BMIPP abnormal findings [53], or even after revascularization [54]. Abnormal findings focally located in the left anterior descending artery area more strongly predict cardiac death than those in the left circumflex or right coronary artery area [55]. These studies were single center studies. According to the accumulated findings described above, a large multicenter prospective cohort study (B-SAFE: BMIPP Single-photon emission computed tomography Analysis for decreasing cardiac Events in HD patients) was performed in Japan [56]. B-SAFE clearly indicated the power of BMIPP for the management of HD patients in regard to cardiac mortality predictions [57] and non-fatal cardiac events [58]. B-SAFE researchers stated that BMIPP is a logical choice for the routine testing of HD patients at high risk of cardiac events [58]. The value of prognosis stratification is also viable in a group of HD patients without obstructive CAD [55, 59]. In these studies, BMIPP scores higher than 12 or focal low uptake in the left anterior descending area were found to be markers of a poor prognosis and cardiac death without obstructive CAD. BMIPP is not only useful for detection and prognostic assessments, but also for monitoring drug effects [60, 61]. Nishimura *et al.* reported that the oral administration of nicorandil to patients with HD improved myocardial BMIPP uptake.

However, it is unrealistic to perform BMIPP on all CKD/HD patients due to their large numbers. Some triaging is required. A study by Nakata *et al.* provided good insights to overcome this issue [62]. They combined ECG, blood tests, and BMIPP imaging and identified an abnormal Q wave on ECG, a C-reactive protein (CRP) level of >2.38, and a BMIPP score of >16 as prognostic markers for these patients. They found that the prognosis of patients was good when they had none or only one of the three markers. On the other hand, patients who had two or three of these markers showed a significantly poorer prognosis than those who did not. This finding indicates that it is possible to select appropriate patients for BMIPP imaging with simple and inexpensive ECG and blood sampling. BMIPP imaging only needs to be performed on patients who exhibit abnormal Q waves or CRP levels of >2.38. When abnormal Q waves and CRP levels of >2.38 were both detected in a patient, this patient was already proven to have a poor prognosis, and, thus, it is not necessary to perform a BMIPP scan (Fig. **2**).

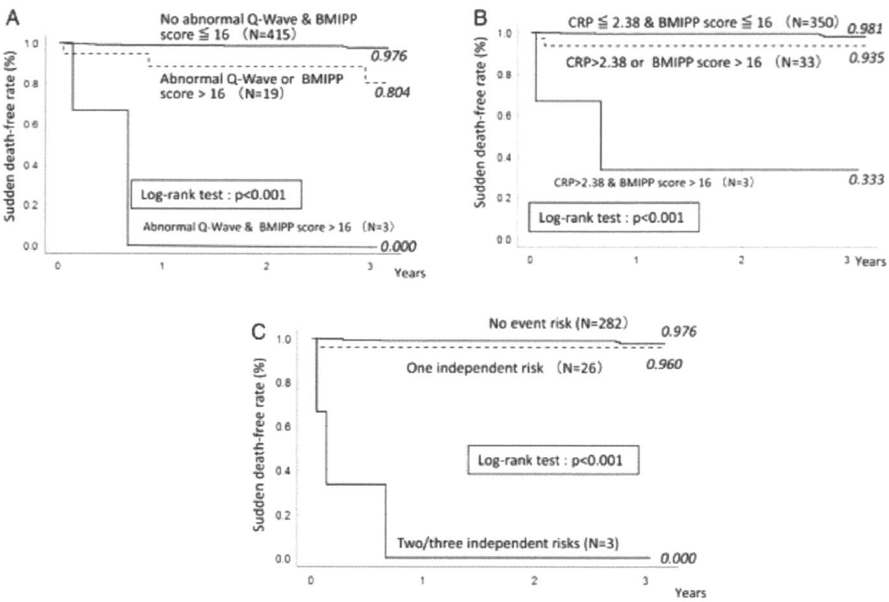

Fig. (2). Sudden death-free survival is stratified by combinations of categorical variables: abnormal Q-wave, increased C-reactive protein (CRP) level, and BMIPP score. Adapted with permission from Reference [62].

In the B-SAFE sub-analysis, another important issue regarding interpretation variability was noted [63]. In the B-SAFE study, image interpretation was performed in an experienced core laboratory and a significant prognostic difference was noted between patients with abnormal and normal BMIPP findings. However, this sub-study proved that when image interpretation was performed by clinical centers, they failed to distinguish the risk of events. Similar findings showing the effects of training were previously reported for MPI with Tl [64] and Tc-99m-labeled tracers [65]. In contrast to perfusion tracers, BMIPP is not yet used worldwide. The provision of training tools to learn how to accurately interpret images of BMIPP is needed in order to promote the wider distribution of BMIPP.

Hypertrophic Cardiomyopathy

BMIPP images myocardial damage itself, not myocardial perfusion. Thus, reductions in BMIPP uptake are not always related to major (macroscopic) coronary arteries; they may be associated with microvascular circulation. Tanabe *et al.* reported a case of microvascular ischemia that resulted in reduced BMIPP uptake [66]. A decrease in the myocardial uptake of BMIPP has been shown to correlate with microvascular obstruction after AMI [67]. Therefore, BMIPP is expected to have the capacity to identify myocardial damage according to cardiomyopathies, such as microvascular damage and early fibrotic changes. Many studies indicated that reduced BMIPP is frequently observed in patients with hypertrophic cardiomyopathy (HCM), particularly in the area of hypertrophy [68, 69], and this finding correlates with a poor prognosis [70, 71]. This reduction in BMIPP uptake in HCM frequently corresponds to the late gadolinium enhancement imaged on MRI [72, 73], which is also related to the poor prognosis of patients with HCM [74, 75].

Dilated Cardiomyopathy

In dilated cardiomyopathy (DCM), mismatch between perfusion and BMIPP, which is a common finding in ischemic cardiomyopathy, is not frequent. Using this difference, DCM and ischemic cardiomyopathy can be differentiated [76]. Ishida examined patients with LVEF of less than 40% and found that the defect scores of Tl at rest and BMIPP were similar in the DCM group, but significantly different (BMIPP>Tl) in the ischemic cardiomyopathy group. When a segmental mismatch was observed in severe heart failure patients, the probability of ischemic cardiomyopathy became very high [77].

However, a minor mismatch may be found in DCM patients. Yazaki indicated that a mismatch in DCM was a strong predictor of short-term prognoses [78]. Yoshida investigated MPI with Tc-99m MIBI, fatty acid metabolism with BMIPP, and myocardial tissue fibrosis with late gadolinium enhancement on MRI

[79]. The findings obtained revealed a correlation between a minor mismatch in BMIPP/perfusion and prognosis in DCM patients. The location of the mismatch did not correspond to that of the late gadolinium enhancement, which suggests that the mechanism responsible for the mismatch in DCM differs from that in myocardial fibrosis.

BMIPP is also useful for evaluating patient prognoses and predicting therapeutic responses. A previous study that evaluated thirty-seven DCM patients receiving beta-blocker therapy revealed that the global myocardial uptake of BMIPP, which was measured from planar anterior images, had very high sensitivity (0.93) and specificity (1.00) to distinguish responders from non-responders [80]. Zavadovsky examined DCM patients receiving cardiac resynchronization therapy (CRT) and found that the defect score of BMIPP strongly predicted beneficial responses to CRT [81]. These findings suggest that BMIPP provides a lot of beneficial information on patients with cardiomyopathy.

Takotsubo Cardiomyopathy

Takotsubo cardiomyopathy is a very specific disease entity and was initially reported by Sato [82]. It is frequently triggered by a strong emotional challenge, such as fury or distress, or physical stress, including a severe cold or subarachnoid hemorrhage, and leads to the sudden onset of heart failure. In typical cases, apical ballooning and dyskinesis in the apex may be recovered in the long term.

Manabe reviewed studies that used FDG PET or BMIPP to investigate Takotsubo cardiomyopathy [83]. He listed 16 studies for FDG PET and 14 for BMIPP. All studies on BMIPP were written by Japanese researchers, while most of those on FDG PET were reported from other countries. In the FDG PET studies, two types of preparations, glucose loading or fasting conditions, were performed. Thus, the findings obtained were not homogenous across studies. Even in a single study performed under overnight fasting conditions, a mixed pattern of a mismatch (FDG higher than perfusion) to an inverse mismatch (FDG lower than perfusion) was detected [84]. This finding indicates the difficulties associated with the interpretation of FDG PET images of Takotsubo cardiomyopathy. On the other hand, most of the BMIPP studies showed a mismatch (BMIPP lower than perfusion) pattern. Similar to ACS with viability, an insulted myocardium showed lower BMIPP uptake than perfusion. Since this pattern indicates viability in ACS, this mismatch pattern, which is commonly detected in Takotsubo cardiomyopathy, is concordant with typical Takotsubo cardiomyopathy having a good prognosis. A study that performed BMIPP, MIBG and MIBI imaging during the acute, sub-acute, and chronic stages of Takotsubo cardiomyopathy also demonstrated that scintigraphic abnormalities generally recovered in the long term [85].

However, this mismatch pattern has also been reported in ACS. Difficulties are associated with making a differential diagnosis between Takotsubo cardiomyopathy and ACS. Approximately 1% of ACS cases were actually Takotsubo cardiomyopathy misdiagnosed as ACS [86]. Thus, the differentiation between these two conditions is very important. Takotsubo cardiomyopathy shows a specific apical ballooning pattern. Thus, the localization of scintigraphic findings may contribute to differentiating between ACS and Takotsubo cardiomyopathy. Matsuo investigated the defect scores of BMIPP on apical and non-apical lesions in patients with Takotsubo cardiomyopathy and ACS [87] and found that BMIPP defects were exclusively located in the apical area in patients with Takotsubo cardiomyopathy. Based on the pathophysiology of Takotsubo cardiomyopathy, which is considered to be microcirculatory and/or neurohormonal, anatomical information on major coronary artery distribution may also contribute to differentiation [88]. A previous study using fusion images of SPECT and coronary CT angiography clearly demonstrated that the location of BMIPP and perfusion defects did not correspond to the coronary artery distribution [89] (Fig. **3**). The differentiation between Takotsubo cardiomyopathy and ACS is facilitated by SPECT/CT hybrid images.

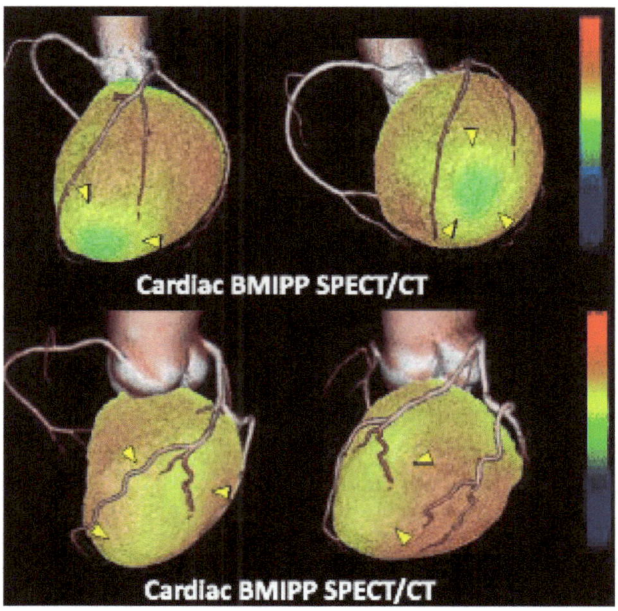

Fig. (3). A fusion image of BMIPP and coronary CTA of Takotsubo cardiomyopathy (top row) and coronary artery disease (bottom row). A defect in a case of coronary artery disease congruent with coronary artery distribution. A defect in a case of Takotsubo cardiomyopathy incongruent with coronary artery distribution. Adapted with permission from reference [89].

Heart Failure

Heart failure and its management is the most important and challenging issue for cardiology. As noted previously, BMIPP is a very useful tool for the risk stratification of patients with DCM. However, its utility for patients with heart failure remains unknown. Hashimoto *et al.* followed up 133 patients with heart failure and a preserved ejection fraction (HFpEF) who underwent BMIPP imaging [90]. They found that the group with a higher BMIPP defect score (threshold =4) had more major adverse cardiac events, indicating that BMIPP is of potential prognostic value, even in HFpEF patients.

The method used in Hashimoto's study was the common scoring technique. Scoring is a basic technique for evaluating focal/regional abnormalities. Since heart failure involves the whole myocardium, a technique to measure global myocardial metabolism quantitatively warrants a more precise evaluation of heart failure. Kida *et al.* revealed that global myocardial uptake and its washout measured on planar images clearly correlated with the condition of heart failure [91]. They revealed that BNP and LVEF were clearly related to the heart to mediastinal ratio (H/M) and washout. They used planar images, not SPECT images, to quantify the myocardial uptake of BMIPP. This is a similar simple and practical technique that is frequently used in studies employing MIBG. However, the range of the H/M ratio of BMIPP was much narrower than that of MIBG. For example, the ADMIRE-HF study evaluated the usefulness of MIBG for NYHA class II and III HF patients, similar to Kida's study. The delayed H/M of MIBG in ADMIRE-HF was 1.46 for patients without events and 1.39 for those with events. These H/M values were markedly smaller than those in Kida's study with BMIPP. This narrow range of normal to abnormal values indicated that the BMIPP analysis is susceptible to measurement errors, such as inter/intra-observer variabilities. Therefore, a more precise quantitative method is needed.

As noted in the DCM section, BMIPP is useful for triaging patients who respond to specific therapeutic interventions, such as CRT [81] and beta-blocker therapy [80]. It is not limited to DCM. Cardiac resynchronization therapy improves the clinical status and survival of patients with severe left ventricular dysfunction. However, due to the high rate of failure and high cost of this therapy [92], triaging patients who will respond to this therapy is essential [81]. Lishmanov *et al.* examined 28 patients who underwent CRT, which was not limited to DCM, using BMIPP and perfusion SPECT [93]. They separated patients into hyper-responders (LVEF improvement of more than 10%), responders (improvement between 10-5%), and non-responders (improvement of less than 5%), and found that hyper-responders had smaller BMIPP defects.

Fewer studies have been conducted on BMIPP than on MIBG. Therefore, further studies with large patient populations are needed to clarify the usefulness of BMIPP for heart failure.

NEW CLINICAL APPLICATIONS

Radiation Injuries in the Myocardium

Reductions in BMIPP uptake are non-specific to ischemic insults. They are caused by any type of myocardial damage. Fig. (**4**) shows reductions in BMIPP uptake and increases in FDG uptake in patients who underwent radiation for lung cancer. Myocardial damage caused by radiation therapy may be evaluated using several nuclear medicine techniques, including FDG PET [94, 95] and resting MIBI with ECG-gated SPECT [96]. BMIPP also showed significant findings with radiotherapy combined with chemotherapy [97] or radiation alone [98]. Studies using FDG, MIBI, and BMIPP revealed that each tracer detected different magnitudes and characteristics of radiation-induced damage. Studies with FDG indicated that 10~20 Gy of radiation induced increases in the uptake of FDG, reflecting myocardial damage [94, 95]. A study using ECG-gated MIBI SPECT revealed that a radiation dose of 40 Gy or higher increased heart rates and other cardiac function parameters [96]. The findings of a prospective BMIPP study showed that myocardial fatty acid metabolism was progressively impaired by chemoradiotherapy during and even after the cessation of therapy [97]. Reductions in BMIPP uptake after radiation therapy were noted, even after one year. Reductions in BMIPP uptake were correlated with the volume of myocardium involved in the radiation field and the radiation dose to the myocardium. However, some cases showed delayed (1 year after radiation therapy) BMIPP reductions, even with low dose radiation and small irradiated myocardial volume [97]. Radiation to the heart increases the subsequent rate of developing ischemic heart disease [99]. Delayed reductions in BMIPP uptake, even one year after radiation, indicate that not only direct myocardial injury, but also indirect/secondary effects, such as radiation-induced atherosclerosis and/or vascular damage, are caused by radiation. However, there is currently no widely accepted study that shows the effects of BMIPP findings on patient prognoses in this population. Therefore, further large-scale follow-up studies are needed.

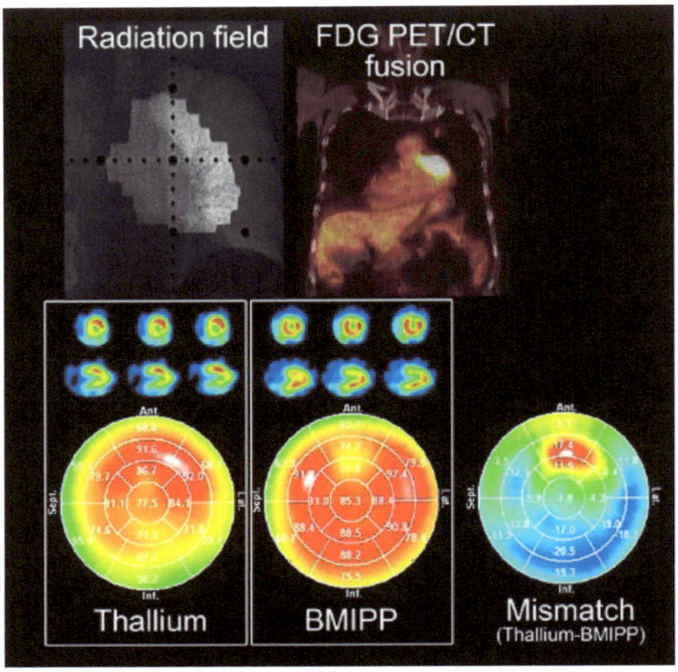

Fig. (4). Radiation therapy for lung cancer. The basal side of the left ventricular anterior wall included in the radiation field showed the decreased myocardial uptake of BMIPP and increased uptake of FDG. Note the Thallium image does not show decreased uptake in the same area, and even shows relatively high perfusion.

Cardiac Sarcoidosis

Sarcoid lesions exhibit extensive metabolic activity, resulting in strong FDG uptake. Thus, FDG PET (or PET/CT) performed under fasting conditions is recommended for the diagnosis of cardiac sarcoidosis. However, based on the physiological uptake of FDG by the healthy myocardium, physiological FDG uptake needs to be suppressed by a very long fasting period, typically 18 hours. This may be too long for some unhealthy patients. Even with long fasting periods, the success rate of suppressing normal myocardial FDG uptake is not 100%. Thus, a simpler and more patient-friendly method to detect cardiac sarcoidosis is required. Momose *et al.* reported that a mismatch between perfusion and BMIPP was frequently detected in cardiac sarcoidosis [100]. They concluded that Tl/BMIPP imaging may be an alternative to FDG PET for the detection of cardiac sarcoidosis. This finding was supported by a recent study that compared Tl/BMIPP findings with FDG PET performed under overnight fasting conditions [101]. They found that FDG uptake evaluated as SUVmax (maximum uptake in the region of interest which is normalized with injected activity and patient's weight) was significantly higher in a Tl/BMIPP mismatch area than in a matched area, indicating that a Tl/BMIPP mismatch is a frequent finding in "active" sarcoid lesions. Due to the difficulties associated with preparing for FDG PET and the ease of BMIPP, BMIPP may serve not as a "poor man's FDG", but as a more practical method and replacement for FDG.

Chronic Thromboembolism Pulmonary Hypertension

Chronic thromboembolism pulmonary hypertension (CTEPH) is chronic pulmonary hypertension that results from chronic pulmonary thromboembolism [102]. It is typically diagnosed with CT and lung perfusion scintigraphy and treated with pulmonary thromboendarterectomy and/or balloon pulmonary angioplasty [102]. Increased right ventricular systolic pressure and right ventricle hypertrophy are observed on echocardiography. A previous study revealed that BMIPP uptake was enhanced in patients with CTEPH and that it decreased after pulmonary thromboendarterectomy [103]. They also performed FDG PET and found that FDG uptake and BMIPP uptake were both elevated. This phenomenon has not been reported for ischemic heart disease or other heart diseases involving the left ventricle. Metabolism in the right ventricle has not yet been studied in detail using nuclear medicine techniques. This field warrants further research.

Triglyceride Deposit Cardiomyovasculopathy

Triglyceride deposit cardiomyovasculopathy (TGCV) is a novel clinical entity that was initially reported by Hirano in 2008 [104]. It is characterized by the inability of the myocardium to utilize long-chain fatty acids. The washout of BMIPP from the myocardium was found to be markedly reduced in patients with TGCV [105]. BMIPP is known to be trapped in the triglyceride pool and is slowly washed out from the myocardium due to beta-oxidation. This delayed washout may be related to the etiology of TGCV and may provide useful information on this newly found disease entity. Further studies are warranted.

Mitochondrial Cardiomyopathy

Mitochondrial cardiomyopathy is a heterogeneous disease entity resulting from abnormalities in mitochondrial DNA and function. Ikawa *et al.* examined five patients with mitochondrial myopathy, encephalopathy, lactic acidosis, and stroke-like episodes (MELAS) using Tc-99m MIBI and BMIPP [106]. They identified two patients with increased BMIPP uptake and the accelerated washout of MIBI. MIBI is known to accumulate in mitochondria, and, thus, is associated with mitochondrion functional abnormalities. Similar findings were reported by Matsuo who found increased BMIPP uptake in the septum and reduced Tc-99m MIBI uptake in MELAS patients [107]. On the other hand, a recent case report showed reduced BMIPP uptake with normal MIBI uptake, which is similar to the mismatch pattern frequently found for ischemic heart disease [108].

Mitochondrial cardiomyopathy is a heterogeneous disease group that involves not only the myocardium, but also vessels. This mixed etiology, which involves the myocardium and vessels, may make the disease phenotype very complex. Further studies are needed to identify the reasons for these complex findings.

METHODOLOGICAL ASPECTS

How to Quantify BMIPP

A proper diagnosis with small inter-observer and intra-observer variabilities requires a method to quantify image parameters. The most frequently used technique is scoring the myocardial uptake of a tracer into 0 (=normal uptake) to 4 (=no uptake). However, the scoring method will still have some subjectivity. In an attempt to reduce this subjectivity, creation of a normal database of BMIPP (and also MIBG) was performed in Japan [109]. In this study, the distribution of BMIPP is significantly higher than that of the Tc-99m perfusion agent in the septum. Decreased uptake in the inferior wall was noted for I-123 MIBG, but not for BMIPP. MIBG and BMIPP are both labeled with the same I-123, and, thus, this difference indicates the different distribution of metabolism and neural function in the left ventricle. Once a normal database is established, an automatic scoring method may be created. The validation of such an automated scoring system has already been performed [110] and proven to be more reliable than expert image interpretation. This scoring is already used in clinical settings and is useful in prognostic assessments of patients with CAD [44].

The second step for quantification is measuring tracer activity. H/M is widely used for this purpose in I-123 MIBG imaging. The same method may be useful for BMIPP imaging. This simple method is based on the lack of the specific uptake of tracers on the mediastinum, with only a non-specific background existing. Thus, specific uptake in the myocardium may be evaluated by dividing myocardial activity by that in the mediastinum. This method is suitable for measuring abnormal uptake involving the whole myocardium, and, thus, is frequently used in studies on heart failure [91, 111], and also ischemic heart diseases [30, 112]. By using this H/M measurement early after a tracer injection and several hours later, the washout rate may also be measured. The accelerated washout of BMIPP has been reported to correlate with the poor condition of heart failure [91, 111]. In AMI patients, accelerated washout is a good indicator of wall motion recovery after revascularization [30]. In patients with angina pectoris, accelerated washout was detected before PCI, but normalized after PCI [112].

A more scientifically precise method to quantify tracer kinetics is a compartment model analysis. Okizaki *et al.* attempted to perform two-compartment model analysis for the group of hypertrophic cardiomyopathies [113]. They demonstrated that k_3 is a sensitive predictor for the early detection of HCM. In their model, k_3 was the transfer ratio from the reversible tissue compartment (C_1) to the irreversible tissue compartment (C_2). It currently remains unclear as to what the "irreversible tissue compartment" actually means. They speculate that C_2 corresponds to the triglyceride pool in the myocardium.

Technical Advances in Imaging Equipment

Diagnoses using BMIPP will become more specific and accurate when performed with perfusion images. As previously described, the BMIPP/perfusion mismatch pattern indicates an ischemic/damaged, but viable myocardium and is useful not only for making a diagnosis, but also for prognostic assessments and monitoring therapeutic responses. However, the gamma-ray energy of I-123, which is used to label BMIPP, is too close to that of Tc-99m (I-123; 159keV, Tc-99m; 141keV), and, thus, these two radioisotopes are indistinguishable when a conventional Anger-camera using Thallium-doped sodium iodide (NaI (Tl)) crystals is used. This is a major issue associated with dual isotope imaging using BMIPP and perfusion agents. A diagnosis using BMIPP relies on the mismatch pattern, which means a lower BMIPP uptake than perfusion. When severe cross-talk occurs (shine through from one tracer to another), the defect area of BMIPP overlaps with perfusion tracer uptake, resulting in the disappearance of the mismatch pattern. This is a critical issue when using BMIPP, and, thus, only Tl-201 may be imaged with BMIPP for simultaneous dual isotope imaging. When a Tc-99--labeled tracer is used as the perfusion agent, perfusion and BMIPP imaging must be performed separately. Based in its long half-life, low photon energy, and high radiation dose, Tl-201 is not ideal for perfusion imaging.

Recent solid state detectors (cadmium-zinc-telluride: CZT is a frequently used material) have very high energy resolution, which is suitable for distinguishing photons from I-123 and Tc-99m. The simultaneous acquisition of BMIPP and Tc-99m-labeled myocardial perfusion agents has become possible with the use of an advanced solid state detector. A preclinical study using the CZT detector clearly confirmed that cross-talk between each tracer was very limited and did not deteriorate image quality [114]. A similar validation was performed for two commercially available clinical scanners: Discovery NM 530c (GE Healthcare, Milwaukee, USA) [115] and D-SPECT (Spectrum-Dynamics, Caesarea, Israel) [116]. Using these scanners, dual isotope imaging was performed easily with excellent image quality, which will be very beneficial for patient care.

GUIDELINES

I-123 BMIPP is only widely available in Japan. Thus, there are currently no globally accepted guidelines. In 2010, the Japanese Circulation Society revised the "Guidelines for Clinical Use of Cardiac Nuclear Medicine" Japanese guidelines. It classified usefulness into three categories (I to III) with three levels of evidence (A to C). The following are a list of recommendations and its categories/levels [117, 118] (Table **1**). As noted in the Table **1**, BMIPP is widely recommended for ischemic heart disease. However, it is important to note that this classification of BMIPP is only accepted in Japan.

Table 1. Recommendations in Japanese guideline

	Class	Level of Evidence
For coronary artery diseases		
Diagnosis of acute coronary syndrome		
For acute myocardial infarction	IIb	C
For unstable angina	I	B
Diagnosis of chronic coronary artery diseases	IIa	C
Diagnosis of vasospastic angina	IIa	C
Prognosis and risk stratification	IIb	C
For cardiomyopathy and heart failure		
Differential diagnosis of cardiomyopathy	IIb	B
Prognosis and risk stratification of cardiomyopathy	IIb	C
Evaluation of myocardial ischemia in hemodialysis hearts	IIb	C

RADIATION DOSE

The typical dose for BMIPP imaging in Japan is 111 MBq. According to the most recent data from ICRP (ICRP pub.128) [119], its effective dose for 1 MBq is 0.016 mSv (/MBq). Thus, a single procedure for BMIPP induces roughly 1.8 mSv per procedure. It is acceptably low. Based on this aspect of radiation burden, BMIPP is considered to be a patient-friendly method for diagnosis.

SUMMARY

BMIPP is a unique tracer that provides data on myocardial damage from the aspect of metabolism. It provides additional information on myocardial damage regardless of perfusion abnormalities (such as the regulation of metabolism and radiation damage) and time (including previous ischemic memory and future prognoses).

BMIPP; more than meets the MPI!

CONSENT FOR PUBLICATION

Not applicable.

CONFLICT OF INTEREST

The authors declare no conflict of interest, financial or otherwise.

ACKNOWLEDGEMENTS

Declared none.

REFERENCES

[1] Knapp FF Jr, Kropp J. Iodine-123-labelled fatty acids for myocardial single-photon emission tomography: current status and future perspectives. Eur J Nucl Med 1995; 22(4): 361-81. [http://dx.doi.org/10.1007/BF00941855]

[2] Fujiwara S, Takeishi Y, Tojo T, *et al.* Fatty acid imaging with 123I-15-(p-iodophenyl)---R,S-methylpentadecanoic acid in acute coronary syndrome. J Nucl Med 1999; 40(12): 1999-2006.

[3] Machulla HJ, Marsmann M, Dutschka K. Biochemical concept and synthesis of a radioiodinated phenylfatty acid for *in vivo* metabolic studies of the myocardium. Eur J Nucl Med 1980; 5(2): 171-3. [http://dx.doi.org/10.1007/BF00252480]

[4] Hock A, Spohr G, Schmitz M, *et al.* 17-Iodine-123 iodoheptadecanoic acid for metabolic liver studies in humans. J Nucl Med 1986; 27(10): 1533-9.

[5] Kudoh T, Tamaki N, Magata Y, *et al.* Metabolism substrate with negative myocardial uptake of iodine-123-BMIPP. J Nucl Med 1997; 38(4): 548-53.

[6] Fukuchi K, Nozaki S, Yoshizumi T, *et al.* Enhanced myocardial glucose use in patients with a deficiency in long-chain fatty acid transport (CD36 deficiency). J Nucl Med 1999; 40(2): 239-43.

[7] Yoshizumi T, Nozaki S, Fukuchi K, *et al.* Pharmacokinetics and metabolism of 123I-BMIPP fatty acid analog in healthy and CD36-deficient subjects. J Nucl Med 2000; 41(7): 1134-8.

[8] Nakatani K, Watabe T, Masuda D, *et al.* Myocardial energy provision is preserved by increased utilization of glucose and ketone bodies in CD36 knockout mice. Metabolism 2015; 64(9): 1165-74. [http://dx.doi.org/10.1016/j.metabol.2015.05.017]

[9] Putri M, Syamsunarno MR, Iso T, *et al.* CD36 is indispensable for thermogenesis under conditions of fasting and cold stress. Biochem Biophys Res Commun 2015; 457(4): 520-5. [http://dx.doi.org/10.1016/j.bbrc.2014.12.124]

[10] Higuchi T, Taki J, Nakajima K, Kinuya S, Namura M, Tonami N. Time course of discordant BMIPP and thallium uptake after ischemia and reperfusion in a rat model. J Nucl Med 2005; 46(1): 172-5.

[11] Noriyasu K, Mabuchi M, Kuge Y, *et al.* Serial changes in BMIPP uptake in relation to thallium uptake in the rat myocardium after ischaemia. Eur J Nucl Med Mol Imaging 2003; 30(12): 1644-50. [http://dx.doi.org/10.1007/s00259-003-1305-z]

[12] Fukushima K, Momose M, Kondo C, Hagiwara N, Sakai S. Accelerated BMIPP uptake immediately after reperfused ischemia in the isolated rat heart model. Ann Nucl Med 2011; 25(8): 560-5. [http://dx.doi.org/10.1007/s12149-011-0510-2]

[13] Hosokawa R, Nohara R, Fujibayashi Y, *et al.* Myocardial kinetics of iodine-123-BMIPP in canine myocardium after regional ischemia and reperfusion: implications for clinical SPECT. J Nucl Med 1997; 38(12): 1857-63.

[14] Hosokawa R, Nohara R, Fujibayashi Y, *et al.* Metabolic fate of iodine-123-BMIPP in canine myocardium after administration of etomoxir. J Nucl Med 1996; 37(11): 1836-40.

[15] Fujiwara S, Takeishi Y, Atsumi H, Takahashi K, Tomoike H. Fatty acid metabolic imaging with iodine-123-BMIPP for the diagnosis of coronary artery disease. J Nucl Med 1997; 38(2): 175-80.

[16] Watanabe K, Ohta Y, Toba K, *et al.* Abnormal fatty acid metabolism in patients with coronary vasospasm. Ann Nucl Med 1999; 13(1): 33-41. [http://dx.doi.org/10.1007/BF03165425]

[17] Yamabe H, Abe H, Yokoyama M, *et al.* Resting 123I-BMIPP scintigraphy in diagnosis of effort angina pectoris with reference to subsets of the disease. Ann Nucl Med 1998; 12(3): 139-44. [http://dx.doi.org/10.1007/BF03164778]

[18] Takeishi Y, Fujiwara S, Atsumi H, Takahashi K, Sukekawa H, Tomoike H. Iodine-123-BMIPP imaging in unstable angina: a guide for interventional strategy. J Nucl Med 1997; 38(9): 1407-11.

[19] Kawai Y, Tsukamoto E, Nozaki Y, Morita K, Sakurai M, Tamaki N. Significance of reduced uptake of iodinated fatty acid analogue for the evaluation of patients with acute chest pain. J Am Coll Cardiol 2001; 38(7): 1888-94. [http://dx.doi.org/10.1016/S0735-1097(01)01634-5]

[20] Nishimura M, Hashimoto T, Kobayashi H, *et al.* Myocardial scintigraphy using a fatty acid analogue detects coronary artery disease in hemodialysis patients. Kidney Int 2004; 66(2): 811-9. [http://dx.doi.org/10.1111/j.1523-1755.2004.00808.x]

[21] Inaba Y, Bergmann SR. Diagnostic accuracy of beta-methyl-p-[123I]-iodophenyl-pentadecanoic acid (BMIPP) imaging: a meta-analysis. J Nucl Cardiol 2008; 15(3): 345-52. [http://dx.doi.org/10.1016/j.nuclcard.2008.02.019]

[22] Saitoh M, Hasegawa K, Hasegawa K, Kondoh T, Yanagawa T. Detection of coronary artery disease using 12-lead electrocardiogram and simultaneous dual myocardial imaging with iodine-123-be-a-methyl iodophenyl- pentadecanoic acid (BMIPP) and thallium-201 in patients with unstable angina. Intern Med 1995; 34(11): 1064-70. [http://dx.doi.org/10.2169/internalmedicine.34.1064]

[23] Fukuoka R, Horita Y, Namura M, *et al.* Serial changes in glucose-loaded 18F-fluoro-2-deoxyglucose positron emission tomography, 99mTc-tetrofosmin and 123I-beta-methyl-p-iodophenyl--enta-decanoic acid myocardial single-photon emission computed tomography images in patients with anterior acute myocardial infarction. Circ J 2013; 77(1): 137-45. [http://dx.doi.org/10.1253/circj.CJ-12-0011]

[24] Fukuoka Y, Nakano A, Uzui H, *et al.* Reverse blood flow-glucose metabolism mismatch indicates preserved oxygen metabolism in patients with revascularised myocardial infarction. Eur J Nucl Med Mol Imaging 2013; 40(8): 1155-62. [http://dx.doi.org/10.1007/s00259-013-2423-x]

[25] Franken PR, Dendale P, De Geeter F, Demoor D, Bossuyt A, Block P. Prediction of functional outcome after myocardial infarction using BMIPP and sestamibi scintigraphy. J Nucl Med 1996; 37(5): 718-22.

[26] Seki H, Toyama T, Higuchi K, *et al.* Prediction of functional improvement of ischemic myocardium with (123I-BMIPP SPECT and 99mTc-tetrofosmin SPECT imaging: a study of patients with large acute myocardial infarction and receiving revascularization therapy. Circ J 2005; 69(3): 311-9. [http://dx.doi.org/10.1253/circj.69.311]

[27] Hashimoto A, Nakata T, Tsuchihashi K, Tanaka S, Fujimori K, Iimura O. Postischemic functional recovery and BMIPP uptake after primary percutaneous transluminal coronary angioplasty in acute myocardial infarction. Am J Cardiol 1996; 77(1): 25-30. [http://dx.doi.org/10.1016/S0002-9149(97)89129-1]

[28] Hambye AS, Vervaet A, Dobbeleir A, Dendale P, Franken P. Prediction of functional outcome by

quantification of sestamibi and BMIPP after acute myocardial infarction. Eur J Nucl Med 2000; 27(10): 1494-500.
[http://dx.doi.org/10.1007/s002590000332]

[29] Christian TF, Schwartz RS, Gibbons RJ. Determinants of infarct size in reperfusion therapy for acute myocardial infarction. Circulation 1992; 86(1): 81-90.
[http://dx.doi.org/10.1161/01.CIR.86.1.81]

[30] Biswas SK, Sarai M, Yamada A, *et al.* The washout rate of (123)I-BMIPP and the evolution of left ventricular function in patients with successfully reperfused ST-segment elevation myocardial infarction: comparisons with the echocardiography. Int J Cardiovasc Imaging 2010; 26 (Suppl. 1): 155-64.
[http://dx.doi.org/10.1007/s10554-009-9575-6]

[31] Nakata T, Kobayashi T, Tamaki N, *et al.* Prognostic value of impaired myocardial fatty acid uptake in patients with acute myocardial infarction. Nucl Med Commun 2000; 21(10): 897-906.
[http://dx.doi.org/10.1097/00006231-200010000-00003]

[32] Nanasato M, Hirayama H, Ando A, *et al.* Incremental predictive value of myocardial scintigraphy with 123I-BMIPP in patients with acute myocardial infarction treated with primary percutaneous coronary intervention. Eur J Nucl Med Mol Imaging 2004; 31(11): 1512-21.
[http://dx.doi.org/10.1007/s00259-004-1556-3]

[33] Hashimoto A, Nakata T, Tamaki N, *et al.* Serial alterations and prognostic implications of myocardial perfusion and fatty acid metabolism in patients with acute myocardial infarction. Circ J 2006; 70(11): 1466-74.
[http://dx.doi.org/10.1253/circj.70.1466]

[34] Fukushima Y, Toba M, Ishihara K, *et al.* Usefulness of 201TlCl/ 123I-BMIPP dual-myocardial SPECT for patients with non-ST segment elevation myocardial infarction. Ann Nucl Med 2008; 22(5): 363-9.
[http://dx.doi.org/10.1007/s12149-007-0126-8]

[35] Ueda T, Toyama T, Seki R, *et al.* Prediction of functional outcome in stunned myocardium after myocardial infarction using BMIPP and tetrofosmin imaging. J Int Med Res 2009; 37(2): 367-77.
[http://dx.doi.org/10.1177/147323000903700211]

[36] Bonow RO, Maurer G, Lee KL, *et al.* Myocardial viability and survival in ischemic left ventricular dysfunction. N Engl J Med 2011; 364(17): 1617-25.
[http://dx.doi.org/10.1056/NEJMoa1100358]

[37] Inaba Y, Bergmann SR. Prognostic value of myocardial metabolic imaging with BMIPP in the spectrum of coronary artery disease: a systematic review. J Nucl Cardiol 2010; 17(1): 61-70.
[http://dx.doi.org/10.1007/s12350-009-9157-y]

[38] Fujita K, Kasama S, Kurabayashi M. Serial dual single-photon emission computed tomography of thallium-201 and iodine-123 beta-methyliodophenyl pentadecanoic acid scintigraphy can predict functional recovery of patients with coronary artery disease after coronary artery bypass graft surgery. Nucl Med Commun 2015; 36(2): 148-55.
[http://dx.doi.org/10.1097/MNM.0000000000000228]

[39] Takeishi Y, Sukekawa H, Saito H, *et al.* Clinical significance of decreased myocardial uptake of 123I-BMIPP in patients with stable effort angina pectoris. Nucl Med Commun 1995; 16(12): 1002-8.
[http://dx.doi.org/10.1097/00006231-199512000-00003]

[40] Nakamura A, Momose M, Kondo C, Nakajima T, Kusakabe K, Hagiwara N. Ability of 201Tl and 123I-BMIPP mismatch to diagnose myocardial ischemia in patients with suspected coronary artery disease. Ann Nucl Med 2009; 23(9): 793-8.
[http://dx.doi.org/10.1007/s12149-009-0307-8]

[41] Tamaki N, Tadamura E, Kudoh T, *et al.* Prognostic value of iodine-123 labelled BMIPP fatty acid analogue imaging in patients with myocardial infarction. Eur J Nucl Med 1996; 23(3): 272-9.

[http://dx.doi.org/10.1007/BF00837625]

[42] Matsuki T, Tamaki N, Nakata T, *et al.* Prognostic value of fatty acid imaging in patients with angina pectoris without prior myocardial infarction: comparison with stress thallium imaging. Eur J Nucl Med Mol Imaging 2004; 31(12): 1585-91. [http://dx.doi.org/10.1007/s00259-004-1551-8]

[43] Chikamori T, Fujita H, Nanasato M, Toba M, Nishimura T. Prognostic value of I-123 15-(--iodophenyl)-3-(R,S) methylpentadecanoic acid myocardial imaging in patients with known or suspected coronary artery disease. J Nucl Cardiol 2005; 12(2): 172-8. [http://dx.doi.org/10.1016/j.nuclcard.2004.12.293]

[44] Nakata T, Hashimoto A, Matsuki T, Yoshinaga K, Tsukamoto K, Tamaki N. Prognostic value of automated SPECT scoring system for coronary artery disease in stress myocardial perfusion and fatty acid metabolism imaging. Int J Cardiovasc Imaging 2013; 29(1): 253-62. [http://dx.doi.org/10.1007/s10554-012-0069-6]

[45] Nakajima K, Shimizu K, Taki J, *et al.* Utility of iodine-123-BMIPP in the diagnosis and follow-up of vasospastic angina. J Nucl Med 1995; 36(11): 1934-40.

[46] Yoneyama K, Akashi YJ, Ashikaga K, *et al.* Severity of myocardial fatty acid dysmetabolism induced by coronary spasm does not differ with Thrombolysis in Myocardial Infarction (TIMI) grade during intracoronary acetylcholine provocation tests. Int Heart J 2014; 55(5): 416-21. [http://dx.doi.org/10.1536/ihj.14-102]

[47] Manske CL, Thomas W, Wang Y, Wilson RF. Screening diabetic transplant candidates for coronary artery disease: identification of a low risk subgroup. Kidney Int 1993; 44(3): 617-21. [http://dx.doi.org/10.1038/ki.1993.289]

[48] K/DOQI Workgroup.. K/DOQI clinical practice guidelines for cardiovascular disease in dialysis patients. Am J Kidney Dis 2005; 45(4) (Suppl. 3): S1-S153.

[49] Nakai S, Masakane I, Shigematsu T, *et al.* An overview of regular dialysis treatment in Japan (as of 31 December 2007). Ther Apher Dial 2009; 13(6): 457-504. [http://dx.doi.org/10.1111/j.1744-9987.2009.00789.x]

[50] Iwasaki M, Joki N, Tanaka Y, *et al.* Declining Prevalence of Coronary Artery Disease in Incident Dialysis Patients Over the Past Two Decades. J Atheroscler Thromb 2014; 21(6): 593-604.

[51] Nishimura M, Murase M, Hashimoto T, *et al.* Influence of diabetes mellitus on diagnostic potential of iodine-123-BMIPP imaging for coronary artery stenosis in hemodialysis patients. J Nephrol 2006; 19(4): 481-91.

[52] Takamura T, Takahashi N, Ishigami T, *et al.* Combining chronic kidney disease with 201thallium/123iodine beta methyliodophenyl pentadecanoic acid dual myocardial single-photon emission computed tomography findings is useful for the evaluation of cardiac event risk. Nucl Med Commun 2009; 30(1): 54-61. [http://dx.doi.org/10.1097/MNM.0b013e328314b879]

[53] Nishimura M, Tsukamoto K, Hasebe N, Tamaki N, Kikuchi K, Ono T. Prediction of cardiac death in hemodialysis patients by myocardial fatty acid imaging. J Am Coll Cardiol 2008; 51(2): 139-45. [http://dx.doi.org/10.1016/j.jacc.2007.08.057]

[54] Nishimura M, Tokoro T, Nishida M, *et al.* Myocardial fatty acid imaging identifies a group of hemodialysis patients at high risk for cardiac death after coronary revascularization. Kidney Int 2008; 74(4): 513-20. [http://dx.doi.org/10.1038/ki.2008.211]

[55] Nishimura M, Hashimoto T, Tamaki N, Kobayashi H, Ono T. Focal impairment in myocardial fatty acid imaging in the left anterior descending artery area, a strong predictor for cardiac death in hemodialysis patients without obstructive coronary artery disease. Eur J Nucl Med Mol Imaging 2015; 42(10): 1612-21.

[http://dx.doi.org/10.1007/s00259-015-3120-8]

[56] Hasebe N, Moroi M, Nishimura M, *et al.* Prognostic study of cardiac events in Japanese high risk hemodialysis patients using I-BMIPP-SPECT: B-SAFE study design. Ther Apher Dial 2008; 12(6): 526-30.
[http://dx.doi.org/10.1111/j.1744-9987.2008.00643.x]

[57] Moroi M, Tamaki N, Nishimura M, *et al.* Association between abnormal myocardial fatty acid metabolism and cardiac-derived death among patients undergoing hemodialysis: results from a cohort study in Japan. Am J Kidney Dis 2013; 61(3): 466-75.
[http://dx.doi.org/10.1053/j.ajkd.2012.09.017]

[58] Zen K, Tamaki N, Nishimura M, *et al.* Cardiac event risk stratification in patients with end-stage renal disease: Sub-analysis of the B-SAFE study. Int J Cardiol 2016; 202: 694-700.
[http://dx.doi.org/10.1016/j.ijcard.2015.09.119]

[59] Nishimura M, Tsukamoto K, Tamaki N, Kikuchi K, Iwamoto N, Ono T. Risk stratification for cardiac death in hemodialysis patients without obstructive coronary artery disease. Kidney Int 2011; 79(3): 363-71.
[http://dx.doi.org/10.1038/ki.2010.392]

[60] Nishimura M, Okamoto Y, Takatani T, *et al.* Improvement of myocardial fatty acid metabolism by oral nicorandil in hemodialysis patients without coronary artery disease. J Nephrol 2015; 28(2): 227-34.
[http://dx.doi.org/10.1007/s40620-014-0125-5]

[61] Nishimura M, Tokoro T, Takatani T, *et al.* Effects of intravenous l-carnitine on myocardial fatty acid imaging in hemodialysis patients: responders or non-responders to l-carnitine. Springerplus 2015; 4: 353.
[http://dx.doi.org/10.1186/s40064-015-1119-z]

[62] Nakata T, Hashimoto A, Moroi M, *et al.* Sudden death prediction by C-reactive protein, electrocardiographic findings, and myocardial fatty acid uptake in haemodialysis patients: analysis of a multicentre prospective cohort sub-study. Eur Heart J Cardiovasc Imaging 2016; 17(12): 1394-404.
[http://dx.doi.org/10.1093/ehjci/jev294]

[63] Kiriyama T, Kumita S, Moroi M, *et al.* Interpretative variability and its impact on the prognostic value of myocardial fatty acid imaging in asymptomatic hemodialysis patients in a multicenter trial in Japan. Circ J 2015; 79(1): 153-60.
[http://dx.doi.org/10.1253/circj.CJ-14-0646]

[64] Wackers FJ, Bodenheimer M, Fleiss JL, Brown M. Factors affecting uniformity in interpretation of planar thallium-201 imaging in a multicenter trial. The Multicenter Study on Silent Myocardial Ischemia (MSSMI) Thallium-201 Investigators. J Am Coll Cardiol 1993; 21(5): 1064-74.
[http://dx.doi.org/10.1016/0735-1097(93)90226-Q]

[65] Suleiman K, Desai D, Raval U, Senior R, Lahiri A. The effect of training on the interpretation of 99Tcm-sestamibi myocardial perfusion SPET in patients with suspected coronary artery disease. Nucl Med Commun 1997; 18(10): 922-6.
[http://dx.doi.org/10.1097/00006231-199710000-00005]

[66] Tanabe Y, Yoneyama K, Izumo M, Kongoji K, Harada T, Akashi YJ. A case of coronary microvascular spasm with slow flow induced by the intracoronary acetylcholine provocation test. Cardiovasc Interv Ther 2015; 30(4): 372-6.
[http://dx.doi.org/10.1007/s12928-014-0308-y]

[67] Mori H, Isobe S, Sakai S, *et al.* Microvascular obstruction on delayed enhancement cardiac magnetic resonance imaging after acute myocardial infarction, compared with myocardial (201)Tl and (123)I-BMIPP dual SPECT findings. Eur J Radiol 2015; 84(8): 1516-24.
[http://dx.doi.org/10.1016/j.ejrad.2015.05.002]

[68] Kurata C, Tawarahara K, Taguchi T, *et al.* Myocardial emission computed tomography with iodine-

123-labeled beta-methyl-branched fatty acid in patients with hypertrophic cardiomyopathy. J Nucl Med 1992; 33(1): 6-13.

[69] Shimonagata T, Nishimura T, Uehara T, *et al.* Discrepancies between myocardial perfusion and free fatty acid metabolism in patients with hypertrophic cardiomyopathy. Nucl Med Commun 1993; 14(11): 1005-13. [http://dx.doi.org/10.1097/00006231-199311000-00012]

[70] Nishimura T, Nagata S, Uehara T, *et al.* Prognosis of hypertrophic cardiomyopathy: assessment by 123I-BMIPP (beta-methyl-p-(123I)iodophenyl pentadecanoic acid) myocardial single photon emission computed tomography. Ann Nucl Med 1996; 10(1): 71-8. [http://dx.doi.org/10.1007/BF03165056]

[71] Ohtsuki K, Sugihara H, Kuribayashi T, Nakagawa M. Impairment of BMIPP accumulation at junction of ventricular septum and left and right ventricular free walls in hypertrophic cardiomyopathy. J Nucl Med 1999; 40(12): 2007-13.

[72] Amano Y, Kumita S, Takayama M, Kumazaki T. Comparison of contrast-enhanced MRI with iodine-123 BMIPP for detection of myocardial damage in hypertrophic cardiomyopathy. AJR Am J Roentgenol 2005; 185(2): 312-8. [http://dx.doi.org/10.2214/ajr.185.2.01850312]

[73] Hashimura H, Kiso K, Yamada N, *et al.* Myocardial impairment detected by late gadolinium enhancement in hypertrophic cardiomyopathy: comparison with 99mTc-MIBI/tetrofosmin and 123I-BMIPP SPECT. Kobe J Med Sci 2013; 59(3): E81-92.

[74] O'Hanlon R, Grasso A, Roughton M, *et al.* Prognostic significance of myocardial fibrosis in hypertrophic cardiomyopathy. J Am Coll Cardiol 2010; 56(11): 867-74. [http://dx.doi.org/10.1016/j.jacc.2010.05.010]

[75] Prinz C, Schwarz M, Ilic I, *et al.* Myocardial fibrosis severity on cardiac magnetic resonance imaging predicts sustained arrhythmic events in hypertrophic cardiomyopathy. Can J Cardiol 2013; 29(3): 358-63. [http://dx.doi.org/10.1016/j.cjca.2012.05.004]

[76] Ishida Y, Yasumura Y, Nagaya N, *et al.* Myocardial imaging with 123I-BMIPP in patients with congestive heart failure. Int J Card Imaging 1999; 15(1): 71-7. [http://dx.doi.org/10.1023/A:1006152804670]

[77] Abe H, Iguchi N, Utanohara Y, *et al.* Non-invasive diagnosis of coronary artery disease by 123I-BMIPP/201TlCl dual myocardial SPECT in patients with heart failure. Int J Cardiol 2014; 176(3): 969-74. [http://dx.doi.org/10.1016/j.ijcard.2014.08.129]

[78] Yazaki Y, Isobe M, Takahashi W, *et al.* Assessment of myocardial fatty acid metabolic abnormalities in patients with idiopathic dilated cardiomyopathy using 123I BMIPP SPECT: correlation with clinicopathological findings and clinical course. Heart 1999; 81(2): 153-9. [http://dx.doi.org/10.1136/hrt.81.2.153]

[79] Yoshida A, Takano H, Asai K, *et al.* Comparison of perfusion-metabolism mismatch in 99mTc-MIBI and 123I-BMIPP scintigraphy with cardiac magnetic resonance in patients with dilated cardiomyopathy. J Card Fail 2013; 19(7): 445-53. [http://dx.doi.org/10.1016/j.cardfail.2013.05.009]

[80] Ito T, Hoshida S, Nishino M, *et al.* Relationship between evaluation by quantitative fatty acid myocardial scintigraphy and response to beta-blockade therapy in patients with dilated cardiomyopathy. Eur J Nucl Med 2001; 28(12): 1811-6. [http://dx.doi.org/10.1007/s00259-001-0668-2]

[81] Zavadovsky KV, Gulya MO, Lishmanov YB, Lebedev DI. Perfusion and metabolic scintigraphy with (123)I-BMIPP in prognosis of cardiac resynchronization therapy in patients with dilated cardiomyopathy. Ann Nucl Med 2016; 30(5): 325-33.

[http://dx.doi.org/10.1007/s12149-016-1064-0]

[82] Sato HUT, Dote K, Ishihara M. Tako-tsubo-like left ventricular dysfunction due to multivessel coronary spasm From ischemia to heart failure. Tokyo: Kagakuhyoronsha Publishing 1990; pp. 56-64.

[83] Manabe O, Naya M, Oyama-Manabe N, Koyanagawa K, Tamaki N. The role of multimodality imaging in takotsubo cardiomyopathy. J Nucl Cardiol 2018. [http://dx.doi.org/10.1007/s12350-018-1312-x]

[84] Kobylecka M, Budnik M, Kochanowski J, *et al.* Takotsubo cardiomyopathy: FDG myocardial uptake pattern in fasting patients. Comparison of PET/CT, SPECT, and ECHO results. J Nucl Cardiol 2017.

[85] Uchida Y, Nanjo S, Fujimoto S, *et al.* Scintigraphic studies on the etiology of Ampulla Cardiomyopathy. J Cardiol 2008; 51(2): 121-30. [http://dx.doi.org/10.1016/j.jjcc.2008.02.002]

[86] Kurowski V, Kaiser A, von Hof K, *et al.* Apical and midventricular transient left ventricular dysfunction syndrome (tako-tsubo cardiomyopathy): frequency, mechanisms, and prognosis. Chest 2007; 132(3): 809-16. [http://dx.doi.org/10.1378/chest.07-0608]

[87] Matsuo S, Nakajima K, Kinuya S, Yamagishi M. Diagnostic utility of 123I-BMIPP imaging in patients with Takotsubo cardiomyopathy. J Cardiol 2014; 64(1): 49-56. [http://dx.doi.org/10.1016/j.jjcc.2013.10.019]

[88] Seko Y, Sasaki K, Kato T, Inoko M. (123)I-BMIPP single-photon emission computed tomography for diagnosing chest pain in patients with nonobstructive coronary angiograms: Takotsubo or vasospasm? Clin Case Rep 2017; 5(10): 1716-7. [http://dx.doi.org/10.1002/ccr3.1134]

[89] Sugihara Y, Fukushima Y, Kumita SI, Takano H, Shimizu W. Diagnostic performance of hybrid cardiac SPECT/CT imaging for patients with takotsubo cardiomyopathy European journal of hybrid imaging 2018; 2(1)

[90] Hashimoto H, Nakanishi R, Mizumura S, *et al.* Prognostic Value of (123)I-BMIPP SPECT in Patients with Nonischemic Heart Failure with Preserved Ejection Fraction. J Nucl Med 2018; 59(2): 259-65. [http://dx.doi.org/10.2967/jnumed.117.195743]

[91] Kida K, Akashi YJ, Yoneyama K, Shimokawa M, Musha H. 123I-BMIPP delayed scintigraphic imaging in patients with chronic heart failure. Ann Nucl Med 2008; 22(9): 769-75. [http://dx.doi.org/10.1007/s12149-008-0180-x]

[92] Abraham WT, Hayes DL. Cardiac resynchronization therapy for heart failure. Circulation 2003; 108(21): 2596-603. [http://dx.doi.org/10.1161/01.CIR.0000096580.26969.9A]

[93] Lishmanov Y, Minin S, Efimova I, *et al.* The possible role of nuclear imaging in assessment of the cardiac resynchronization therapy effectiveness in patients with moderate heart failure. Ann Nucl Med 2013; 27(4): 378-85. [http://dx.doi.org/10.1007/s12149-013-0696-6]

[94] Evans JD, Gomez DR, Chang JY, *et al.* Cardiac (1)(8)F-fluorodeoxyglucose uptake on positron emission tomography after thoracic stereotactic body radiation therapy. Radiother Oncol 2013; 109(1): 82-8. [http://dx.doi.org/10.1016/j.radonc.2013.07.021]

[95] Ghobadi G, van der Veen S, Bartelds B, *et al.* Physiological interaction of heart and lung in thoracic irradiation. Int J Radiat Oncol Biol Phys 2012; 84(5): e639-46. [http://dx.doi.org/10.1016/j.ijrobp.2012.07.2362]

[96] Zhang P, Hu X, Yue J, *et al.* Early detection of radiation-induced heart disease using (99m)Tc-MIBI SPECT gated myocardial perfusion imaging in patients with oesophageal cancer during radiotherapy. Radiother Oncol 2015; 115(2): 171-8.

[http://dx.doi.org/10.1016/j.radonc.2015.04.009]

[97] Takanami K, Arai A, Umezawa R, *et al.* Association between radiation dose to the heart and myocardial fatty acid metabolic impairment due to chemoradiation-therapy: Prospective study using I-123 BMIPP SPECT/CT. Radiother Oncol 2016; 119(1): 77-83. [http://dx.doi.org/10.1016/j.radonc.2016.01.024]

[98] Umezawa R, Takase K, Jingu K, *et al.* Evaluation of radiation-induced myocardial damage using iodine-123 beta-methyl-iodophenyl pentadecanoic acid scintigraphy. J Radiat Res (Tokyo) 2013; 54(5): 880-9. [http://dx.doi.org/10.1093/jrr/rrt011]

[99] Darby SC, Ewertz M, McGale P, *et al.* Risk of ischemic heart disease in women after radiotherapy for breast cancer. N Engl J Med 2013; 368(11): 987-98. [http://dx.doi.org/10.1056/NEJMoa1209825]

[100] Momose M, Fukushima K, Kondo C, *et al.* Diagnosis and Detection of Myocardial Injury in Active Cardiac Sarcoidosis--Significance of Myocardial Fatty Acid Metabolism and Myocardial Perfusion Mismatch. Circ J 2015; 79(12): 2669-76. [http://dx.doi.org/10.1253/circj.CJ-15-0681]

[101] Kataoka S, Momose M, Fukushima K, *et al.* Regional myocardial damage and active inflammation in patients with cardiac sarcoidosis detected by non-invasive multi-modal imaging. Ann Nucl Med 2017; 31(2): 135-43. [http://dx.doi.org/10.1007/s12149-016-1136-1]

[102] Mahmud E, Madani MM, Kim NH, *et al.* Chronic Thromboembolic Pulmonary Hypertension: Evolving Therapeutic Approaches for Operable and Inoperable Disease. J Am Coll Cardiol 2018; 71(21): 2468-86. [http://dx.doi.org/10.1016/j.jacc.2018.04.009]

[103] Sakao S, Daimon M, Voelkel NF, *et al.* Right ventricular sugars and fats in chronic thromboembolic pulmonary hypertension. Int J Cardiol 2016; 219: 143-9. [http://dx.doi.org/10.1016/j.ijcard.2016.06.010]

[104] Hirano K, Ikeda Y, Zaima N, Sakata Y, Matsumiya G. Triglyceride deposit cardiomyovasculopathy. N Engl J Med 2008; 359(22): 2396-8. [http://dx.doi.org/10.1056/NEJMc0805305]

[105] Higashi M, Ikeda Y, Miyauchi H, *et al.* Imaging Modalities for Triglyceride Deposit Cardiomyovasculopathy. Annals of Nuclear Cardiology 2017; 3(1): 94-102. [http://dx.doi.org/10.17996/anc.17-00028]

[106] Ikawa M, Kawai Y, Arakawa K, *et al.* Evaluation of respiratory chain failure in mitochondrial cardiomyopathy by assessments of 99mTc-MIBI washout and 123I-BMIPP/99mTc-MIBI mismatch. Mitochondrion 2007; 7(1-2): 164-70. [http://dx.doi.org/10.1016/j.mito.2006.11.008]

[107] Matsuo S, Nakajima K, Kinuya S, Sato Y, Matsumoto N, Horie M. Cardiac scintigraphic findings of mitochondrial myopathy, encephalopathy, lactic acidosis and stroke-like episodes: A case report. Exp Clin Cardiol 2008; 13(2): 93-5.

[108] Tashiro R, Onoue N, Rikimaru H, *et al.* Mitochondrial Cardiomyopathy with a Unique (99m)Tc-MIBI/(123)I-BMIPP Mismatch Pattern. Intern Med 2017; 56(3): 321-5. [http://dx.doi.org/10.2169/internalmedicine.56.7525]

[109] Matsuo S, Nakajima K, Yamashina S, *et al.* Characterization of Japanese standards for myocardial sympathetic and metabolic imaging in comparison with perfusion imaging. Ann Nucl Med 2009; 23(6): 517-22. [http://dx.doi.org/10.1007/s12149-009-0269-x]

[110] Yoshinaga K, Matsuki T, Hashimoto A, Tsukamoto K, Nakata T, Tamaki N. Validation of automated

quantitation of myocardial perfusion and fatty acid metabolism abnormalities on SPECT images. Circ J 2011; 75(9): 2187-95.
[http://dx.doi.org/10.1253/circj.CJ-10-1272]

[111] Akashi YJ, Kida K, Suzuki K, *et al.* The significance of 123I-BMIPP delayed scintigraphic imaging in cardiac patients. Int J Cardiol 2007; 117(2): 145-51.
[http://dx.doi.org/10.1016/j.ijcard.2006.04.056]

[112] Koyama K, Akashi YJ, Kida K, *et al.* Relevance of I-BMIPP delayed scintigraphic imaging for patients with angina pectoris - a pilot study. Archives of medical science. AMS 2011; 7(3): 428-32.

[113] Okizaki A, Shuke N, Sato J, *et al.* A compartment model analysis for investigation of myocardial fatty acid metabolism in patients with hypertrophic cardiomyopathy. Nucl Med Commun 2007; 28(9): 726-35.
[http://dx.doi.org/10.1097/MNM.0b013e32828da1c7]

[114] Kobayashi M, Matsunari I, Nishi K, *et al.* Simultaneous acquisition of (99m)Tc- and (123)I-labeled radiotracers using a preclinical SPECT scanner with CZT detectors. Ann Nucl Med 2016; 30(4): 263-71.
[http://dx.doi.org/10.1007/s12149-015-1055-6]

[115] Takahashi Y, Miyagawa M, Nishiyama Y, Kawaguchi N, Ishimura H, Mochizuki T. Dual radioisotopes simultaneous SPECT of (99m)Tc-tetrofosmin and (123)I-BMIPP using a semiconductor detector. Asia Ocean J Nucl Med Biol 2015; 3(1): 43-9.

[116] Ko T, Utanohara Y, Suzuki Y, *et al.* A preliminary feasibility study of simultanecus dual-isotope imaging with a solid-state dedicated cardiac camera for evaluating myocardial perfusion and fatty acid metabolism. Heart Vessels 2016; 31(1): 38-45.
[http://dx.doi.org/10.1007/s00380-014-0578-4]

[117] JCS Joint Working Group. 2010. JCS Joint Working Group. Guidelines for clinical use of cardiac nuclear medicine (JCS 2010) Available from: 2010 http://www.j-circ.or.jp/guideline/pdf/JCS2010tamaki.h.pdf

[118] JCS Joint Working Group. Guidelines for clinical use of cardiac nuclear medicine (JCS 2010) - digest version. Circ J 2012; 76(3): 761-7.
[http://dx.doi.org/10.1253/circj.CJ-88-0019]

[119] Mattsson S, Johansson L, Leide Svegborn S, *et al.* Radiation Dose to Patients from Radiopharmaceuticals: a Compendium of Current Information Related to Frequently Used Substances. Ann ICRP 2015; 44(2) (Suppl.): 7-321.
[http://dx.doi.org/10.1177/0146645314558019]

CHAPTER 9

Potential Uses of ^{123}*m*IBG and Analogous PET Tracers to Guide Use of Cardiac Implantable Electronic Devices in Heart Failure and Associated Arrhythmias

Mark I. Travin*

Department of Radiology, Division of Nuclear Medicine, Montefiore Medical Center, Albert Einstein College of Medicine, Bronx, NY, USA

Abstract: Heart failure has become a worldwide pandemic, with high morbidity and mortality, and also high costs. While better therapies are improving outcomes, many of the treatments are invasive and expensive, particularly cardiac implantable electronic devices (CIEDs). As the effectiveness of many pharmacologic therapies are attributed to their addressing the neurohormonal pathophysiology underlying heart failure, one would expect that using CIEDs based on neurohormonal parameters would provide more effective use of them. An important component of the neurohormonal system is cardiac adrenergic innervation that can be imaged with single photon radiotracers such as iodine-123 *meta*iodobenzylguanidine (^{123}I-*m*IBG) and analogous positron emission (PET) tracers such as carbon-11-metahydroxyephedrine (^{11}C-HED). Adrenergic imaging has consistently been shown to effectively risk stratify patients with heart failure with reduced ejection fraction (HFrEF), and it does so independently of, and in many cases better than, customarily used parameters. In addition, adrenergic imaging has been shown to effectively and independently stratify HFrEF patients in terms of the risk of a lethal ventricular arrhythmic event. For therapeutic guidance, while adrenergic imaging is unlikely to influence institution of guidelines directed pharmacologic treatments, there is much evidence of a potential to help guide use of CIEDs such as biventricular pacemakers for cardiac resynchronization therapy (CRT), ventricular assist devices for end-stage HFrEF (LVAD), and implantable cardioverter defibrillators (ICDs). In particular, ^{123}I-*m*IBG imaging parameters appear to follow a patient's clinical response to CRT and perhaps could better identify which patients are more likely to benefit. ^{123}I-*m*IBG imaging parameters, by identifying when pharmacologic therapy is failing, could show earlier in the disease course when LVAD would be beneficial, and then later help determine when or if patients who already have the device have achieved reverse ventricular remodeling sufficient to consider LVAD explantation. Finally, evidence indicates that adrenergic imaging should be able to more effectively guide use of ICDs than current recommendations that are based largely on ejection fraction, with imaging especially able to identify patients who are

* **Corresponding author Mark I. Travin:** Department of Radiology, Division of Nuclear Medicine, Montefiore Medical Center, 111 East 210th St. Bronx, NY 10467-2490, USA; Tel: 7189205014; Fax: 7189205014; Email: mtravin@montefiore.org

Shinro Matsuo (Ed.)

very unlikely to benefit from this device that has underappreciated morbidities. In addition, with regard to addressing ventricular arrhythmias, there are studies reporting benefits of adrenergic imaging for guidance of invasive electrophysiological therapeutic procedures. Thus, while CIEDs have provided tremendous benefit to people with advanced heart failure, with technologic advances continuously occurring, radionuclide adrenergic imaging shows much promise in more effectively guiding use of these devices.

Keywords: Adrenergic Innervation, Autonomic Nervous System, Cardiac Resynchronization Therapy (CRT), Cardiac Implantable Electronic Device (CIED), Heart Failure, ^{123}I-*m*IBG, Implantable Cardioverter Defibrillator (ICD), Left Ventricular Assist Device (LVAD), Radionuclide Adrenergic Imaging, Ventricular Arrhythmias.

INTRODUCTION

Heart failure (HF) is considered by many to be a pandemic, affecting more than 26 million people worldwide, with an anticipated dramatically increased future prevalence as populations age [1]. In the United States (US), data from 2011-2014 estimated that 6.5 million people 20 years of age or older had HF, up from about 5.7 million in 2009-2012 [2]. By 2030, it is predicted that >8 million people 18 or older will have HF. While survival after HF onset has been improving, the US mortality rate remains high at 35% - 37% in 1 year [3], and 39% to about 50% in 5 years [2]. HF is also an expensive condition, with the total cost in 2012 estimated to be $30.7 billion and projected to be $69.7 billion by 2030 [2]. It is therefore crucial that preventive efforts be enhanced and for new therapies to be developed. It is also important that treatments, both new ones and those currently used, be effectively targeted to appropriate patients, especially the more invasive and costly cardiac implantable electronic devices (CIEDs). There is evidence that radionuclide imaging with adrenergic tracers may be useful in this regard.

NEUROHORMONAL REGULATION OF CARDIOVASCULAR FUNCTION

While in the distant past, the approach to HF was primarily directed towards the hemodynamic effects of decreased cardiac output (CO), much current focus is on neurohormonal (also known as "neurohormonal") mechanisms and molecular pathophysiology for patients with both abnormal and preserved ejection fractions (EF) [4]. Neurohormonal pathophysiology includes both circulating hormones, such as epinephrine, norepinephrine (NE), arginine vasopressin, B-type natriuretic peptide (BNP) and mediators of the renin-angiotensin-aldosterone system (RAAS), and direct cardiac and vascular innervation by autonomic neurons, all serving to regulate CO, blood volume and vascular tone for maintenance of sufficient circulation to body organs and tissues [5, 6]. Cardiovascular autonomic innervation consists of complex arrangements of afferent and efferent sympathetic and parasympathetic fibers coursing between the brain, spinal cord, relay points, and cardiovascular structures and other organs, described in detail in a recent review by Jamali *et al.* [7]. The mediator of the sympathetic system is norepinephrine (NE), and that of the parasympathetic system is acetylcholine. Radionuclide analogues of these mediators and of target organ receptors have been developed and studied. As clinical investigations and patient use have been limited mostly to NE radiotracer analogues, this review will focus on assessment of cardiac pre-sympathetic (adrenergic) innervation.

RADIONUCLIDE IMAGING OF CARDIAC SYMPATHETIC INNERVATION

Cardiac autonomic sympathetic imaging focuses on the synaptic junction [8, 9]. In the presynaptic terminal, NE is synthesized from tyrosine and stored in vesicles. In response to stimuli, NE is released from the vesicles into the synaptic spaces and binds to post-synaptic α, β1 and β2-receptors on the myocyte membrane, producing physiologic changes. Most NE is then taken back into the pre-synaptic terminal *via* an energy dependent protein-mediated norepinephrine transporter-1 (NET-1) process for catabolic disposal. A false neurotransmitter NE analogue, guanethidine, can be radiolabelled with iodine-123, best in the meta-position, to create I-123 *meta*-iodobenzylguanidine (^{123}I-*m*IBG) [10, 11]. When administered intravenously to a patient, ^{123}I-*m*IBG diffuses into synaptic spaces and is taken up similar to NE *via* NET-1 into the presynaptic terminal. However, as a false neurotransmitter, the compound is not metabolized and therefore accumulates, allowing imaging with a conventional gamma or newer solid-state camera. The finding of satisfactory myocardial tracer uptake signifies both intact anatomic neuronal innervation and satisfactory neuronal physiologic function [12] (although reduced tracer uptake could also occur because of competition from increased circulating or synaptic NE).

Positron emission tomography (PET) tracers have also been studied, but none are US Food and Drug Administration (FDA) approved for clinical use at the time of this writing [13]. PET yields higher counts, and thus better image quality than ^{123}I-*m*IBG. PET tracers also have a variety of biologic properties that lead to differing uptake characteristics in both normal situations and disease states [14]. The most commonly studied PET adrenergic tracer, ^{11}C-meta-hydroxyephedrine (HED), has better NET-1 selectivity than ^{123}I-*m*IBG, thus better differentiating innervated *versus* denervated myocardium [15]. Other PET radiotracers that have been investigated include ^{11}C-epinpehrine and ^{11}C-phenylephrine, as well as an ^{18}F-based adrenergic tracer ([^{18}F]LMI1195) [16].

As a SPECT tracer, ^{123}I-*m*IBG can be imaged with both planar and single photon emission tomographic (SPECT) techniques. Acquisition methodology and image results for interpretation are described in detail in published guidelines of the European Association of Nuclear Medicine (EANM) Cardiovascular Committee/European Council of Nuclear Cardiology [17] and the American Society of Nuclear Cardiology (ASNC) [18]. The major focus of image interpretation has been global cardiac tracer uptake in reference to mediastinal uptake on an anterior planar image, termed the "heart to mediastinum ratio" (HMR). Normal HMRs (for Anger cameras) range from 1.9-2.8, a mean of 2.2 ± 0.3, with a value ≥1.6 (within 2 standard deviations of the mean) used as a threshold for risk stratification studies (higher values being better) [19]. In addition, the change in cardiac counts between the initial (early) and 4-hour (late) anterior planar images, termed washout (WO) or washout rate (WR), that reflects both cellular retention of tracer and competition from circulating catecholamines, has been shown to reflect integrity and function of sympathetic innervation, with a reported value for controls subject of 10% ± 9% (lower values being better) [20].

Tomographic imaging allows better visualization and quantitative analysis of differences in regional tracer uptake. As the autonomic nervous system plays a key role in the genesis and propagation of cardiac arrhythmias, and because innervation injury is thought to create regions of electrical heterogeneity, there has been much focus on using adrenergic imaging to assess risk of lethal ventricular arrhythmias and potentially guide therapy, especially use of the implantable cardiac defibrillator (ICD) [21, 22]. In addition to tracer uptake heterogeneity, it has been proposed that preserved uptake of a perfusion tracer in a region with dysinnervation (neural dysfunction) or denervation (anatomic loss of sympathetic nerves), termed a "perfusion/adrenergic mismatch," have been shown to produce a regions of denervation supersensitivity [23].

CLINICAL APPLICATIONS OF ADRENERGIC IMAGING IN HEART FAILURE

Risk Stratification Power in Patients with Heart Failure

The ability of ^{123}I-*m*IBG imaging to risk stratify patients with heart failure was first illustrated by Schofer *et al.* [24] who showed that a lower HMR was associated with a lower left ventricular ejection fraction (LVEF) and lower myocardial NE content, both parameters associated with worsened clinical HF. Shortly thereafter a key study by Merlet *et al.* [25] reported that HMR was extremely effective in risk stratifying patients with advanced systolic HF (New York Heart Association (NYHA) Class II – IV, LVEF <45%) that was independent of customarily used risk stratification variables such as LVEF and cardiac size, with patients having a relatively high HMR having a 98% negative predictive value for death over 25 months. Subsequently, following many single-center studies confirming risk stratification power of ^{123}I-*m*IBG imaging in HF [26], the landmark AdreView Myocardial Imaging for Risk Evaluation in Heart Failure (ADMIRE-HF, AdreView = ^{123}I-*m*IBG) trial was undertaken [27]. In this international multicenter observational cohort study of 961 patients with NYHA Class II-III HF and LVEF ≤35%, it was found that in relation to patients with an HMR <1.6, those with a value ≥1.6 had a decreased (37% to 15%) occurrence of worsening NYHA class, life-threatening ventricular arrhythmias, and cardiac death over a 17-month median follow-up. Of note, for these patients who by conventional criteria were considered high risk, those with HMR ≥1.6 had a <1% mortality. ADMIRE-HF findings were confirmed by a 6 center Japanese consortium study that re-analyzed previously collected ^{123}I-*m*IBG data on 1322 patients with HF, with late HMR at approximately a threshold of 1.68 effectively risk stratifying patients in terms of all-cause mortality independently from conventional HF variables that included NYHA class, BNP, LVEF, and age [28]. Based on the aforementioned studies, and numerous others not described here showing consistent findings, one can rightly claim that the ability of ^{123}I-*m*IBG imaging to effectively risk stratify patients with HFrEF independently of conventional risk stratification conventional parameters has been established. Data has also been generated showing risk stratification power in patients with higher EFs [28, 29].

Risk Stratification for Risk of Ventricular Arrhythmias and Sudden Cardiac Death

Shortly after the development of ^{123}I-*m*IBG, Donald Wieland, the principle investigator, often commented that "although perfusion tracers like ^{201}Tl provided information on the 'plumbing of the heart,' *m*IBG provided clinicians with insights into the 'wiring' of the heart" [10]. It is understood that abnormalities of cardiac autonomic innervation can lead to the development of sustained cardiac atrial and ventricular arrhythmias *via* several mechanisms, including creation of abnormal electrical heterogeneity in cardiac substrate, by acting as an arrhythmic trigger, and by propagating an otherwise self-terminating arrhythmia [30, 31]. Therefore, abnormalities of cardiac autonomic innervation increase the likelihood of arrhythmic sudden cardiac death (SCD).

Numerous animal and clinical investigations have demonstrated that ^{123}I-*m*IBG cardiac uptake abnormalities are associated with increased susceptibility to ventricular arrhythmias. Working in the laboratory of Dr. Douglas Zipes, Kammerling *et al.* [23] observed that creation of sympathetic efferent denervation in dogs increased vulnerability to programmed ventricular stimulation induced ventricular fibrillation, termed "denervation supersensitivity". In the same institution, Stanton *et al.* [32] reported that in patients one week or more after myocardial infarction (MI), the finding of ^{123}I-*m*IBG defects in regions of perfused myocardium were associated with spontaneous ventricular tachyarrhythmias. Working under the direction of Michael Dae, Yoshioka *et al.* [33] found that ^{123}I-*m*IBG regional defects created in rabbits were associated with an electrophysiologically demonstrated shortening or dispersion of activation recovery intervals that could increase the likelihood of a fatal arrhythmia. Finally working under James Willerson, McGhie *et al.* [34] saw that ^{123}I-*m*IBG defects that were more extensive than ^{201}Tl perfusion defects 1-2 weeks after MI were associated with increased ventricular ectopy including tachycardia.

In Japan, for patients with LVEF <40% Tamaki *et al.* [35] compared arrhythmia associated ECG parameters such as heart rate variability (HRV), QT dispersion and signal-averaged electrocardiography (SAECG) with ^{123}I-*m*IBG image findings, and found that those with SCD had a lower HMR and greater WR, with only WR and LVEF independently predictive of SCD, while the ECG parameters showed no independent predictive power.

In ADMIRE-HF [27], with non-fatal arrhythmic events (separate from SCD) defined as documented spontaneous sustained (>30s) ventricular tachycardia, resuscitated cardiac arrest, or an appropriate ICD discharge (antitachycardia pacing or defibrillation), an HMR ≥1.6 was associated with a significantly lower combined arrhythmic and SCD event rate than those with HMR < 1.6 (3.5% *versus* 10.4% $p < 0.01$). The highest rate of 13.1% was in patients with HMR 1.30 to 1.39, and the highest HMR of a subject experiencing a fatal arrhythmic event was 1.60. In a subsequent analysis of tomographic images of 471 ADMIRE-HF patients whose heart failure was classified as ischemic in origin [36], as shown in Fig. (**1**) patients with higher summed dysinnervation scores (^{123}I-*m*IBG summed scores >14) had significantly higher arrhythmic and SCD outcomes ($p = 0.042$), but most high at 21.1% in patients with intermediately (^{123}I-*m*IBG summed scores 14-28) abnormal dysinnervation. The planar and tomographic findings of intermediate abnormality severities being associated with the highest arrhythmic event rates may indicate that such patients have the most electrical heterogeneity, as well as being more likely to die from arrhythmic than pump failure causes in relation to patients with the severest abnormalities. In addition, as in nearly all analyses of ^{123}I-*m*IBG imaging, risk stratification was independent of other commonly used variables, in this case BNP and LVEF.

As discussed before, adrenergic PET tracers, while in some ways similar to ^{123}I-*m*IBG, also have different physical and biologic properties. For example, Luisi *et al.* [15] demonstrated that in a porcine model ^{11}C-HED yields an improved signal to noise ratio that improves the ability to determine defect severity. The ability of this PET tracer to perform arrhythmic risk stratification was investigated in the Prediction of ARrhythmic Events with Positron Emission Tomography trial (PAREPET) study, in which in 204 subjects with an ischemic cardiomyopathy were followed for more than 4 years, ^{11}C-HED image findings effectively predicted the occurrence of sudden cardiac arrest define as arrhythmic death, an ICD shock for VT >240/minute or ventricular fibrillation, and did so independently of symptoms, infarct volume, LVEF, or BNP [37]. Further analyses by this group showed that variables associated with an increased likelihood of sudden cardiac death (SCD) were different from those associated with non-sudden cardiac death (NSCD). A greater extent of ^{11}C-HED denervation was independently associated with SCD while other variables were predictive of NSCD. Importantly, after statistically adjusting for competing risks, neither LVEF nor NYHA class – the key variables used in guidelines for ICD use – was independently associated with either outcome [38, 39].

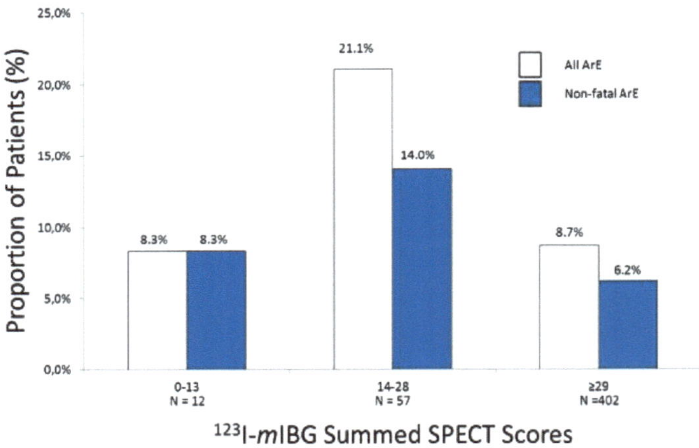

Fig. (1). Proportion of arrhythmic events (ArE) and non-fatal arrhythmic events in relation to low, intermediate, and high 17-segment ^{123}I-*m*IBG scores. Note: Non-fatal ArEs include only spontaneous sustained (>30 seconds) ventricular tachycardia, resuscitated cardiac arrest and appropriate ICD activation. Reprinted by permission from Springer Nature, Journal of Nuclear Cardiology, Travin MI, Henzlova MJ, van Eck-Smit BLF, Jain J, Carrió I, Folks RD, Garcia EV, Jacobson AF, Verberne HJ. Assessment of ^{123}I-*m*IBG and ^{99m}Tc-tetrofosmin single-photon emission computed tomographic images for the prediction of arrhythmic events in patients with ischemic heart failure. J Nucl Cardiol; 2017; 24: 377-91 [36].

In summary, in the studies discussed here and in numerous others [40], the value of ^{123}I-*m*IBG imaging to predict the risk of lethal or potential lethal ventricular arrhythmias beyond that of other commonly used parameters has been consistently shown in diverse patient groups. It is therefore reasonable to assert that the independent arrhythmic risk stratification ability of adrenergic imaging is established.

USE OF CARDIAC ADRENERGIC IMAGING TO GUIDE THERAPY

In the current era in which costs of medical care are high, it is no longer considered sufficient for an imaging technique to solely risk stratify a patient. Professional societies and payers are demanding that imaging techniques, particularly those that are most expensive, be clinically effective. As per Shaw *et al.*, the utility of a cardiovascular imaging technique depends on its results leading to "appropriate and targeted therapies that improve symptom burden and long-term outcomes [that] are not offset by high upfront procedural and induced costs, [and the clinical benefit] must significantly outweigh any untoward risks associated with imaging [41].

At the current time, the US FDA approval for cardiac ^{123}I-*m*IBG imaging is limited to helping to "identify patients with lower one and two-year mortality risks, as indicated by an HMR ≥1.6" with the advisory that, "[in] patients with congestive heart failure, AdreView utility has not been established for: selecting a therapeutic intervention or for monitoring the response to therapy; [or] using the HMR to identify a patient with a high risk for death [42]". Nevertheless, numerous studies have demonstrated that ^{123}I-*m*IBG imaging can effectively track the effectiveness of HF pharmacologic therapies, with HMR consistently improving in response to guidelines directed HF medical management [43, 44]. In response to β-blockers, Gerson *et al.* [45] reported that the ^{123}I-*m*IBG HMR improved, particularly if the initial value was lower, and Kasama *et al.* found that such improvement was associated with favorable LV remodeling [46]. Toyoma *et al.* [47] showed that HMR improvement with β-blocker therapy was associated with improved NYHA functional class and in ventricular function. Guidelines recommended medications directed at the RAAS, including ACE-I, ARBs, and mineralocorticoids, have also been shown to improve the ^{123}I-*m*IBG HMR [48 - 50].

Nevertheless, despite these consistent observations of an association between better ^{123}I-*m*IBG image findings and improved clinical condition in response to guidelines directed pharmacologic therapies, with some evidence [51, 52] that adrenergic imaging could potentially help guide initiation of such therapies, because the benefits to risk and cost ratios are very high it is unlikely that imaging will be used in this regard [53]. An alternative potential role of ^{123}I-*m*IBG here was suggested by a study of Matsui *et al.* [54] who found that patients whose HMR did not improve after 6 months of comprehensive pharmacologic therapy were less likely to survive. For such patients the appropriate approach could be to more readily consider more aggressive, invasive therapies. Thus, adrenergic imaging may help to better and earlier select patients for whom high risk, expensive device therapies, such as pacemaker cardiac resynchronization therapy (CRT), a left ventricular assist device (LVAD) and an implantable cardiac defibrillator (ICD), should be instituted, *versus* those for whom minimal benefit would be expected.

^{123}I-*m*IBG Imaging to Guide Use of Cardiac Resynchronization Therapy (CRT)

While CRT with a biventricular pacemaker (BiV) can improve outcome in HF patients who meet guideline criteria, 30% - 40% of those receiving CRT do not benefit [55, 56]. There is evidence that ^{123}I-*m*IBG imaging can improve patient selection and help follow response to CRT therapy. Scholtens *et al.* [57] reviewed 9 studies, a total of 225 patients, between 2005 and 2011 who underwent CRT and who also had an ^{123}I-*m*IBG imaging study [58 - 66] As in Table (**1**) despite methodological and patient differences among these studies, they consistently showed that improvements in ^{123}I-*m*IBG sympathetic image parameters in response to CRT were associated with improved LVEF. In some of the studies, the baseline HMR predicted response. D'Orio Nishioka *et al.* [61], studying 30 patients with NYHA Class III-IV HFrEF and QRS duration >120 milliseconds undergoing CRT therapy, observed that in relation to ventricular dimensions on echocardiography and QRS duration, by multivariate analysis HMR was the only independent predictor of improvements in NYHA class, LV dimensions and LVEF. An ROC derived optimal threshold of 1.36 (higher value more likely to respond) yielded a sensitivity of 75% and specificity of 71%. Tanaka *et al.* [66], evaluating 50 patients with NYHA III-IV ischemic cardiomyopathy and QRS >120 milliseconds begun on CRT therapy, saw that those with both baseline mechanical dyssynchrony by echocardiography and an HMR ≥1.6 were more likely at 7 months to have a favorable response to CRT in terms of reverse myocardial remodeling (≥ 15% reduction in end-systolic volume) and improved 3-year survival with freedom from clinical HF progression, illustrated in Fig. (**2**).

Table 1. Response of ^{123}I-*m*IBG Parameters to Cardiac Resynchronization Therapy.

				Late HMR			**Washout (%)**			**Change in LVEF**	
Study Authors	**Publication Year**	**# of Patients**	**Patient Cohort**	**Pre-CRT**	**Post-CRT**	**p**	**Pre-CRT**	**Post CRT**	**p**		**p**
Erol-Yilmaz *et al.* [58]	2005	13	All patients[I]	1.3 ± 0.2	1.4 ± 0.2	0.03	40.2 ± 12.0	28.3 ± 1.6	0.001	14% to 21%	0.007
Higuchi *et al.* [59]	2006	9	Responders[II]	1.40 ± 0.28	1.56 ± 0.23	<0.05	50.30 ± 3.13	46.60 ± 1.11	NS	16% to 17.7%	NS
		9	Non-responders	1.62 ± 0.23	1.55 ± 0.22	NS	46.90 ± 1.14	49.40 ± 8.13	NS	22.2% to 23%	NS

(Table 1) cont.....

				Late HMR			Washout (%)			Change in LVEF	
Study Authors	**Publication Year**	**# of Patients**	**Patient Cohort**	**Pre-CRT**	**Post-CRT**	**p**	**Pre-CRT**	**Post CRT**	**p**		**p**
Gould *et al.* [60]	2007	19	All patients [III]	1.45 ± 0.06	1.54 ± 0.08	0.03	28 ± 2	29 ± 2	NS	25% to 33%	<0.001
Nishioka *et al.* [61]	2007	21	Responders[I]	1.50 ± 0.23	1.64 ± 0.21	0.03	38 ± 20	32 ± 13	NS	24% to 29%	0.01
		9	Non-responders	1.22 ± 0.23	1.27 ± 0.23	NS	59 ± 30	70 ± 43	NS	22% to 21%	NS
Burri *et al.* [62]	2008	8	Responders[IV]	1.36 ± 0.20	1.44 ± 0.24	NS	49 ± 19	39 ± 12	0.036	24.7% to 30%	0.034
		8	Non-responders	1.31 ± 0.18	1.28 ± 0.11	NS	50 ± 13	57 ± 5	NS		
Cha *et al.* [63]	2008	16	All patients	1.8 ± 0.7	2.1 ± 0.7	0.04	54 ± 22	34 ± 24	0.01	23% to 33%	<0.001
Cha *et al.* [64]	2011	45	All patients	1.82 ± 0.58	1.97 ± 0.59	0.03	48 ± 19	37 ± 22	0.01	25.8% to 33.4%	<0.01
		22	Responders[V]	2.04	2.30	0.04	39	21	0.004	NR	
		23	Non-responders	1.49	1.57	NS	61	56	NS	NR	
Shinohara *et al.* [65]	2011	19	Responders[V]	1.83 ± 0.34	1.98 ± 0.52	0.047	57.7 ± 15.7	51.9 ± 18.0	NS	30.8% to 36.8%	NS
		8	Non-responders	1.55 ± 0.46	1.58 ± 0.39	NS	63.9 ± 18.6	62.1 ± 18.9	NS	25.8% to 30.7%	NS
Tanaka *et al.* [66]	2011	50	All patients	31 patients with baseline dyssynchrony [VI] For baseline HMR ≥1.6, 94% responded. For baseline HMR <1.6, 57% responded (p = 0.03).							
		35	Responders[V]	19 patients without baseline dyssynchrony For baseline HMR ≥1.6, 64% responded. For baseline HMR <1.6, 0% responded (p = 0.03).							
		15	Non-responders								

CRT = cardiac resynchronization therapy; HMR = heart to mediastinum ratio; LVEF = left ventricular ejection fraction; NR = not reported; NS = non-significant.

I. Improvement in NYHA class.

II. Improvement in dyssynchrony index on quantitative gated SPECT.

III. Assessed response to biventricular pacing.

IV. Improvement in NYHA class and LVEF ≥ 5%.

V. ≥15% reduction in left ventricular end-systolic volume.

VI. Speckle-tracking radial strain anteroseptal/posterior wall time difference ≥130ms.

Data extracted from Scholtens AM, Braat AJ, Tuinenburg A, Meine M, Verberne HJ. Cardiac sympathetic innervation and cardiac resynchronization therapy. Heart Fail Rev 2014; 19: 567-73 [57], and individual references.

As would be expected, for patients with different HF pathophysiology, the relation of ^{123}I-*m*IBG images results to CRT response varies. Cha *et al.* [64] and D'Orio Nishioka *et al.* [61] both observed that patients with non-ischemic cardiomyopathy (NICM) are more likely than those with ischemic cardiomyopathy (ICM) to respond favorably to CRT. In addition, as per the study by Tanaka *et al.*, combining innervation imaging with another parameter, such as baseline mechanical dyssynchrony, is likely to better select patients likely to benefit from CRT. Also, as there are reportedly 20 definitions of response to CRT [67] that include LV structural and functional improvement, symptomatic clinical response and event occurrence, in order to be able to effectively assess the ability of imaging to best select appropriate patients for CRT, criteria for response to therapy will need to be standardized. Finally, it will be important to set standard procedural details for ^{123}I-*m*IBG imaging, including the ideal radiotracer dose to administer, the most suitable collimator for imaging, and image interpretation methods that may also include tomographic analysis of regions where the LV pacer wire may be best placed.

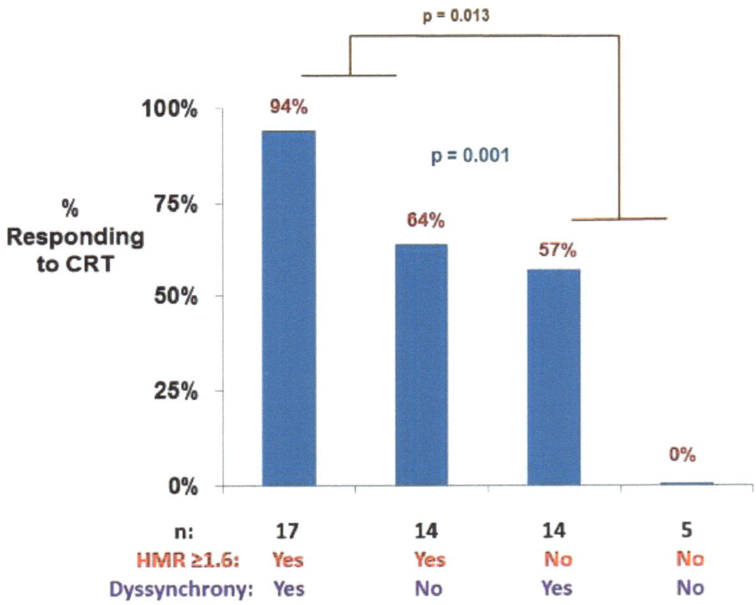

Fig. (2). Response to cardiac resynchronization therapy (CRT), defined as ≥15% relative reduction in echocardiographic end-systolic volume, in relation to cardiac ^{123}I-*m*IBG heart to mediastinum ratio (HMR, late images) and baseline dyssynchrony. Patients with HMR ≥ 1.6 were more likely to respond to CRT. Data extracted from Tanaka H, Tatsumi K, Fujiwara S, Tsuji T, Kaneko A, Ryo K, Fukuda Y, Matsumoto K, Shigeru M, Yoshida A, Kawai H, Hirata K. Effect of left ventricular dyssynchrony on cardiac sympathetic activity in heart failure patients with wide QRS duration. Circ J. 2012; 76: 382-9 [66].

^{123}I-*m*IBG Imaging to Guide Use of a Left Ventricular Assist Device (LVAD)

In the past 10 years, left ventricular assist devices (LVAD) have become increasingly used in patients with advanced HF, with approximately 20,000 devices implanted in the US during this period [68]. In general, patients receive LVADs either as a bridge to heart transplant or as destination “lifelong support”

[69] therapy if transplant is not a viable option. While improvements in device technology, such as the recently introduced HeartMate3 LVAD, that promise to improve patient comfort, decrease risk of pump thrombosis and improve survival free of disabling strokes or the need to repair or replace a device [70], better guidance in the use of an LVAD is essential. While there are published clinical criteria describing when LVADs should be considered in end stage HF [71], there is potential benefit of using adrenergic imaging to better help decide when LVAD therapy should be undertaken. In addition, as recent pilot clinical trials [72 - 74] report that after a period of ventricular unloading from LVAD therapy, 25% - 30% of patients have ventricular functional improvement sufficient for device explantation, adrenergic imaging should also have value in this regard.

A study by Imamura *et al.* [75] described how ^{123}I-*m*IBG imaging might help predict beneficial reverse LV remodeling in response to LVAD therapy, illustrated in Fig. (**3**). In 27 NICM patients with an LVEF of 17% ± 7%, the 6 who exhibited reverse remodeling, defined as an EF ≥35% after 6 months of LVAD use, had a lower baseline tracer washout rate (WR) than the 21 patients who did not (31.0 ± 6.1 *versus* 41.9 ± 5.8, respectively, $p < 0.001$). By logistic regression analyses, only cumulative β-blocker dose and WR predicted reverse remodeling, with WR ≤ 39% being the only independent predictor. Patients with a WR ≤ 39 also had a larger decrease in LV diastolic diameter. There was a trend towards a higher HMR predicting reverse remodeling, with insufficient statistical power from a small cohort likely precluding statistical significance.

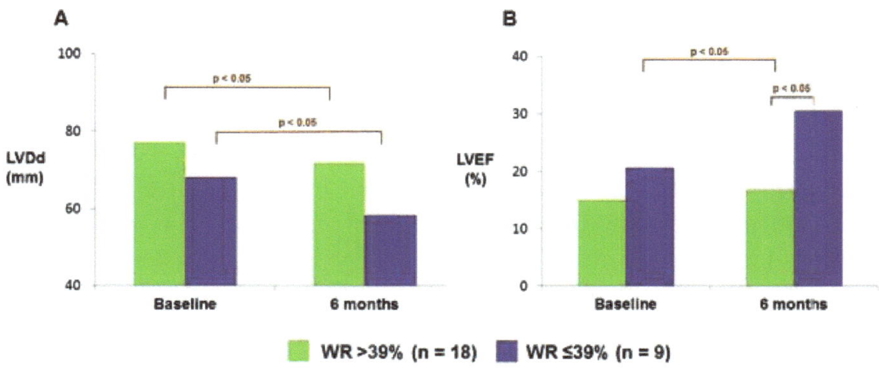

Fig. (3). Postoperative left ventricular remodeling in relation to pre-left ventricular assist device (LVAD) washout rate (WR) levels. After 6 months of LVAD use: A). The mean left ventricular diastolic diameter (LVDd) decreased for patients with or without lower WR levels (p <0.05), B). The mean left ventricular ejection fraction (LVEF) improved only for patients with WR ≤39%, at 6 months significantly higher than for patients with WR >39%. Data extracted from Imamura T, Kinugawa K, Nitta D, Kinoshita O, Nawata K, Ono M. Preoperative iodine-123 meta-iodobenzylguanidine imaging is a novel predictor of left ventricular reverse remodeling during treatment with a left ventricular assist device. J Artif Organs. 2016; 19: 29-36 [75].

At the time of this writing the author is unaware of other investigation using adrenergic imaging to predict response to an LVAD. However, several studies have explored how ^{123}I-*m*IBG imaging could potentially help determine which patients on therapy might have successful device explanation. A study by Miyagawa *et al.* from 2001 [76] was unable to detect any improvement in ^{123}I-*m*IBG imaging parameters after 2 months of therapy, but patient cohort size was only 10, and all were implanted by "old-fashioned" devices [77]. In contrast, in 12 patients with end-stage HF, Drakos *et al.* found that after 3 months of LVAD therapy, most with continuous flow devices, there was an increase in late HMR from 1.25 ± 0.18 to 1.43 ± 0.13 ($p=0.01$) and a significant decrease in WR from 51.0 ± 23.2% to 30.6 ± 8.7% ($p < 0.02$), associated with an improved EF, peak oxygen consumption, LV size, hemodynamics and serum sodium and creatinine, and a fall in BNP [78]. Improvement appeared to favor patients whose cardiomyopathies were nonischemic in etiology. George *et al.* [79] observed that after 208 ± 86 days of LVAD use in 14 patients with NICM, there was a 54.7% increase in HMR. The 10 patients who were able to have their devices explanted had better improvements in HMR, WR, and NE levels.

For sure, there appears to be much potential for adrenergic imaging to guide LVAD use. As more patients with end-stage HF receive this device, there is opportunity for larger investigatory studies to be performed.

^{123}I-*m*IBG Imaging to Guide Use of an Implantable Cardioverter Defibrillator (ICD)

A feared outcome of advanced HF is sudden cardiac death (SCD), most often from a ventricular tachyarrhythmia, frequently occurring in a patient who is otherwise clinically stable and has a reasonably good quality of life on medical therapies. Based on a series of large, prospective randomized clinical trials - MADIT-2 (Multicenter Automatic Defibrillator Implantation Trial-II) [80], DINAMIT (Defibrillator in Acute Myocardial Infarction Trial) [81], DEFINITE (Defibrillators in Non-ischemic Cardiomyopathy Treatment Evaluation) [82] and SCD-HeFT (Sudden Cardiac Death in Heart Failure Trial) [83], prophylactic primary prevention implantation of an ICD is a Class IA recommendation "to reduce total mortality in selected patients with nonischemic [dilated cardiomyopathy] or ischemic heart disease at least 40 days post-MI with LVEF ≤ 35%, and NYHA class II or III symptoms on [guideline directed medical therapy], who have reasonable expectation of meaningful survival for more than 1 year" [84].

Nevertheless, basing ICD use predominantly on EF is widely considered to be inadequate. Buxton *et al.* reported that a patient's clinical status is often more important than LVEF in predicting SCD, with the understanding that LVEF bears no direct relation to the mechanisms of lethal ventricular arrhythmias [85]. Myerburg explained that while an LVEF of 35% was often the threshold for patient entry into the randomized clinical trials, patient in the 30% -35% range were underrepresented and thus received uncertain or no benefit from an ICD [86]. More recently for patients with NICM, Køber *et al.* [87], while finding a small absolute decrease (8.2% to 4.3%, $p < 0.005$) in SCD after 67.6 months (median) of an ICD, observed no significant decrease in cardiovascular death or death from any cause. Barsheshet *et al.* [88] reported that more than 80% of patients receiving an ICD for primary prevention do not use the device for as long as 8 years. Clearly, the majority of patients who receive an ICD do not use it. At the same time, potential serious complications and discomforts from an ICD – infections, device malfunction, lead problems, and recalls - are underappreciated [89 - 91], with an estimated cost of $325,000 per year-of life saved [92].

Thus, a better method of selecting patients who would most benefit from prophylactic ICD implantation is desirable. As in Fig. (**4**), the genesis of lethal ventricular arrhythmias is multifactorial, involving abnormal myocardial substrate, an acute trigger and modulating factors [31, 93], and thus assessing a parameter common to all of these components, such as cardiac adrenergic innervation, would be expected to effectively contribute to deciding the appropriateness of an ICD in a particular patient [21, 30]. The first study addressing the potential for ^{123}I-*m*IBG imaging to select patients who might best benefit from ICD therapy was by Arora *et al.* [94], in which, for 17 patients with advanced HF who had ICDs and 2 controls, those an HMR <1.54 was more likely to have had prior device discharges than those without, shown in Fig. (**5**) Representative images from this study are shown in Fig. (**6**). A follow-up prospective investigation by Nagahara *et al.* [95] of 54 patients with an ICD reported that SCD or an arrhythmic induced ICD discharge correlated with HMR independent of LVEF and other variables. Recently, Verschure *et al.* [96] followed 135 stable HF subjects with a mean LVEF of 25% for a median of 30 months, and found that a combination of the late HMR ratio and LVEF was significantly associated with freedom from appropriate ICD therapy.

In a sub-analysis of 777 patients in the ADMIRE-HF study who initially did not have an ICD, Hachamovitch and associates [97] found that while an HMR did not identify improved survival after later ICD implantation, HMR could determine the number of additional lived saved per 100 treated, with effectiveness in this regard peaking at an HMR of ≈1.5, suggesting that ^{123}I-*m*IBG imaging might optimize the cost-effectiveness of ICD use. In a cost-effective analysis of ADMIRE-HFX (an extended follow-up study of ADMIRE-HF) [98] patients based on an HMR threshold of 1.6, O'Day *et al.* [99] it was determined that use of ^{123}I-*m*IBG imaging could, with minimal impact on survival, reduce ICD use by 21%, with savings of $5,248,404 and $513,036 per quality-adjusted life-year lost over 2 and 10 years, respectively, more effective in patients with LVEFs 25%-35% than in those at <25%.

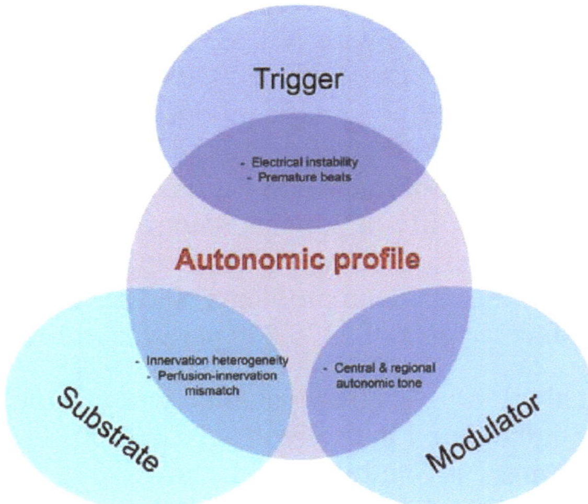

Fig. (4). Mechanisms of arrhythmia: importance of the autonomic profile. Reprinted with permission from Borgquist R, Singh JP. An electrophysiologist perspective on risk stratification in heart failure: can better understanding of the condition of the cardiac sympathetic nervous system help. J Nucl Med 2015; 56: 59S-64S [93].

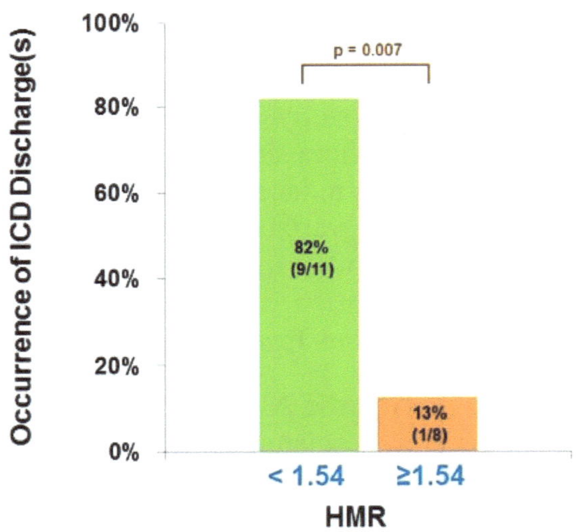

Fig.(5). Occurrence of implantable cardioverter defibrillator (ICD) discharges in relation to heart to mediastinum ratio (HMR). Data from Arora R, Ferrick KJ, Nakata T, Kaplan RC, Rozengarten M, Latif F, Ng K, Marcano V, Heller S, Fisher JD, Travin MI. I-123 MIBG imaging and heart rate variability analysis to predict the need for an implantable cardioverter defibrillator. J Nucl Cardiol 2003; 10: 121-131 [94].

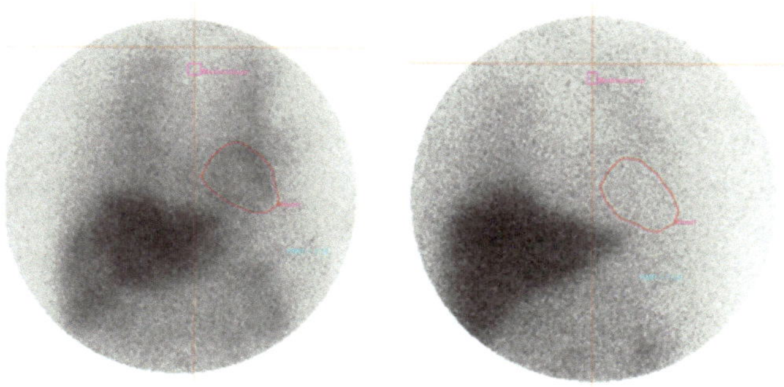

Fig. (6). Two patients with HFrEF with previously implanted ICDs who underwent ^{123}I-*m*IBG imaging. A). 80-year-old man with non-ischemic cardiomyopathy, LVEF of 35%. The heart to mediastinum ratio (HMR) was 1.79. There were no ICD discharges over the 2-year period prior to and during the 6 year period after imaging. B). 50-year-old woman with ischemic cardiomyopathy, LVEF of 32%. The HMR was 1.04. There were a reported 7 ICD discharges in the 2 year-period prior to imaging (although none over the following 6 years) [94].

For tomographic ^{123}I-*m*IBG imaging, Boogers *et al.* [100] prospectively followed 116 patients with a mean LVEF of 28% referred for ICD implantation, finding that at 3-year follow-up, those with a summed innervation defect score >26 were more than 10x likely to have appropriate ICD therapy than patients with scores ≤26. In 27 patients with LVEF ≤35% followed a mean of 16 months after ICD implantation, Marshall *et al.* [101] observed that occurrence of an ICD discharge in response to ventricular fibrillation or sustained rapid ventricular tachycardia, or sudden death likely to have been arrhythmic in nature, was associated with lower HMRs on planar images, and higher summed dysinnervation higher adrenergic/perfusion mismatch scores.

While much focus has been on using ^{123}I-*m*IBG imaging to identify patients who would not benefit from an ICD despite meeting guidelines criteria indications to undergo implantation, the majority of patients who suffer sudden arrhythmic cardiac death do not meet guideline criteria to receive the device [102]. In a sub-analysis of ADMIRE-HF data that included patients found on core-lab review to have higher EFs than initially reported, HMR was as predictive of death or a potentially lethal arrhythmic event in patients with EFs >35% as it was in those with EFs ≤ 35%, with adjusted hazard ratios of 5.28 and 2.39, respectively [29].

While the aforementioned provides evidence that use of ^{123}I-*m*IBG imaging could help better select patients who should receive an ICD, thereby not subjecting those who are very unlikely to benefit to the underappreciated risks and high cost, the lack of a prospective randomized trial akin to MADIT-2, DINAMIT, DEFINITE, and SCD-HeFT has precluded clinical use of adrenergic imaging in this setting. Recently an international multicenter prospective industry sponsored study was undertaken that planned to randomize >2000 HF subjects with NYHA Class II-II HF and LVEF 25% - 35%, to ^{123}I-*m*IBG HMR guided ICD implantation *versus* a guidelines directed approach, comparing over a 2.75 to 3-year follow-up period the occurrences of all-cause mortality and various secondary outcomes that include ventricular arrhythmias [103]. Unfortunately, the study was discontinued in March 2018 because of insufficient patient and site recruitment. Subsequent studies remain uncertain at this time.

Currently, the only published societal guideline document addressing the matter is the "American Society of Nuclear Cardiology/Society of Nuclear Medicine and Molecular Imaging Model Coverage Policy: Myocardial sympathetic innervation imaging: Iodine-123 *meta*-iodobenzylguanidine (^{123}I-mIBG)" [104]. This document, that represents an expert consensus evaluation of current literature, states at a "Specific Indication" that ^{123}I-*m*IBG imaging is recommended "for patients with NYHA Class II-III HF with LVEF ≤35% to help stratify risk and to promote more informed clinical decision-making when the result of ^{123}I-*m*IBG study is likely to influence the decision regarding ICD implant". A circumstance labeled a "Potential/Emerging" indication was, "For patients who received an ICD for primary and or secondary prevention of SCD who subsequently underwent complete device and lead removal due to definite infection and there is uncertainty on the part of treating physician to proceed with ICD replacement, when the result of ^{123}I-*m*IBG study is likely to influence the decision regarding device placement".

^{123}I-*m*IBG Imaging as a Potential Tool for Guiding Electrophysiological Procedures

Patients with an ICD have an approximately 5% annual occurrence of ventricular tachyarrhythmias that require device discharges [83]. ICD discharges are extremely uncomfortable and thus associated with a lower quality of life and a higher mortality. While antiarrhythmic medical therapies are initially attempted, their efficacy is limited, and there are frequent side effects. This problem is customarily addressed with an electrophysiologic (EP) procedure that attempts to ablate the arrhythmic focus. There is evidence that radionuclide imaging, including with adrenergic tracers, can assist in this process [105].

Several studies have found that global and regional ^{123}I-*m*IBG uptake can predict arrhythmic inducibility during an EP study. In 50 patients with prior MI and LVEF <40% who were referred for EP testing, Bax *et al*. reported that the summed ^{123}I-*m*IBG dysinnervation score, adjusted for global uptake (*i.e.*, HMR), was higher in patients who had an inducible ventricular tachyarrhythmia [106]. Zhou *et al.* [107] assessed ^{123}I-*m*IBG uptake in infarct border zones that are mixtures of scar and viable tissue, which have increased susceptibility to ventricular arrhythmias [108]. Decreased ^{123}I-*m*IBG counts in this border zone, below a threshold ratio (to the mediastinum) of 2.2, was a better predictor of tachyarrhythmia inducibility than the extent of the border zone or of the infarct scar.

3D mapping of ^{123}I-*m*IBG uptake has shown potential for helping to identify specific locations to ablate. In a feasibility study of 15 patients with ischemic heart disease and drug-refractory VT referred for EP ablation, Klein *et al.* [109] compared the utility of customary electroanatomic voltage maps with ^{123}I-*m*IBG image denervation maps. Denervation zones were found to be ~2.5x larger than bipolar voltage-defined scar, and while only 64% of successful ablation sites were within electroanatomic scar or border zones, 100% were within ^{123}I-*m*IBG denervation or transition zones. Additional work by this group led by Abdulghani *et al.* [110] showed that denervation characteristics associated with drug-refractory VT differ between ischemic and non-ischemic cardiomyopathies, with the former having larger areas of denervation, and that EP ablations change ^{123}I-*m*IBG uptake distant from the ablation site. Thus, further exploration of ^{123}I-*m*IBG innervation changes associated with ablation procedures promises to provide improved understanding of arrhythmic mechanisms that could help better guide future patient management including more selective use of ICDs, such as if imaging directed ablation procedures could preclude their need in some patients. The use of adrenergic imaging in this regard would likely be enhanced by more exact image depiction of tracer distribution through use of PET tracers [111] or by use of ^{123}I-*m*IBG if imaged by solid state cameras that have demonstrated enhanced tracer localization [112].

CONCLUDING REMARKS

Since the advent of adrenergic imaging in 1981 with ^{123}I-*m*IBG and later developed analogous PET tracers, its ability to evaluate patients with heart failure and associated arrhythmias beyond conventional assessment methods has been well established by a wealth of investigatory studies. An area in which adrenergic imaging could have a dramatic impact in patient management is through better guidance of use of cardiac implantable electronic devices, specifically biventricular pacemakers for cardiac synchronization therapy to improve LV function and patient symptoms, initiation of and potential discontinuation of left ventricular assist devices, and use of implantable cardiac defibrillators to prevent sudden arrhythmic deaths. More focused use of CIEDs would decrease the morbidities related to them as well as reduce costs. At the same time, adrenergic imaging would likely find additional patients who might benefit but do not meet clinical criteria to receive these devices. Currently, clinical use of adrenergic imaging for this purpose has been hampered by lack of the large randomized prospective clinical studies that are needed for the technique to be incorporated into societal guidelines. Perhaps smaller prospective studies, such as for situations in which current guidelines are considered equivocal or deficient, would be the way to proceed.

CONSENT FOR PUBLICATION

Not applicable.

CONFLICT OF INTEREST

The author (editor) declares no conflict of interest, financial or otherwise.

ACKNOWLEDGEMENTS

Declared none.

REFERENCES

[1] Savarese G, Lund LH. Global public burden of heart failure Card Fail Rev 2017; 3: 7–11. https://www.cfrjournal.com/articles/global-public-health-burden-heart-failure accessed 7/10/18) [http://dx.doi.org/10.15420/cfr.2016:25:2]

[2] Benjamin EJ, Virani SS, Callaway CW, *et al.* American Heart Association Council on Epidemiology and Prevention Statistics Committee and Stroke Statistics Subcommittee. Heart Disease and Stroke Statistics-2018 Update: A Report From the American Heart Association. Circulation 2018; 137: e67-e492.
[http://dx.doi.org/10.1161/CIR.0000000000000558]

[3] Cheng RK, Cox M, Neely ML, *et al.* Outcomes in patients with heart failure with preserved, borderline, and reduced ejection fraction in the Medicare population. Am Heart J 2014; 168: 721-30. [http://dx.doi.org/10.1016/j.ahj.2014.07.008]

[4] Braunwald E. Heart failure. J Am Coll Cardiol Heart Fail 2013; 1: 1-20.

[5] Bell DR. Control mechanisms in circulatory function. Medical Physiology: Principles of Clinical Medicine. 4th ed. Philadelphia: Lippincott, Williams & Wilkins 2013; pp. 317-20.

[6] Colucci WS. 2018. Pathophysiology of heart failure: Neurohumoral adaptations. http://www.uptodate.com/contents/pathophysiology-of-heart-failure-neurohumoral-adaptationsaccessed 7/10/2018; topic last updated January 29, 2018

[7] Jamali HK, Waqar F, Gerson MC. Cardiac autonomic innervation. J Nucl Cardiol 2017; 24: 1558-70. [http://dx.doi.org/10.1007/s12350-016-0725-7]

[8] Travin MI. Current clinical applications and next steps for cardiac innervation imaging. Curr Cardiol Rep 2017; 19(1): 1.
[http://dx.doi.org/10.1007/s11886-017-0817-2]

[9] Flotats A, Carrió I. Cardiac neurotransmission SPECT imaging. J Nucl Cardiol 2004; 11: 587-602. [http://dx.doi.org/10.1016/j.nuclcard.2004.07.007]

[10] Raffel DM, Wieland DM. Development of mIBG as a cardiac innervation imaging agent. J Am Coll Cardiol Img 2010; 3: 111-6.
[http://dx.doi.org/10.1016/j.jcmg.2009.09.015]

[11] Kline RC, Swanson DP, Wieland DM, *et al.* Myocardial imaging in man with I-123 meta-iodobenzylguanidine. J Nucl Med 1981; 22: 129-32.

[12] Hattori N, Schwaiger M. Metaiodobenzylguanidine scintigraphy of the heart. What have we learned clinically? Eur J Nucl Med 2000; 27: 1-6.
[http://dx.doi.org/10.1007/s002590050505]

[13] Bengel FM, Schwaiger M. Assessment of cardiac sympathetic neuronal function using PET imaging. J Nucl Cardiol 2004; 11: 603-16.
[http://dx.doi.org/10.1016/j.nuclcard.2004.06.133]

[14] Lautamäki. Sasano T, Higuchi T, Nekolla SG, Lardo AC, Holt DP, Dannals RF, Roselle Abraham M, Bengel FM. Multiparametric molecular imaging provides mechanistic insights into sympathetic impairment in the viable infarct zone. J Nucl Med 2015; 56: 457-63.
[http://dx.doi.org/10.2967/jnumed.114.149971]

[15] Luisi AJ, Suzuki G, deKemp R, Haka MS, Toorongian SA, Canty JM. Regional ^{11}C-hydroxyephedrine retention in hibernating myocardium: chronic inhomogeneity of sympathetic innervation in the absence of infarction. J Nucl Med 2005; 46: 1368-74.

[16] Sinusas AJ, Lazewatsky J, Brunetti J, *et al.* Biodistribution and radiation dosimetry of LMI1195: first-in-human study of a novel ^{18}F-labeled tracer for imaging myocardial innervation. J Nucl Med 2014; 55: 1-7.
[http://dx.doi.org/10.2967/jnumed.114.140137]

[17] Flotats A, Carrió I, Agostini D, *et al.* Proposal for standardization of 123I-metaiodobenzylguanidine (MIBG) cardiac sympathetic imaging by the EANM Cardiovascular Committee and the European Council of Nuclear Cardiology. Eur J Nucl Med Mol Imaging 2010; 37: 1802-12.
[http://dx.doi.org/10.1007/s00259-010-1491-4]

[18] Henzlova MJ, Duvall WL, Einstein AJ, Travin MI, Verberne HJ. ASNC imaging guidelines for SPECT nuclear cardiology procedures: stress, protocols, and tracers. J Nucl Cardiol 2016; 23: 606-39.
[http://dx.doi.org/10.1007/s12350-015-0387-x]

[19] Jacobson AF, Lombard J, Banerjee G, Camici PG. 123I-mIBG scintigraphy to predict risk for adverse cardiac outcomes in heart failure patients: design of two prospective multicenter international trials. J Nucl Cardiol 2009; 16: 113-21.
[http://dx.doi.org/10.1007/s12350-008-9008-2]

[20] Morozumi T, Kusuoka H, Fukuchi K, *et al.* Myocardial iodine-123-metaiodobenzylguanidine images and autonomic nerve activity in normal subjects. J Nucl Med 1997; 38: 49-52.

[21] Tomaselli GF, Zipes DP. What causes sudden death in heart failure? Circ Res 2004; 95: 754-76.
[http://dx.doi.org/10.1161/01.RES.0000145047.14691.db]

[22] Kelesidis I, Travin MI. Use of cardiac radionuclide imaging to identify patients at risk for arrhythmic sudden cardiac death. J Nucl Cardiol 2012; 19: 142-52.
[http://dx.doi.org/10.1007/s12350-011-9482-9]

[23] Kammerling JJ, Green FJ, Watanabe AM, *et al.* Denervation supersensitivity of refractoriness in noninfarcted areas apical to transmural myocardial infarction. Circulation 1987; 76: 383-93.
[http://dx.doi.org/10.1161/01.CIR.76.2.383]

[24] Schofer J, Spielmann R, Schuchert A, Weber K, Schlüter M. Iodine-123 meta-iodobenzylguanidine scintigraphy: a noninvasive method to demonstrate myocardial adrenergic nervous system disintegrity in patients with idiopathic dilated cardiomyopathy. J Am Coll Cardiol 1988; 12: 1252-8.
[http://dx.doi.org/10.1016/0735-1097(88)92608-3]

[25] Merlet P, Valette H, Dubois-Randé J, *et al.* Prognostic value of cardiac metaiodobenzylguanidine in patients with heart failure. J Nucl Med 1992; 33: 471-7.

[26] Verberne HJ, Brewster LM, Somsen GA, van Eck-Smit BL. Prognostic value of myocardial 123I-metaiodobenzylguanidine (MIBG) parameters in patients with heart failure: a systematic review. Eur Heart J 2008; 29: 1147-59. [http://dx.doi.org/10.1093/eurheartj/ehn113]

[27] Jacobson AF, Senior R, Cerqueira MD. Myocardial iodine 123 meta-iodobenzylguanidine imaging and cardiac events in heart failure: results of the prospective ADMIRE-HF (Adreview myocardial imaging for risk evaluation in heart failure). J Am Coll Cardiol 2010; 55: 2212-22. [http://dx.doi.org/10.1016/j.jacc.2010.01.014]

[28] Nakata T, Nakajima K, Yamashina S, *et al.* A pooled analysis of multicenter cohort studies of I-12--mIBG cardiac sympathetic innervation imaging for assessment of long-term prognosis in chronic heart failure. J Am Coll Cardiol Img 2013; 6: 772-84. [http://dx.doi.org/10.1016/j.jcmg.2013.02.007]

[29] Shah AM, Bourgoun M, Narula J, Jacobson AF, Solomon SD. Influence of ejection fraction on the prognostic value of sympathetic innervation imaging with Iodine-123 MIBG in heart failure. J Am Coll Cardiol Img 2012; 5: 1139-46. [http://dx.doi.org/10.1016/j.jcmg.2012.02.019]

[30] Verrier RL, Antzelevich C. Autonomic aspects of arrhythmogenesis: the enduring and the new. Curr Opin Cardiol 2004; 19: 2-11. [http://dx.doi.org/10.1097/00001573-200401000-00003]

[31] Travin MI. Feng DaLi, Taub CC. Novel imaging approaches for predicting arrhythmic risk. Circ Cardiovasc Imaging 2015; 8: e003019. [http://dx.doi.org/10.1161/CIRCIMAGING.115.003019]

[32] Stanton MS, Tuli MM, Radtke NL, *et al.* Regional sympathetic denervation after MI in humans detected noninvasively using I-123-MIBG. J Am Coll Cardiol 1989; 14: 1519-26. [http://dx.doi.org/10.1016/0735-1097(89)90391-4]

[33] Yoshioka K, Gao D, Chin M, *et al.* Heterogeneous sympathetic innervation influences local myocardial repolarization in normally perfused rabbit hearts. Circulation 2000; 101: 1060-6. [http://dx.doi.org/10.1161/01.CIR.101.9.1060]

[34] McGhie AI, Corbett JR, Akers MS, *et al.* Regional cardiac adrenergic function using I-123 MIBG SPECT imaging after acute myocardial infarction. Am J Cardiol 1991; 67: 236-42. [http://dx.doi.org/10.1016/0002-9149(91)90552-V]

[35] Tamaki S, Yamada T, Okuyama Y, *et al.* Cardiac iodine-123 metaiodobenzylguanidine imaging predicts sudden cardiac death independently of left ventricular ejection fraction in patients with chronic heart failure and left ventricular systolic dysfunction: results from a comparative study with signal-averaged electrocardiogram, heart rate variability, and QT dispersion. J Am Coll Cardiol 2009; 53: 426-35. [http://dx.doi.org/10.1016/j.jacc.2008.10.025]

[36] Travin MI, Henzlova MJ, van Eck-Smit BLF, *et al.* Assessment of 123I-mIBG and 99mTc-tetrofosmin single-photon emission computed tomographic images for the prediction of arrhythmic events in patients with ischemic heart failure. J Nucl Cardiol 2017; 24: 377-91. [http://dx.doi.org/10.1007/s12350-015-0336-8]

[37] Fallavollita JA, Heavey BM, Luisi AJ Jr, *et al.* Regional myocardial sympathetic denervation predicts the risk of sudden cardiac arrest in ischemic cardiomyopathy. J Am Coll Cardiol 2014; 63: 141-9. [http://dx.doi.org/10.1016/j.jacc.2013.07.096]

[38] Fallavollita JA, Dare JD, Carter RL, Baldwa S, Canty JM. Denervated myocardium is preferentially associated with sudden cardiac arrest in ischemic cardiomyopathy. A pilot competing risks analysis of

cause-specific mortality. Circ Cardiovasc Imaging 2017; 10: e006446. [http://dx.doi.org/10.1161/CIRCIMAGING.117.006446]

[39] Khakpour H, Vaseghi M. Risk stratification and sudden cardiac death. Is it time to include autonomic variables? Circ Cardiovasc Imaging 2017; 10: e006819. [http://dx.doi.org/10.1161/CIRCIMAGING.117.006819]

[40] Klein T, Dilsizian V, Cao Q, Chen W, Dickfeld T. The potential role of iodine-123 *meta*iodobenzylguanidine imaging for identifying sustained ventricular tachycardia in patients with cardiomyopathy. Curr Cardiol Rep 2013; 15: 359. [http://dx.doi.org/10.1007/s11886-013-0359-1]

[41] Shaw LJ, Min JK, Hachamovitch R, *et al.* Cardiovascular imaging research at the crossroads. J Am Coll Cardiol Imaging 2010; 3: 316-24. [http://dx.doi.org/10.1016/j.jcmg.2009.11.010]

[42] FDA adreview use http://medlibrary.org/lib/rx/meds/adreview-1/ accessed5/10/18

[43] Treglia G, Stefanelli A, Bruno I, Giordano A. Clinical usefulness of myocardial innervation imaging using Iodine-123-meta-iodobenzylguanidine scintigraphy in evaluating the effectiveness of pharmacological treatments in patients with heart failure: an overview. Eur Rev Med Pharmacol Sci 2013; 17: 56-68.

[44] Travin MI. Clinical applications of myocardial innervation imaging. Cardiol Clin 2016; 34: 133-47. [http://dx.doi.org/10.1016/j.ccl.2015.06.003]

[45] Gerson MC, Craft LL, McGuire N, Suresh DP, Abraham WT, Wagoner LE. Carvedilol improves left ventricular function in heart failure with idiopathic dilated cardiomyopathy and a wide range of sympathetic nervous system function as measured by iodine 123 metaiodobenzylguanidine. J Nucl Cardiol 2002; 9: 608-15. [http://dx.doi.org/10.1067/mnc.2002.127717]

[46] Kasama S, Toyama T, Hatori T, *et al.* Evaluation of cardiac sympathetic nerve activity and left ventricular remodeling in patients with dilated cardiomyopathy on the treatment containing carvedilol. Eur Heart J 2007; 28: 989-95. [http://dx.doi.org/10.1093/eurheartj/ehm048]

[47] Toyama T, Aihara Y, Iwasaki T, *et al.* Cardiac sympathetic activity estimated by 123I-MIBG myocardial imaging in patients with dilated cardiomyopathy after β-blocker or angiotensin-converting enzyme inhibitor therapy. J Nucl Med 1999; 40: 217-23.

[48] Somsen GA, Vlies BV, de Milliano PA, *et al.* Increased myocardial [123-I]-metaiodobenzylguanidine uptake after enalapril treatment in patients with chronic heart failure. Heart 1996; 76: 218-22. [http://dx.doi.org/10.1136/hrt.76.3.218]

[49] Kasama S, Toyama T, Kumakura H, *et al.* Effect of spironolactone on cardiac sympathetic nerve activity and left ventricular remodeling in patients with dilated cardiomyopathy. J Am Coll Cardiol 2003; 41: 574-81. [http://dx.doi.org/10.1016/S0735-1097(02)02855-3]

[50] Kasama S, Toyama T, Kumakura H. Effects of candesartan on cardiac sympathetic nerve activity in patients with congestive heart failure and preserved LVEF. J Am Coll Cardiol 2005; 45: 661-7. [http://dx.doi.org/10.1016/j.jacc.2004.11.038]

[51] Suwa M, Otake Y, Moriguchi A, *et al.* Iodine-123 metaiodobenzylguanidine myocardial scintigraphy for prediction of response to β-blocker therapy in patients with dilated cardiomyopathy. Am Heart J 1997; 133: 353-8. [http://dx.doi.org/10.1016/S0002-8703(97)70232-1]

[52] Choi JY, Lee KH, Hong KP, *et al.* Iodine-123 MIBG imaging before treatment of heart failure with carvedilol to predict improvement of left ventricular function and exercise capacity. J Nucl Cardiol 2001; 8: 4-9.

[http://dx.doi.org/10.1067/mnc.2001.109452]

[53] Udelson JE, Shafer CD, Carrió I. Radionuclide imaging in heart failure: assessing etiology and outcomes and implications for management. J Nucl Cardiol 2002; 9: S40-52. [http://dx.doi.org/10.1067/mnc.2002.128461]

[54] Matsui T, Tsutamoto T, Maeda K, Kusukawa J, Kinoshita M. Prognostic value of repeated 123I-metaiodobenzylguanidine imaging in patients with dilated cardiomyopathy with congestive heart failure before and after optimized treatments – comparison with neurohumoral factors. Circ J 2002; 66: 537-43. [http://dx.doi.org/10.1253/circj.66.537]

[55] Abraham WT, Fisher WG, Smith AL, *et al.* Cardiac resynchronization in chronic heart failure. N Engl J Med 2002; 346: 1845-53. [http://dx.doi.org/10.1056/NEJMoa013168]

[56] Tracy CM, Epstein AE, Darbar D, *et al.* 2012 ACCF/AHA/HRS focused update of the 2008 guidelines for device-based therapy of cardiac rhythm abnormalities: a report of the American College of Cardiology Foundation/American Heart Association Task Force on Practice Guidelines. J Am Coll Cardiol 2012; 60: 1297-313. [http://dx.doi.org/10.1016/j.jacc.2012.07.009]

[57] Scholtens AM, Braat AJ, Tuinenburg A, Meine M, Verberne HJ. Cardiac sympathetic innervation and cardiac resynchronization therapy. Heart Fail Rev 2014; 19: 567-73. [http://dx.doi.org/10.1007/s10741-013-9400-0]

[58] Erol-Yilmaz A, Verberne HJ, Schrama TA, *et al.* Cardiac resynchronization induces favorable neurohumoral changes. Pacing Clin Electrophysiol 2005; 28: 304-10. [http://dx.doi.org/10.1111/j.1540-8159.2005.09508.x]

[59] Higuchi K, Toyama T, Tada H, Naito S, Ohshima S, Kurabayashi M. Usefulness of biventricular pacing to improve cardiac symptoms, exercise capacity and sympathetic nerve activity in patients with moderate to severe chronic heart failure. Circ J 2006; 70: 703-70. [http://dx.doi.org/10.1253/circj.70.703]

[60] Gould PA, Kong G, Kalff V, *et al.* improvement in cardiac adrenergic function post biventricular pacing for heart failure. Europace 2007; 9: 751-6. [http://dx.doi.org/10.1093/europace/eum081]

[61] D'Orio Nishioka SA, Filho MM, Soares Brandão SC, *et al.* Cardiac sympathetic activity pre and post resynchronization therapy evaluated by ^{123}I-MIBG myocardial scintigraphy. J Nucl Cardiol 2007; 14: 852-9. [http://dx.doi.org/10.1016/j.nuclcard.2007.08.004]

[62] Burri H, Sunthorn H, Somsen A, *et al.* Improvement in cardiac sympathetic nerve activity in responders to resynchronization therapy. Europace 2008; 10: 374-8. [http://dx.doi.org/10.1093/europace/eun017]

[63] Cha YM, Oh J, Miyazaki C, *et al.* Cardiac resynchronization therapy upregulates cardiac autonomic control. J Cardiovasc Electrophysiol 2008; 19: 1045-52. [http://dx.doi.org/10.1111/j.1540-8167.2008.01190.x]

[64] Cha YM, Chareonthaitawee P, Dong YX, *et al.* Cardiac sympathetic reserve and response to cardiac resynchronization therapy. Circ Heart Fail 2011; 4: 339-44. [http://dx.doi.org/10.1161/CIRCHEARTFAILURE.110.959858]

[65] Shinohara T, Takahashi N, Saito S, *et al.* Effect of cardiac resynchronization therapy on cardiac sympathetic nervous dysfunction and serum C-reactive protein level. Pacing Clin Electrophysiol 2011; 34: 1225-30. [http://dx.doi.org/10.1111/j.1540-8159.2011.03156.x]

[66] Tanaka H, Tatsumi K, Fujiwara S, *et al.* Effect of left ventricular dyssynchrony on cardiac sympathetic

activity in heart failure patients with wide QRS duration Circ J

[67] Kandala J, Altman R, Park M. Singh. Clinical, laboratory, and pacing predictors of CRT response. J Cardiovasc Transl Res 2012; 5: 196-212. [http://dx.doi.org/10.1007/s12265-012-9352-0]

[68] Miller LW, Rogers JG. Evolution of left ventricular assist device therapy for advanced heart failure. A Review. JAMA Cardiol 2018; 3: 650-8. [http://dx.doi.org/10.1001/jamacardio.2018.0522]

[69] Pinney SP, Anyanwu AC, Lala A, Teuteberg JJ, Uriel N, Mehra MR. Left ventricular assist devices for lifelong support. J Am Coll Cardiol 2017; 69: 2845-61. [http://dx.doi.org/10.1016/j.jacc.2017.04.031]

[70] Mehra MR, Goldstein DJ, Uriel N, *et al.* MOMENTUM 3 Investigators. Two-Year Outcomes with a Magnetically Levitated Cardiac Pump in Heart Failure. N Engl J Med 2018; 378: 1386-95. [http://dx.doi.org/10.1056/NEJMoa1800866]

[71] Yancy CW, Jessup M, Bozkurt B, *et al.* 2017 ACC/AHA/HFSA Focused Update of the 2013 ACCF/AHA guideline for the management of heart failure: A report of the American College of Cardiology/American Heart Association Task Force on Clinical Practice Guidelines and the Heart Failure Society of America. Circulation 2017; 136: e137-61. [http://dx.doi.org/10.1161/CIR.0000000000000509]

[72] Wever-Pinzon O, Drakos SG, McKellar SH, *et al.* Cardiac recovery during long-term ventricular assist device support. J Am Coll Cardiol 2016; 68: 1540-53. [http://dx.doi.org/10.1016/j.jacc.2016.07.743]

[73] Drakos SG, Mehra MR. Clinical myocardial recovery during long-term mechanical support in advanced heart failure: insights into moving the field forward. J Heart Lung Transplant 2016; 35: 413-20. [http://dx.doi.org/10.1016/j.healun.2016.01.001]

[74] Ferrin PC, McCreath L, Navankasattusas S, Drakos SG. Recovery *versus* remission: clinical insights. Heart Fail Clin 2016; 12: 449-59. [http://dx.doi.org/10.1016/j.hfc.2016.03.007]

[75] Imamura T, Kinugawa K, Nitta D, Kinoshita O, Nawata K, Ono M. Preoperative iodine-123 meta-iodobenzylguanidine imaging is a novel predictor of left ventricular reverse remodeling during treatment with a left ventricular assist device. J Artif Organs 2016; 19: 29-36. [http://dx.doi.org/10.1007/s10047-015-0857-6]

[76] Miyagawa S, Sawa Y, Fukushima N, *et al.* Analysis of sympathetic nerve activity in end-stage cardiomyopathy patients receiving left ventricular support. J Heart Lung Transplant 2001; 20: 1181-7. [http://dx.doi.org/10.1016/S1053-2498(01)00347-3]

[77] Coutance G1. Besson FL, Manrique A, Belin A, Agostini D. Myocardial innervation and perfusion imaging during LVAD implantation: a nuclear imaging approach. Heart Fail Clin 2014; 10(1) (Suppl.): S75-84. [http://dx.doi.org/10.1016/j.hfc.2013.08.008]

[78] Drakos SG, Athanasoulis T, Malliaras KG, *et al.* Myocardial sympathetic innervation and long-term left ventricular mechanical unloading. J Am Coll Cardiol Img 2010; 3: 64-70. [http://dx.doi.org/10.1016/j.jcmg.2009.10.008]

[79] George RS, Birks EJ, Cheetham A, *et al.* The effect of long-term left ventricular assist device support on myocardial sympathetic activity in patients with non-ischaemic dilated cardiomyopathy. Eur J Heart Fail 2013; 15: 1035-43. [http://dx.doi.org/10.1093/eurjhf/hft059]

[80] Moss AJ, Zareba W, Hall WJ, *et al.* Prophylactic implantation of a defibrillator in patients with myocardial infarction and reduced ejection fraction. N Engl J Med 2002; 346: 877-83.

[http://dx.doi.org/10.1056/NEJMoa013474]

[81] Hohnloser SH, Connolly SJ, Kuck KH, *et al.* The defibrillator in acute myocardial infarction trial (DINAMIT): study protocol. Am Heart J 2000; 140: 735-9.
[http://dx.doi.org/10.1067/mhj.2000.110088]

[82] Kadish A, Dyer A, Daubert JP, *et al.* Prophylactic defibrillator implantation in patients with nonischemic dilated cardiomyopathy. N Engl J Med 2004; 350: 2151-8.
[http://dx.doi.org/10.1056/NEJMoa033088]

[83] Bardy GH, Lee KL, Mark DB, *et al.* Amiodarone or an implantable cardioverter-defibrillator for congestive heart failure. N Engl J Med 2005; 352: 225-37.
[http://dx.doi.org/10.1056/NEJMoa043399]

[84] Yancy CW, Jessup M, Bozkurt B, *et al.* 2013 ACCF/AHA guideline for the management of heart failure: a report of the American College of Cardiology Foundation/American Heart Association Task Force on Practice Guidelines. Circulation 2013; 128: e240-327.

[85] Buxton AE, Lee KL, Hafley GE, *et al.* Limitations of ejection fraction for prediction of sudden death risk in patients with coronary artery disease: lessons from the MUSTT study. J Am Coll Cardiol 2007; 50: 1150-7.
[http://dx.doi.org/10.1016/j.jacc.2007.04.095]

[86] Myerburg RJ. Implantable cardioverter-defibrillators after myocardial infarction. N Engl J Med 2008; 359: 2245-53.
[http://dx.doi.org/10.1056/NEJMra0803409]

[87] Køber L, Thune JJ, Nielsen JC, *et al.* DANISH Investigators. Defibrillator Implantation in Patients with Nonischemic Systolic Heart Failure. N Engl J Med 2016; 375: 1221-30.
[http://dx.doi.org/10.1056/NEJMoa1608029]

[88] Barsheshet A, Moss AJ, Huang DT, McNitt S, Zareba W, Goldenberg I. Applicability of a risk score for prediction of the long-term (8-year) benefit of the implantable cardioverter-defibrillator. J Am Coll Cardiol 2012; 59: 2075-9.
[http://dx.doi.org/10.1016/j.jacc.2012.02.036]

[89] Lee DS, Krahn AD, Healey JS, *et al.* Evaluation of early complications related to De Novo cardioverter defibrillator implantation insights from the Ontario ICD database. J Am Coll Cardiol 2010; 55: 774-82.
[http://dx.doi.org/10.1016/j.jacc.2009.11.029]

[90] Maisel WH, Moynahan M, Zuckerman BD, *et al.* Pacemaker and ICD generator malfunctions: analysis of Food and Drug Administration annual reports. JAMA 2006; 295: 1901-6.
[http://dx.doi.org/10.1001/jama.295.16.1901]

[91] Voigt A, Shalaby A, Saba S. Rising rates of cardiac rhythm management device infections in the United States: 1996 through 2003. J Am Coll Cardiol 2006; 48: 590-1.
[http://dx.doi.org/10.1016/j.jacc.2006.05.016]

[92] Zwanziger J, Hall WJ, Dick AW, *et al.* The cost effectiveness of implantable cardioverter-defibrillators: results from the Multicenter Automatic Defibrillator Implantation Trial (MADIT)-II. J Am Coll Cardiol 2006; 47: 2310-8.
[http://dx.doi.org/10.1016/j.jacc.2006.03.032]

[93] Borgquist R, Singh JP. An electrophysiologist perspective on risk stratification in heart failure: can better understanding of the condition of the cardiac sympathetic nervous system help. J Nucl Med 2015; 56: 59S-64S.
[http://dx.doi.org/10.2967/jnumed.114.148452]

[94] Arora R, Ferrick KJ, Nakata T, *et al.* I-123 MIBG imaging and heart rate variability analysis to predict the need for an implantable cardioverter defibrillator. J Nucl Cardiol 2003; 10: 121-31.
[http://dx.doi.org/10.1067/mnc.2003.2]

[95] Nagahara D, Nakata T, Hashimoto A, *et al.* Predicting the need for an implantable cardioverter defibrillator using cardiac metaiodobenzylguanidine activity together with plasma natriuretic peptide concentration or left ventricular function. J Nucl Med 2008; 49: 225-33. [http://dx.doi.org/10.2967/jnumed.107.042564]

[96] Verschure DO, de Groot JR, Mirzaei S, *et al.* Cardiac 123I-mIBG scintigraphy is associated with freedom of appropriate ICD therapy in stable chronic heart failure patients. Int J Cardiol 2017; 248: 403-8. [http://dx.doi.org/10.1016/j.ijcard.2017.08.003]

[97] Hachamovitch R, Nutter B, Menon V, Cerqueira MD. Predicting risk *versus* potential survival benefit using 123I-mIBG imaging in patients with systolic dysfunction eligible for implantable cardiac defibrillator implantation. Analysis of data from the prospective ADMIRE-HF study. Circ Cardiovasc Imaging 2015; 8: e003110. [http://dx.doi.org/10.1161/CIRCIMAGING.114.003110]

[98] Narula J, Gerson M, Thomas GS, Cerqueira MD, Jacobson AF. 123I-MIBG imaging for prediction of mortality and potentially fatal events in heart failure: The ADMIRE-HFX Study. J Nucl Med 2015; 56: 1011-8. [http://dx.doi.org/10.2967/jnumed.115.156406]

[99] O'Day K. Levy, Johnson, Jacobson AF. Cost-effectiveness analysis of iodine-123 metaiodobenzylguanidine imaging for screening heart failure patients eligible for an implantable cardioverter defibrillator in the USA. Appl Health Econ Health Policy 2016; 14: 8361-73.

[100] Boogers MJ, Borleffs CJ, Henneman MM, *et al.* Cardiac sympathetic denervation assessed with 123-Iodine metaiodobenzylguanidine imaging predicts ventricular arrhythmias in implantable cardioverter-defibrillator patients. J Am Coll Cardiol 2010; 55: 2769-7. [http://dx.doi.org/10.1016/j.jacc.2009.12.066]

[101] Marshall A1. Cheetham A, George RS, Mason M, Kelion AD. Cardiac iodine-123 metaiodobenzylguanidine imaging predicts ventricular arrhythmia in heart failure patients receiving an implantable cardioverter-defibrillator for primary prevention. Heart 2012; 98: 1359-65. [http://dx.doi.org/10.1136/heartjnl-2012-302321]

[102] Exner DV, Klein GJ, Prystowsky EN. Primary prevention of sudden death with implantable defibrillator therapy in patients with cardiac disease. Can we afford to do it? (Can we afford not to?). Circulation 2001; 104: 1564-70. [http://dx.doi.org/10.1161/hc3801.096395]

[103] International Study to Determine if AdreView Heart Function Scan Can be Used to Identify Patient s With M ild or M oderate Heart Failure (HF) That Benefit From Implanted M edical Device,ADM IRE-ICD, at Clin trialshttps://www.clinicaltrials.gov/ct2/show/NCT02656329 accessed 12/26/17

[104] Sciammarella MG, Gerson M, Buxton AE, *et al.* ASNC/SNMMI model coverage policy: Myocardial sympathetic innervation imaging: iodine-123 meta- iodobenzylguanidine (123I-mIBG). J Nucl Cardiol 2015; 22: 804-11. [http://dx.doi.org/10.1007/s12350-015-0202-8]

[105] Duell J, Dilsizian V, Smith M, Chen W, Dickfeld T. Nuclear imaging guidance for ablation of ventricular arrhythmias. Curr Cardiol Rep 2016; 18: 19. [http://dx.doi.org/10.1007/s11886-015-0697-2]

[106] Bax JJ, Kraft O, Buxton AE, *et al.* 123 I-MIBG scintigraphy to predict inducibility of ventricular arrhythmias on cardiac electrophysiology testing: a prospective multicenter pilot study. Circ Cardiovasc Imaging 2008; 1: 131-40. [http://dx.doi.org/10.1161/CIRCIMAGING.108.782433]

[107] Zhou Y, Zhou W, Folks RD, *et al.* I-123 mIBG and Tc-99m myocardial SPECT imaging to predict inducibility of ventricular arrhythmia on electrophysiology testing: a retrospective analysis. J Nucl Cardiol 2014; 21: 913-20.

[http://dx.doi.org/10.1007/s12350-014-9911-7]

[108] Roes SD, Borleffs XJ, van der Geest RJ, *et al.* Infract tissue heterogeneity assessed with contrast-enhanced MRI predicts spontaneous ventricular arrhythmia in patients with ischemic cardiomyopathy and implantable cardioverter-defibrillator. Circ Cardiovasc Imaging 2009; 2: 183-90. [http://dx.doi.org/10.1161/CIRCIMAGING.108.826529]

[109] Klein T, Abdulghani M, Smith M, *et al.* Three-Dimensional 123I-Meta-Iodobenzylguanidine Cardiac Innervation Maps to Assess Substrate and Successful Ablation Sites for Ventricular Tachycardia: A Feasibility Study for a Novel Paradigm of Innervation Imaging. Circ Arrhythm Electrophysiol 2015; 8: 583-91. [http://dx.doi.org/10.1161/CIRCEP.114.002105]

[110] Abdulghani M, Duell J, Smith M, *et al.* Global and regional myocardial innervation before and after ablation of drug-refractory ventricular tachycardia assessed with ^{123}I-MIBG. J Nucl Med 2015; 56: 52S-8S. [http://dx.doi.org/10.2967/jnumed.115.155143]

[111] Sasano T, Abraham R, Chang KC, *et al.* Abnormal sympathetic innervation of viable myocardium and the substrate of ventricular tachycardia after myocardial infarction. J Am Coll Cardiol 2008; 51: 2266-75. [http://dx.doi.org/10.1016/j.jacc.2008.02.062]

[112] D'estanque E, Hedon C, Lattuca B, *et al.* Optimization of a simultaneous dual-isotope 201Tl/123I-MIBG myocardial SPECT imaging protocol with a CZT camera for trigger zone assessment after myocardial infarction for routine clinical settings: Are delayed acquisition and scatter correction necessary? J Nucl Cardiol 2017; 24: 1361-9. [http://dx.doi.org/10.1007/s12350-016-0524-1]

CHAPTER 10

Neurotransmitter Imaging for Cardiomyopathy and Takotsubo Syndrome

Takayuki Warisawa[1,2] and **Yoshihiro J. Akashi**[*,2]

[1] *International Center for Circulatory Health, National Heart and Lung Institute, Imperial College London, Hammersmith Hospital, London, United Kingdom*

[2] *Division of Cardiology, Department of Internal Medicine, St. Marianna University School of Medicine, Kawasaki, Japan*

Abstract: Although the guidelines of the Japanese Circulation Society recommend Iodine-123 meta-iodobenzylguanidine (^{123}I-MIBG) myocardial scintigraphy in patients with heart failure, this scintigraphy can be applied to evaluate cardiac sympathetic activity in hypertrophic cardiomyopathy (HCM) and takotsubo syndrome (TTS). Increased cardiac sympathetic activity in HCM is associated with the various clinical features, the advancement of disease stage, and the prognosis. However, it has not been fully studied whether this neurotransmitter imaging function as a monitor of the therapeutic effect in HCM.

^{123}I-MIBG myocardial scintigraphy has been taken an important role to explore the underlying pathophysiological mechanism in TTS. TTS is a novel cardiac syndrome involving acute onset of ST-segment elevation on electrocardiography, mimicking acute myocardial infarction without coronary artery flow limitation. Although over 25-years have passed since the first description, the details of the underlying pathophysiology are still unclear. Of great interest now is whether it could be utilized to stratify the cardiac risk in patients with TTS using ^{23}I-MIBG myocardial scintigraphy.

In this chapter, we focus on the clinical value of ^{123}I-MIBG myocardial scintigraphy in these patients.

Keywords: Hypertrophic Cardiomyopathy, ^{123}I-MIBG Myocardial Scintigraphy, Takotsubo Syndrome.

[*] **Corresponding author Yoshihiro J. Akashi:** Division of Cardiology, Department of Internal Medicine, St. Marianna University School of Medicine, 2-16-1 Sugao, Miyamae-Ku, Kawasaki City, Kanagawa prefecture, 216-8511, Japan; Tel: 81449778111, Fax: +81449767093; E-mail: yoakashi-circ@umin.ac.jp

Shinro Matsuo (Ed.)

INTRODUCTION

Cardiomyopathy is the collective term which is defined by structural and functional abnormalities of the ventricular myocardium that is unexplained by flow limiting coronary artery disease or abnormal loading conditions [1]. Iodine-123 meta-iodobenzylguanidine (^{123}I-MIBG) myocardial scintigraphy plays an important role in this field as well.

With regard to dilated cardiomyopathy, there are abundant evidences about disease severity, prognosis and effect of treatment in the context of heart failure. Most of these evidences are reviewed in the previous chapter. Briefly, the late heart-to-mediastinum ratio (H/M) and washout rate (WR) are strong predictors of cardiac death and ventricular arrhythmias [2 - 5] and also can be used for monitoring the effect of medical therapy, such as beta-blockers and renin-angiotensin-aldosterone system inhibitors [6 - 10]. Hence, the guidelines of the Japanese Circulation Society recommend ^{123}I-MIBG myocardial scintigraphy in patients with heart failure [11].

In this chapter, in order to avoid repeated description, we will focus on clinical value of ^{123}I-MIBG myocardial scintigraphy in hypertrophic cardiomyopathy and Takotsubo Syndrome.

HYPERTROPHIC CARDIOMYOPATHY

Hypertrophic cardiomyopathy (HCM) is defined by the presence of increased left ventricular (LV) wall thickness which is not solely explained by abnormal loading conditions [12]. This is the most common genetic cardiovascular disease with a prevalence in general population of 1:500 and is characterized by extreme heterogeneity with regard to phenotypic expression, pathophysiology, and clinical course [12 - 14]. HCM could cause several symptoms such as dyspnea, chest pain and syncope, impaired tolerance of exercise, heart failure, lethal arrythmias and sudden cardiac death. Histopathologically, HCM shows myocyte disarray which causes LV hypertrophy with diastolic dysfunction. The prognosis of HCM is associated with the degree of hypertrophy and the severity of left ventricular outflow tract (LVOT) obstruction which is caused by asymmetric septal myocardial hypertrophy.

Relationship Between Cardiac Sympathetic Activity and Clinical Features in HCM

Before the introduction of ^{123}I-MIBG myocardial scintigraphy, impaired cardiac sympathetic activity in HCM had been reported: impaired norepinephrine (NE) uptake at synaptic cleft causes increased spillover of NE with increased plasma level of NE [15].

Several reports demonstrated impaired cardiac sympathetic system in HCM which is characterized by decreased late H/M and increased WR on ^{123}I-MIBG scintigraphy [16 - 19]. Decreased late H/M can be observed in the early stage of HCM without either LV systolic dysfunction or LV dilatation [16]. Nakajima *et al.* and Taki *et al.* reported correlation between WR and severity of hypertrophy, respectively [17 - 18]. Other report showed WR was significantly associated with septum thickness and LVOT obstruction [19]. These data indicate that the impairment of cardiac sympathetic activity in HCM starts in the early stage of disease and correlates to the degree of septal hypertrophy and thus, correlates to LVOT obstruction and diastolic dysfunction.

Terai *et al.* evaluated the changes of cardiac sympathetic activity throughout the clinical course from early to end-stage HCM [16]. In this study, 46 patients with HCM were divided into three different stage of HCM: preserved LV systolic function, LV systolic dysfunction without LV dilatation, and LV systolic dysfunction with LV dilatation. The reduced regional early uptake and increased WR were magnified progressively through the advancement of the disease stage. These results suggested that cardiac sympathetic impairment in HCM could advance with the development of LV systolic dysfunction and dilatation, and that ^{123}I-MIBG myocardial scintigraphy might be a useful modality for the evaluation of pathophysiologic changes in HCM.

Other report showed relationship between ^{123}I-MIBG scintigraphy and laboratory data and echocardiographical findings [20]. The plasma level of brain natriuretic peptide and left ventricular mass index was independent and significant predictors of late H/M ($p=0.0001$ and $p=0.0009$, respectively). The plasma level of NE was an independent and significant predictor of WR ($p=0.0018$). These findings indicate that impairments of cardiac sympathetic activity might reflect the progression of myocardial damage or dysfunction in HCM.

Usefulness of ^{123}I-MIBG Scintigraphy for Prognosis in HCM

In patients with HCM, congestive heart failure (CHF), lethal arrhythmias and sudden cardiac death are major prognostic determinants [12 - 13].

Hiase *et al.* investigated whether cardiac sympathetic activity was useful for predicting the onset of CHF in HCM [21]. In this study, 84 patients were followed up for 9-86 months. The prevalence of CHF during follow-up period was 0% in patients with normal H/M (>2.11), 3.3% in patients with mildly-decreased H/M (1.86-2.11), and 55.0% in patients with highly-decreased H/M (<1.86), respectively. Multivariate analysis also showed late H/M was the most powerful predictor of CHF in comparison with other conventional prognostic variables.

Regarding the lethal arrythmias, Terai *et al.* evaluated the relationship between cardiac sympathetic activity and the occurrence of ventricular tachycardia (VT) in HCM [22]. They compared the HCM patients with VT (n=15) to those without VT (n=29), defined as a run of ≥ 3 consecutive beats at a rate of ≥ 120 beats/min on Holter monitoring. WR was significantly higher in the patients with VT compared to those without VT (26.8 ± 6.4% *vs* 17.4 ± 5.7%, $p<0.0001$). The logistic multiple regression analysis also demonstrated WR was the most powerful predictor of occurrence of VT in patients with HCM.

Other report also suggested that both WR >40% and late H/R <2.00 could be useful prognostic predictors of CHF and sudden cardiac death [23].

Role as a Monitor for Medical Therapy in HCM

It is well known that beta-blockers are efficient for controlling symptoms in HCM and transcatheter septal ablation is also effective for HCM with significant LVOT gradient [12 - 13]. Currently, however, clinical evidences with ^{123}I-MIBG scintigraphy regarding medical therapy in HCM are very limited.

One case report demonstrated gradual increase of late H/M and decrease of WR at 6 and 18 months after the transcatheter septal ablation compared with baseline levels of pre-procedure, which indicated that regional cardiac morphologic change in LVOT reduction could improve global cardiac sympathetic activity over a long period of time [24].

TAKOTSUBO SYNDROME

Takotsubo syndrome (TTS) is a cardiac syndrome involving acute onset of ST-segment elevation on electrocardiography, mimicking acute myocardial infarction, but with a normal coronary artery [25]. TTS was first described in Japan and was named after an octopus trap: a fishing jar with a narrow neck and wide base, the appearance of which is similar to the apical ballooning seen on left ventriculography in the typical case [26] (Fig. **1**). The prognosis of TTS was initially reported to be favorable compared with that for ST-segment elevation myocardial infarction [27], but recent studies demonstrated that acute and long-term mortalities are both higher than previously recognized: 4-5% for in-hospital mortality and 5% for recurrence [28 - 29]. Therefore, TTS is now receiving more and more attentions in cardiovascular medicine. Although over 25-years have passed since the first description, the details of the underlying pathophysiology are still unclear. Multivessel epicardial coronary spasm, microvascular dysfunction, catecholamine toxicity, and a combination of them have been suggested as a cause of the characteristic ventricular wall motion abnormality [30 - 31].

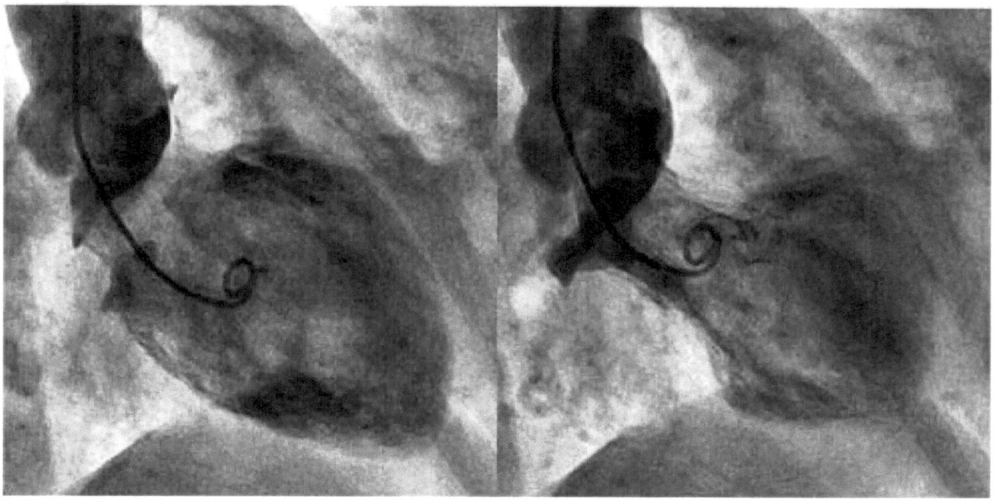

Fig. (1). Typical left ventriculography of Takotsubo syndrome. Left ventriculography during diastolic phase (left) and systolic phase (right) demonstrating the classic appearance of Takotsubo syndrome.

Evidences and Roles of ^{123}I-MIBG Scintigraphy in TTS

Emotional or physical stress is frequently, but not always present prior to the onset of TTS, and could trigger the onset of this syndrome [25]. It has been suggested that epinephrine is a key factor in this pathophysiology [32 - 33]. In the acute phase of TTS, it is known that plasma epinephrine level is more elevated than that of acute myocardial infarction [34].

There are many case reports showing decreased H/M and increased WR in the acute or sub-acute phase of TTS on ^{123}I-MIBG scintigraphy, which are concordant findings with those in heart failure [35 - 41]. The single-photon emission computed tomography (SPECT) imaging is useful to demonstrate regional uptake defect in the myocardial apex, which correlates with impaired LV segments [36]. This has been also confirmed in variants of TTS; the midventricular type and the basal or inverted type [37]. Thus, ^{123}I-MIBG scintigraphy can define the areas of impaired LV segments corresponding to the abnormalities in the cardiac sympathetic activity in TTS.

Akashi *et al.* investigated the serial change of ^{123}I-MIBG scintigraphy findings in 8 patients with TTS [38]. Three-months after the onset, late H/M was significantly increased (1.89 ± 0.25 *vs.* 2.13 ± 0.17, $p<0.05$) and WR was significantly decreased ($39.1 \pm 10.3\%$ *vs.* $25.4 \pm 6.3\%$, $p<0.05$). The SPECT imaging showed impaired uptake of ^{123}I-MIBG mainly in the apex and inferior region both in the acute phase and in 3-months follow-up. In addition, although LV function and epinephrine level are normalized after a few weeks, several case reports showed persistent decrease in ^{123}I-MIBG uptake on SPECT imaging in the apical myocardium [39 - 40]. Other report demonstrated hypokinetic LV segments were characterized by normal perfusion but impaired sympathetic activity on ^{99m}Tc-tetrofosmin/ ^{201}Thallium and ^{123}I-MIBG SPECT imaging and concluded that transient coronary microvascular dysfunction might be an associated phenomenon secondary to acute catecholamine release [41]. These results suggested that neurogenic myocardial stunning could be central causative mechanism of TTS.

Future Prospects of ^{123}I-MIBG Scintigraphy in TTS

Although ^{123}I-MIBG myocardial scintigraphy has taken an important role to elucidate that enhanced sympathetic stimulation is central to TTS, the mechanism by which catecholamine excess causes myocardial stunning in the variety of regional ballooning patterns which characterize this syndrome is still unknown. In addition, whether ^{123}I-MIBG scintigraphy could contribute to quick and useful diagnostic process is doubtful because ^{123}I-MIBG scintigraphy was usually performed over one week after the onset in many of the previous reports as recently pointed out [42]. In principle, urgent invasive diagnostic coronary angiography is mandatory in patients with acute chest pain and ST-segment elevation [30]. On the other hand, one of the current interest in this field is whether ^{123}I-MIBG myocardial scintigraphy can be used for the risk stratification in patients with TTS, particularly about the recurrence, the persistent LV dysfunction, and the treatment strategy.

CONCLUSION

In summary, ^{123}I-MIBG myocardial scintigraphy can be used to evaluate cardiac sympathetic activity in HCM and TTS. Increased cardiac sympathetic activity in HCM is associated with the various clinical features, the advancement of disease stage, and the prognosis. Whether this neurotransmitter imaging could work as a monitor for the effect of treatment in HCM is an issue to be addressed in the future. ^{123}I-MIBG myocardial scintigraphy has been taken an important role to explore the underlined pathophysiological mechanism in TTS. Of great interest now is whether it could be utilized to stratify the cardiac risk in patients with TTS (Fig. **2**).

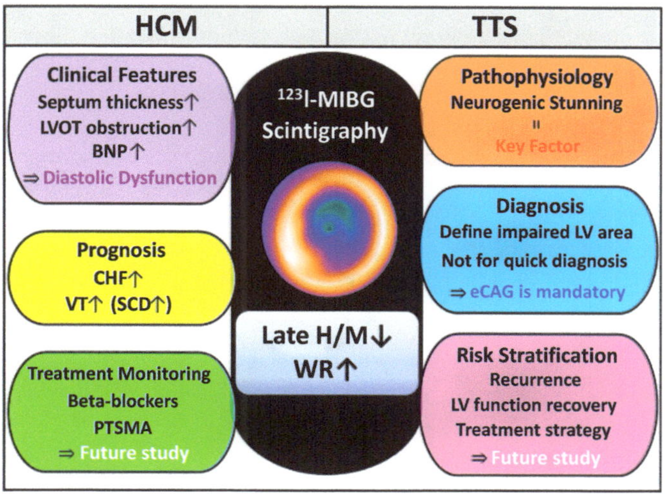

Fig. (2). Roles of neurotransmitter imaging in HCM and TTS ^{123}I-MIBG myocardial scintigraphy is useful to evaluate cardiac sympathetic activity in HCM and TTS. BNP: brain natriuretic peptide; CHF: congestive heart failure; eCAG: emergent coronary angiography; HCM: hypertrophic cardiomyopathy; H/R: heart-t--mediastinum ratio; ^{123}I-MIBG: Iodine-123 meta-iodobenzylguanidine; LV: left ventricular; LVOT: left ventricular outflow tract; PTSMA: percutaneous transluminal septal myocardial ablation; SCD: sudden cardiac death; TTS: takotsubo syndrome; VT: ventricular tachycardia; WR: washout rate.

CONSENT FOR PUBLICATION

Not applicable.

CONFLICT OF INTEREST

The authors declare no conflict of interest, financial or otherwise.

ACKNOWLEDGEMENTS

Declared none.

REFERENCES

[1] Elliott P, Andersson B, Arbustini E, *et al.* Classification of the cardiomyopathies: a position statement from the European Society Of Cardiology Working Group on Myocardial and Pericardial Diseases. Eur Heart J 2008; 29(2): 270-6. [http://dx.doi.org/10.1093/eurheartj/ehm342] [PMID: 17916581]

[2] Merlet P, Valette H, Dubois-Randé JL, *et al.* Prognostic value of cardiac metaiodobenzylguanidine imaging in patients with heart failure. J Nucl Med 1992; 33(4): 471-7. [PMID: 1552326]

[3] Jacobson AF, Senior R, Cerqueira MD, *et al.* Myocardial iodine-123 meta-iodobenzylguanidine imaging and cardiac events in heart failure. Results of the prospective ADMIRE-HF (AdreView Myocardial Imaging for Risk Evaluation in Heart Failure) study. J Am Coll Cardiol 2010; 55(20): 2212-21. [http://dx.doi.org/10.1016/j.jacc.2010.01.014] [PMID: 20188504]

[4] Nakata T, Nakajima K, Yamashina S, *et al.* A pooled analysis of multicenter cohort studies of (123)I-mIBG imaging of sympathetic innervation for assessment of long-term prognosis in heart failure. JACC Cardiovasc Imaging 2013; 6(7): 772-84.
[http://dx.doi.org/10.1016/j.jcmg.2013.02.007] [PMID: 23845574]

[5] Verschure DO, Veltman CE, Manrique A, *et al.* For what endpoint does myocardial 123I-MIBG scintigraphy have the greatest prognostic value in patients with chronic heart failure? Results of a pooled individual patient data meta-analysis. Eur Heart J Cardiovasc Imaging 2014; 15(9): 996-1003.
[http://dx.doi.org/10.1093/ehjci/jeu044] [PMID: 24686260]

[6] Suwa M, Otake Y, Moriguchi A, *et al.* Iodine-123 metaiodobenzylguanidine myocardial scintigraphy for prediction of response to beta-blocker therapy in patients with dilated cardiomyopathy. Am Heart J 1997; 133(3): 353-8.
[http://dx.doi.org/10.1016/S0002-8703(97)70232-1] [PMID: 9060806]

[7] Toyama T, Aihara Y, Iwasaki T, *et al.* Cardiac sympathetic activity estimated by 123I-MIBG myocardial imaging in patients with dilated cardiomyopathy after beta-blocker or angiotensin-converting enzyme inhibitor therapy. J Nucl Med 1999; 40(2): 217-23.
[PMID: 10025826]

[8] Kakuchi H, Sasaki T, Ishida Y, Komamura K, Miyatake K. Clinical usefulness of 123I meta-iodobenzylguanidine imaging in predicting the effectiveness of beta blockers for patients with idiopathic dilated cardiomyopathy before and soon after treatment. Heart 1999; 81(2): 148-52.
[http://dx.doi.org/10.1136/hrt.81.2.148] [PMID: 9922349]

[9] Agostini D, Belin A, Amar MH, *et al.* Improvement of cardiac neuronal function after carvedilol treatment in dilated cardiomyopathy: a 123I-MIBG scintigraphic study. J Nucl Med 2000; 41(5): 845-51.
[PMID: 10809201]

[10] Nakata T, Wakabayashi T, Kyuma M, Takahashi T, Tsuchihashi K, Shimamoto K. Cardiac metaiodobenzylguanidine activity can predict the long-term efficacy of angiotensin-converting enzyme inhibitors and/or beta-adrenoceptor blockers in patients with heart failure. Eur J Nucl Med Mol Imaging 2005; 32(2): 186-94.
[http://dx.doi.org/10.1007/s00259-004-1624-8] [PMID: 15452671]

[11] Guidelines for clinical use of cardiac nuclear medicine (JCS 2010) – digest version –. Circ J 2012; 76(3): 761-7.
[http://dx.doi.org/10.1253/circj.CJ-88-0019] [PMID: 22293456]

[12] Elliott PM, Anastasakis A, Borger MA, *et al.* 2014 ESC Guidelines on diagnosis and management of hypertrophic cardiomyopathy: the Task Force for the Diagnosis and Management of Hypertrophic Cardiomyopathy of the European Society of Cardiology (ESC). Eur Heart J 2014; 35(39): 2733-79.
[http://dx.doi.org/10.1093/eurheartj/ehu284] [PMID: 25173338]

[13] Geske JB, Ommen SR, Gersh BJ. Hypertrophic Cardiomyopathy: Clinical Update. JACC Heart Fail 2018; 6(5): 364-75.
[http://dx.doi.org/10.1016/j.jchf.2018.02.010] [PMID: 29655825]

[14] Cecchi F, Olivotto I, Montereggi A, Santoro G, Dolara A, Maron BJ. Hypertrophic cardiomyopathy in Tuscany: clinical course and outcome in an unselected regional population. J Am Coll Cardiol 1995; 26(6): 1529-36.
[http://dx.doi.org/10.1016/0735-1097(95)00353-3] [PMID: 7594081]

[15] Brush JE Jr, Eisenhofer G, Garty M, *et al.* Cardiac norepinephrine kinetics in hypertrophic cardiomyopathy. Circulation 1989; 79(4): 836-44.
[http://dx.doi.org/10.1161/01.CIR.79.4.836] [PMID: 2924414]

[16] Terai H, Shimizu M, Ino H, *et al.* Changes in cardiac sympathetic nerve innervation and activity in pathophysiologic transition from typical to end-stage hypertrophic cardiomyopathy. J Nucl Med 2003; 44(10): 1612-7.

[PMID: 14530475]

[17] Nakajima K, Bunko H, Taki J, Shimizu M, Muramori A, Hisada K. Quantitative analysis of 123I-meta-iodobenzylguanidine (MIBG) uptake in hypertrophic cardiomyopathy. Am Heart J 1990; 119(6): 1329-37.
[http://dx.doi.org/10.1016/S0002-8703(05)80183-8] [PMID: 2353619]

[18] Taki J, Nakajima K, Bunko H, Simizu M, Muramori A, Hisada K. Whole-body distribution of iodine 123 metaiodobenzylguanidine in hypertrophic cardiomyopathy: significance of its washout from the heart. Eur J Nucl Med 1990; 17(5): 264-8.
[http://dx.doi.org/10.1007/BF00812368] [PMID: 2128050]

[19] Pace L, Betocchi S, Losi MA, *et al.* Sympathetic nervous function in patients with hypertrophic cardiomyopathy assessed by [123I]-MIBG: relationship with left ventricular perfusion and function. Q J Nucl Med Mol Imaging 2004; 48(1): 20-5.
[PMID: 15195000]

[20] Matsuo S, Nakamura Y, Tsutamoto T, Kinoshita M. Impairments of myocardial sympathetic activity may reflect the progression of myocardial damage or dysfunction in hypertrophic cardiomyopathy. J Nucl Cardiol 2002; 9(4): 407-12.
[http://dx.doi.org/10.1067/mnc.2002.122765] [PMID: 12161717]

[21] Hiasa G, Hamada M, Saeki H, *et al.* Cardiac sympathetic nerve activity can detect congestive heart failure sensitively in patients with hypertrophic cardiomyopathy. Chest 2004; 126(3): 679-86.
[http://dx.doi.org/10.1378/chest.126.3.679] [PMID: 15364742]

[22] Terai H, Shimizu M, Ino H, *et al.* Cardiac sympathetic nerve activity in patients with hypertrophic cardiomyopathy with malignant ventricular tachyarrhythmias. J Nucl Cardiol 2003; 10(3): 304-10.
[http://dx.doi.org/10.1016/S1071-3581(03)00362-3] [PMID: 12794630]

[23] Nagamatsu H, Momose M, Kobayashi H, Kusakabe K, Kasanuki H. Prognostic value of 123I-metaiodobenzylguanidine in patients with various heart diseases. Ann Nucl Med 2007; 21(9): 513-20.
[http://dx.doi.org/10.1007/s12149-007-0062-7] [PMID: 18030583]

[24] Okayama S, Uemura S, Horii M, Kawata H, Saito Y. Continuing improvement of cardiac sympathetic activity on I-123 MIBG scintigraphy in a patient with hypertrophic obstructive cardiomyopathy after percutaneous transluminal septal myocardial ablation. J Nucl Cardiol 2008; 15(5): e31-4.
[http://dx.doi.org/10.1016/j.nuclcard.2008.06.015] [PMID: 18761260]

[25] Ghadri JR, Wittstein IS, Prasad A, *et al.* International Expert Consensus Document on Takotsubo Syndrome (Part I): Clinical Characteristics, Diagnostic Criteria, and Pathophysiology. Eur Heart J 2018; 39(22): 2032-46.
[http://dx.doi.org/10.1093/eurheartj/ehy076] [PMID: 29850871]

[26] Sato H. Tako-tsubo-like left ventricular dysfunction due to multivessel coronary spasm.Kodama K, Hori Haze M. Clinical Aspect of Myocardial Injury: From Ischemia to Heart Failure. Tokyo: Kagakuhyoronsha Publishing Co 1990; pp. 56-64. (Article in Japanese)

[27] Elesber AA, Prasad A, Lennon RJ, Wright RS, Lerman A, Rihal CS. Four-year recurrence rate and prognosis of the apical ballooning syndrome. J Am Coll Cardiol 2007; 50(5): 448-52.
[http://dx.doi.org/10.1016/j.jacc.2007.03.050] [PMID: 17662398]

[28] Deshmukh A, Kumar G, Pant S, Rihal C, Murugiah K, Mehta JL. Prevalence of Takotsubo cardiomyopathy in the United States. Am Heart J 2012; 164(1): 66-71.e1.
[http://dx.doi.org/10.1016/j.ahj.2012.03.020] [PMID: 22795284]

[29] Templin C, Ghadri JR, Diekmann J, *et al.* Clinical features and outcomes of takotsubo (stress) cardiomyopathy. N Engl J Med 2015; 373(10): 929-38.
[http://dx.doi.org/10.1056/NEJMoa1406761] [PMID: 26332547]

[30] Akashi YJ, Nef HM, Lyon AR. Epidemiology and pathophysiology of Takotsubo syndrome. Nat Rev Cardiol 2015; 12(7): 387-97.

[http://dx.doi.org/10.1038/nrcardio.2015.39] [PMID: 25855605]

[31] Ghadri JR, Wittstein IS, Prasad A, *et al.* International expert consensus document on takotsubo syndrome (part II): diagnostic workup, outcome, and management. Eur Heart J 2018; 39(22): 2047-62. [http://dx.doi.org/10.1093/eurheartj/ehy077] [PMID: 29850820]

[32] Paur H, Wright PT, Sikkel MB, *et al.* High levels of circulating epinephrine trigger apical cardiodepression in a β2-adrenergic receptor/Gi-dependent manner: a new model of Takotsubo cardiomyopathy. Circulation 2012; 126(6): 697-706. [http://dx.doi.org/10.1161/CIRCULATIONAHA.112.111591] [PMID: 22732314]

[33] Verschure DO, Somsen GA, van Eck-Smit BL, Knol RJ, Booij J, Verberne HJ. Tako-tsubo cardiomyopathy: how to understand possible pathophysiological mechanism and the role of (123)I-MIBG imaging. J Nucl Cardiol 2014; 21(4): 730-8. [PMID: 24464623]

[34] Wittstein IS, Thiemann DR, Lima JAC, *et al.* Neurohumoral features of myocardial stunning due to sudden emotional stress. N Engl J Med 2005; 352(6): 539-48. [http://dx.doi.org/10.1056/NEJMoa043046] [PMID: 15703419]

[35] Verberne HJ, van der Heijden DJ, van Eck-Smit BL, Somsen GA. Persisting myocardial sympathetic dysfunction in takotsubo cardiomyopathy. J Nucl Cardiol 2009; 16(2): 321-4. [http://dx.doi.org/10.1007/s12350-008-9017-1] [PMID: 19156479]

[36] Owa M, Aizawa K, Urasawa N, *et al.* Emotional stress-induced 'ampulla cardiomyopathy': discrepancy between the metabolic and sympathetic innervation imaging performed during the recovery course. Jpn Circ J 2001; 65(4): 349-52. [http://dx.doi.org/10.1253/jcj.65.349] [PMID: 11316138]

[37] Moriya M, Naito K, Takahashi M, *et al.* A case of transient mid-ventricular akinesia (a variant form of Takotsubo cardiomyopathy) followed with I-123-beta-metyl-iodophenyl pentadecanoic acid and I-123-meta-iodobenzyl-guanidine myocardial scintigraphy. J Cardiol 2009; 53(1): 140-5. [http://dx.doi.org/10.1016/j.jjcc.2008.06.008] [PMID: 19167650]

[38] Akashi YJ, Nakazawa K, Sakakibara M, Miyake F, Musha H, Sasaka K. 123I-MIBG myocardial scintigraphy in patients with "takotsubo" cardiomyopathy. J Nucl Med 2004; 45(7): 1121-7. [PMID: 15235057]

[39] Akashi YJ, Takano M, Miyake F. Scintigraphic imaging in Tako-Tsubo cardiomyopathy. Herz 2010; 35(4): 231-8. [http://dx.doi.org/10.1007/s00059-011-3445-4] [PMID: 22086475]

[40] Moriya M, Mori H, Suzuki N, Hazama M, Yano K. Six-month follow-up of takotsubo cardiomyopathy with I-123-beta-metyl-iodophenyl pentadecanoic acid and I-123-meta-iodobenzyl-guanidine myocardial scintigraphy. Intern Med 2002; 41(10): 829-33. [http://dx.doi.org/10.2169/internalmedicine.41.829] [PMID: 12413004]

[41] Cimarelli S, Sauer F, Morel O, Ohlmann P, Constantinesco A, Imperiale A. Transient left ventricular dysfunction syndrome: patho-physiological bases through nuclear medicine imaging. Int J Cardiol 2010; 144(2): 212-8. [http://dx.doi.org/10.1016/j.ijcard.2009.04.025] [PMID: 19443060]

[42] Madias JE. Do we need MIBG in the evaluation of patients with suspected Takotsubo syndrome? Diagnostic, prognostic, and pathophysiologic connotations. Int J Cardiol 2016; 203: 783-4. [http://dx.doi.org/10.1016/j.ijcard.2015.11.046] [PMID: 26595783]

CHAPTER 11

Evaluation of Cardiac Sympathetic Nerve Function using Iodine-123 Metaiodobenzylguanidine Scintigraphy

Hiroshi Mori and **Shinro Matsuo***

Department of Nuclear Medicine, Kanazawa University Hospital, 13-1 Takaramachi, Kanazawa, Ishikawa, Japan 920-8641

Abstract: A heart is controlled by sympathetic and parasympathetic nerve system. The synapse mediator of sympathetic nerve ending is norepinephrine, and the mediator of parasympathetic nerve ending is acetylcholine. In the case of heart failure, infarction or various heart diseases, the abnormality of cardiac sympathetic nerve appears. Iodine-123 metaiodobenzylguanidine (^{123}I-MIBG) is widely used for radiopharmaceutical in the world. ^{123}I-MIBG is proven as a specific radiolabeled tracer of sympathetic innervation heart because of high accumulation ratio compared with normal sympathetic nerve heart. The material is taken up in a sympathetic nerve ending and stored in synapse granular vesicles like uptake-mechanism of norepinephrine. Cardiovascular diseases have a relation with activity of the sympathetic cardiac nerves. To evaluate cardiac sympathetic activity, ^{123}I-MIBG scintigraphy is commonly used. ^{123}I-MIBG scintigraphy is performed at 10 to 15 minutes (early image) and 3 to 4 hours (delayed image) after intravenous injection. Cardiac ^{123}I-MIBG uptake is commonly assessed by viewing the planar images. ^{123}I-MIBG SPECT has been used to evaluate regional denervation and for better quantification of the size and severity of innervation abnormalities. Therefore, ^{123}I-MIBG scintigraphy is very useful and widely available nuclear imaging method for assessing myocardial sympathetic innervation.

Keywords: Coronary artery disease, Heart-to-mediastinum ratio, Iodine-123 metaiodobenzylguanidine.

RADIONUCLIDE AND UPTAKE MECHANISM

Iodine-123 is widely used for radiopharmaceutical in the world. The half-life of ^{123}I is approximately 13 hours, gamma energy is 159 keV. Iodine-123 metaiodobenzylguanidine (^{123}I-MIBG) is similar to a sympathetic nerve mediator. ^{123}I-MIBG is proven as a specific radiolabeled tracer of sympathetic innervation

* **Corresponding author Shinro Matsuo:** Department of Nuclear Medicine, Kanazawa University Hospital, 13-1 Takara-machi, Kanazawa 920-8641, Japan; Tel: 81-76-265-2333; Fax: 81-76-234-4257; E-mail: smatsuo@med.kanazawa-u.ac.jp

heart because of high accumulation ratio compared with normal sympathetic nerve heart by animal experiment [1]. The material is taken up in a sympathetic nerve ending and stored in synapse granular vesicles like uptake-mechanism of norepinephrine (uptake-1 mechanism). Some studies have shown that non-neuronal uptake (uptake-2 mechanism) of ^{123}I-MIBG by the myocardium is not usually significant [2]. Uptake-2 mechanism has been shown to be significant at high plasma ^{123}I-MIBG concentrations by mechanism of passive diffusion. As small amount of ^{123}I-MIBG is injected in the clinical use, the uptake-1 mechanism predominates in ^{123}I-MIBG imaging. ^{123}I-MIBG depends on energy-dependent uptake mechanism by neuroendocrine cells. After intravenous injection, ^{123}I-MIBG concentration increases and reaches plateau within a few minutes [3]. The majority of the material is taken up again, it is stored in synapse granular vesicles and not metabolized by monoamine oxidase (MAO) and catechol-O-methyltransferase (COMT). Taken ^{123}I-MIBG in a sympathetic nerve ending stays for a while, and is excreted gradually. The washout ratio reflects sympathetic nerve activity. Some of the material is flowed out to a blood flow. The material does not combine with beta 1 receptor and has no pharmacological activity. The redundancy of material is excreted by the kidneys. In the clinical field, ^{123}I-MIBG has been used as a radioactive test agent to investigate sympathetic nerve function. In the cardiac field, ^{123}I-MIBG provides us information for cardiac innervation and cardiac function. A cardiac sympathetic nerve function has a relation with heart function, ^{123}I-MIBG imaging enables to assess the severity and prognosis of heart failure [4].

PATIENT PREPARATION

^{123}I-MIBG is contraindicated in patients with known hypersensitivity to iobenguane or iobenguane sulfate. Before ^{123}I-MIBG examination, we must ask for patients about allergies of iodine-containing materials, shellfish, strawberries, or cranberries [5]. It is widely known that various clinical medicines affect to MIBG kinetics. As a preparation for ^{123}I-MIBG examination, health care workers must pay attention to medication history and drug withdrawal (opioid, cocaine, tramadol, tricyclic antidepressants, sympathicomimetics, antihypertensive or cardiovascular agents, antipsychotics), foods and drinks contained catecholamine analogs (caffeinated drinks, chocolate, cocoa, banana, citrus fruit, vanilla, blue cheese, and so on). Especially, such as uptake-1 inhibitor (tricyclic antidepressant, antipsychotics), antihypertensive drugs (adrenergic neuron blocker, reserpine, calcium antagonist) affect to ^{123}I-MIBG imaging due to the decrease of MIBG uptake. In all cases, it is recommended to stop the drugs more than one or two weeks - if feasible.

EXAMINATION METHODS

^{123}I-MIBG scintigraphy is performed at 10 to 15 minutes (early image) and 3 to 4 hours (delayed image) after intravenous injection. Cardiac ^{123}I-MIBG uptake is commonly assessed by viewing the planar images [6]. Initial uptake is considered to be a measure of the number and function of norepinephrine transporters in the heart [7]. In addition, semi-quantitative measures of uptake and washout have been used. Heart-to-mediastinum ratio (HMR) and washout ratio (WR) are calculated. In order to calculate HMR and WR, region of interest (ROI) is drawn around the heart (a circular ROI) and the superior mediastinum (a rectangular ROI) in a planar imaging. The circular ROI is determined on the cardiac region for evaluating the heart count. The rectangular mediastinal ROI is set by automated software. The HMR is calculated from both the early and the delayed planar images. A recent review has reported an average HMR of 2.5 ± 0.3 for healthy subjects [8]. The WR is calculated from the decrease in myocardial counts between the early and the delayed images, normalized to the mediastinal counts. The WR is considered to reflect sympathetic nerve activity. Average WR of 20% ± 10% has been found in healthy subjects. A SPECT imaging enable to detect regional cardiac sympathetic nerve function. Early and delayed ^{123}I-MIBG SPECT images were scored with 17-segment or 20-segment regional quantitative perfusion or gated SPECT, segmental accumulation counts were calculated. The various studies demonstrated that a statistical significant improvement in ^{123}I-MIBG total defect scores (TDS) after medical treatment [9 - 11]. Especially, the regional abnormal findings at inferior wall appear in aged persons or diabetes mellitus patients. It is reported that regional ^{123}I-MIBG accumulation markedly decrease in the case of diabetes mellitus [12].

NORMAL FINDINGS

^{123}I-MIBG is taken in normal thyroid cell, hence a thyroid block is needed. 500 mg of potassium perchlorate is used to protect this gland. The patients have to take this orally 30 min before ^{123}I-MIBG injection [6]. ^{123}I-MIBG is injected intravenously 111MBq in Japan [4], between 148MBq to 370MBq in United States and Europe [13]. Both planar and SPECT images are acquired in an early image (15-20 minutes) and delayed phase (3-4 hours) after injection. In normal myocardium, good uptake of the ^{123}I-MIBG and a high HMR is observed. The uptake in the inferior wall may be heterogeneous or be slightly lower, because the distribution of cardiac sympathetic nerve fiber may be less in that area [13 - 15]. Activity may also be lower at the apex of the left ventricle than at the base because of the partial-volume effect and, possibly, an imbalance of sympathetic and parasympathetic fibers [16]. Homogeneous uniform uptake has also been reported [14]. Cardiac MIBG uptake and cardiac function decrease with age, which should be taken into consideration when assessing regional ^{123}I-MIBG uptake [17]. Sympathetic nerve dysfunction is related closely with severe damage of myocardial and decreased MIBG uptake [7, 18].

CORONARY ARTERY DISEASES

Cardiac sympathetic dysfunction is related with the pathophysiological state of heart failure, infarction, and various other cardiac diseases. ^{123}I-MIBG imaging is well-known to investigate sympathetic nerve dysfunction non-invasively. In coronary artery diseases, cardiac sympathetic function is more sensitive for the detection of ischemia or infarction. For example, in the case of cardiac infarction, cardiac sympathetic dysfunction with MIBG shows larger defect than perfusion imaging. The defect area of MIBG reflects the ischemic area at risk [19]. Even in absence of an infarction, ^{123}I-MIBG imaging can show accumulation defect at ischemic area as shown in Fig. (**1**). The imaging has proved to be a good predictor of prognosis in patients with impaired left ventricular function. In the case of the severity of left ventricular dysfunction and myocardial ischemia, the accumulation of ^{123}I-MIBG is impaired [20]. The WR is increased in patients with acute myocardial infarction (AMI) compared with the normal value [21]. The global WR of ^{123}I-MIBG and left ventricular ejection fraction are correlated significantly. And other studies have reported a significant correlation between the global WR of ^{123}I-MIBG and diastolic ventricular function or cardiac index in ischemic heart failure [7]. ^{123}I-MIBG imaging is widely used to evaluate heart failure severity, prognosis, therapy. In the case of ischemic heart failure, it shows HMR decrease and WR acceleration. Especially, meta-analysis and clinical trials reveal prognosis aggravation, heart failure death, sudden death by the decrease of delayed HMR [22, 23]. Several studies are reported the effectiveness of ^{123}I-MIBG imaging to diagnose and investigate prognosis in patient with ischemic heart failure [23, 24]. Heart failure shows sympathetic hyperactivity, which aggravates. This applies to non-ischemic heart failure [25]. Fatal arrhythmia has a close relation with cardiac sympathetic nerve, the decrease of the delayed HMR or WR acceleration worse the risk of sudden death by fatal arrhythmia. ^{123}I-MIBG imaging will be helpful for decision-making for implantable cardioverter-defibrillator (ICD). ^{123}I-MIBG SPECT imaging is expected to find an arrhythmic event risk and aggravation of the size of the denervated area. HMR and WR are associated with increased fatal arrhythmia and cardiac mortality. It has been reported that HMR less than 1.6 is associated with poor outcome [22]. Meta-analyses showed that in patients with CHF, late HMR is not only useful predictor of events, but also has prognostic implication over the full range of the outcome value for all event categories except arrhythmias [26].

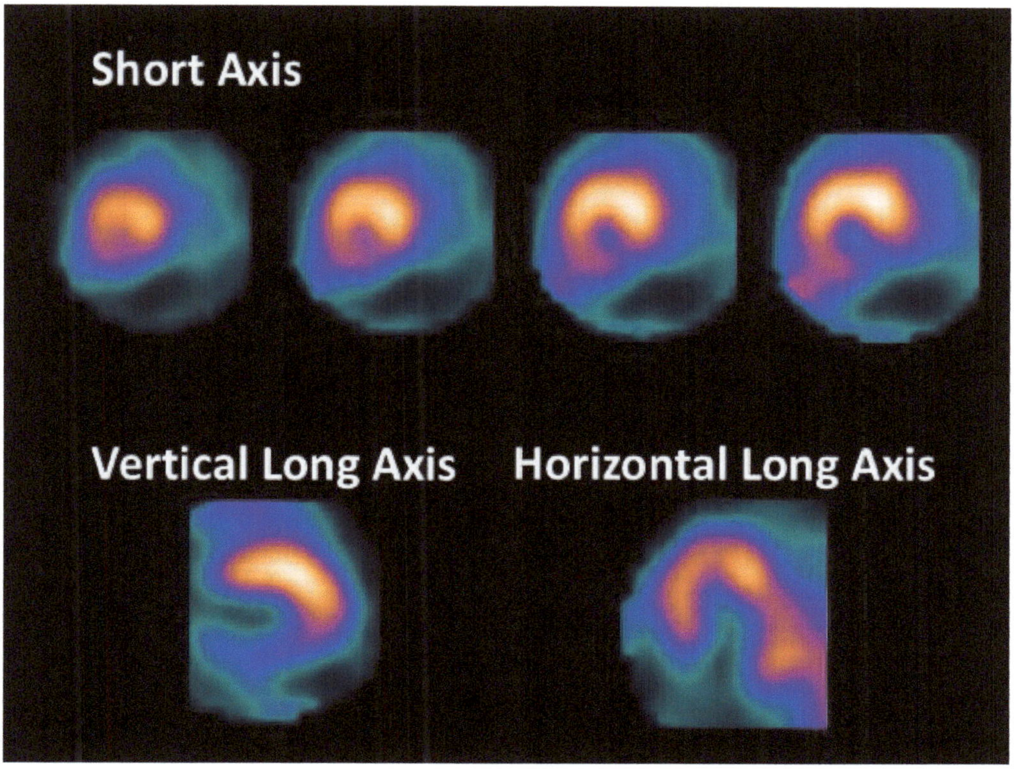

Fig. (1). The patient with ischemic heart disease shows a decreased uptake of MIBG in the inferolateral region of the left ventricle, indicating ischemic denervation.

TRANSPLANTED HEART

Transplanted heart is denervated after operation because cardiac sympathetic nerve is transected during heart transplantation. Sympathetic cardiac reinnervation is needed for 2 to 12 years after post-transplantation. To assess the incidence of early vasculopathy, ^{123}I-MIBG imaging is useful for sympathetic nerve denervation and reinnervation after heart transplantation. Heart-transplanted patients often have possibility of acute ischemic events or left ventricular dysfunction and are considered to be high risk [27, 28]. Coronary artery disease develops in approximately 50% of heart transplanted patients within 5 years after heart transplantation. Therefore, surveillance angiography is performed every year to detect coronary involvement early [27, 29]. In addition, denervation of the sinus node causes inadequate acceleration of heart rate and increase of cardiac output during stress [30]. Furthermore, loss of vasomotor tone may adversely affect the physiologic alternations in coronary blood flow, produce altered hemodynamic performance at rest and during exercise and decrease exercise capacity [31, 32].

DIABETES MELLITUS

The sympathetic nervous system is stimulated in the early stages of diabetes [6, 33], and the adrenergic receptors are exposed for a long time in accordance with catecholamine levels, hyperglycemia and insulin deficiency. As a result, diabetic cardiac autonomic neuropathy appears [6]. In a diabetes mellitus patient, cardiac MIBG accumulation decreases and WR increases following the progression of sympathetic nerve dysfunction. MIBG SPECT shows heterogeneous cardiac accumulation. The accumulation at inferior wall often decrease. Delayed HMR decrease and WR acceleration reflect poor prognosis factor of severe cardiac disease [34]. Although increased washout has been observed in diabetic patients [12, 35], the clinical importance in diabetes is not clear [36]. A diabetic cardiac autonomic neuropathy causes silent myocardial ischemia, infarction, and sudden cardiac death [15]. However, the reasons are not completely understood [37]. A sympathetic dysfunction causes the impaired regulation of coronary blood flow in response to stress. This vascular dysfunction is assumed to play a role in progressive left ventricular dysfunction in diabetic patients without apparent coronary artery stenosis assessed by angiographic examination [38]. Cardiac autonomic neuropathy has also been related to an abnormal left ventricular response to exercise in the absence of ischemic heart disease. Such the response may contribute to left ventricular dysfunction before the expression of irreversible damage [33, 39]. ^{123}I-MIBG abnormal uptake is detected in diabetic patients with silent myocardial ischemia. This suggests a relation between perception of chest pain and diabetic cardiac autonomic neuropathy [15, 37, 40]. Proximal hyperinnervation together with distal denervation may be associated with arrhythmias and sudden cardiac death in diabetic patients [15]. Long-term poor glycemic control is a major factor in the progression of diabetic cardiac autonomic neuropathy [40]. Satisfactory glycemic control in patients with early cardiac denervation may prevent the aggravation of cardiac sympathetic denervation [35]. ^{123}I-MIBG imaging can visualize cardiac defects in diabetic patients [37].

CONCLUSION

^{123}I-MIBG scintigraphy and SPECT are less-invasive examination, and widely available nuclear imaging method for assessing myocardial sympathetic innervation.

CONSENT FOR PUBLICATION

Not applicable.

CONFLICT OF INTEREST

The author (editor) declares no conflict of interest, financial or otherwise.

ACKNOWLEDGEMENTS

Declared none.

REFERENCES

[1] Matsuo S, Nakajima K. Assessment of cardiac sympathetic nerve function using ^{123}i-met--iodobenzylguanidine scintigraphy: technical aspects and standardization. Ann Nucl Cardiol 2015; 1: 27-34.
[http://dx.doi.org/10.17996/ANC.01.01.27]

[2] Dae MW, De Marco T, Botvinick EH, O'Connell JW, Hattner RS, Huberly RS. Scintigraphic assessment of MIBG uptake in globally denervated human and canine hearts: implications for clinical studies. J Nucl Med 1992; 33: 1444-50.

[3] Nakajima K, Okuda K, Matsuo S, Yoshita M, Taki J, Yamada M. Standardization of metaiodobenzylguanidine heart to mediastinum ratio using a calibration phantom:effects of correction on normal databases and a multicenter study. Eur J Nucl Med Mol Imaging 2012; 39: 113-9.
[http://dx.doi.org/10.1007/s00259-011-1963-1]

[4] Nakajima K, Nakata T. Cardiac ^{123}I-MIBG Imaging for Clinical Decision Making: 22-Year Experience in Japan. J Nucl Med 2015; 56: 11S-9S.
[http://dx.doi.org/10.2967/jnumed.114.142794]

[5] Van Vickle SS, Thompson RC. ^{123}I-MIBG Imaging: Patient Preparation and Technologist's Role. J Nucl Med Technol 2015; 43: 82-6.
[http://dx.doi.org/10.2967/jnmt.115.158394]

[6] Carrió I. Cardiac neurotransmission imaging. J Nucl Med 2001; 42: 1062-76.

[7] Glowniak JV. Cardiac studies with metaiodobenzylguanidine: a critique of methods and interpretation of results. J Nucl Med 1995; 36: 2133-7.

[8] Patel AD, Iskandrian AE. MIBG imaging. J Nucl Cardiol 2002; 9: 75-94.
[http://dx.doi.org/10.1067/mnc.2002.121471]

[9] Somsen GA, van Viles B, de Milliano PA, Borm JJ, van Royen EA, Endert E. Increased myocardial ^{123}I-metaiodobenzylguanidine uptake after enalapril treatment in patients with chronic heart failure. Heart 1996; 76: 218-22.
[http://dx.doi.org/10.1136/hrt.76.3.218]

[10] Lotze U, Kaepplinger S, Kober A, Richartz BM, Gottschild D, Figulla HR. Recovery of the cardiac adrenergic nervous system after long-term beta-blocker therapy in idiopathic dilated cardiomyopathy:assessment by increase in myocardial ^{123}I-metaiodobenzylguanidine. J Nucl Med 2001; 42: 49-54.

[11] de Milliano PA, de Groot AC, Tijssen JG, van Eck-Smit BL, Van Zwieten PA, Lie KI. Beneficial effects of metoprolol on myocardial sympathetic function:evidence from a randomized, placebo-controlled study in patients with congestive heart failure. Am Heart J 2002; 144: A14-22.
[http://dx.doi.org/10.1067/mhj.2002.121807]

[12] Hattori N, Tamaki N, Hayashi T, Masuda I, Kudoh T, Tateno M. Regional abnormality of iodine-12--MIBG in diabetic hearts. J Nucl Med 1996; 37: 1985-90.

[13] Flotats A, Carrio I, Agostini D, Marcassa C, Schafers M, Somsen GA. Proposal for standardization of ^{123}I-metaiodobenzylguanidine (MIBG) cardiac sympathetic imaging by the EANM Cardiovascular

Committee and the European Council of Nuclear Cardiology. Eur J Nucl Med Mol Imaging 2010; 37: 1802-12. [published correction appears in Eur J Nucl Med Mol Imaging. 2011; 38: 190.]. [http://dx.doi.org/10.1007/s00259-010-1491-4]

[14] Langer A, Freeman MR, Josse RG, Armstrong PW. Metaiodobenzylguanidine imaging in diabetes mellitus: assessment of cardiac sympathetic denervation and its relation to autonomic dysfunction and silent myocardial ischemia. J Am Coll Cardiol 1995; 25: 610-8. [http://dx.doi.org/10.1016/0735-1097(94)00459-4]

[15] Matsuo S, Takahashi M, Nakamura Y, Kinoshita M. Evaluation of cardiac sympathetic innervation with iodine-123-metaiodobenzylguanidine imaging in silent myocardial ischemia. J Nucl Med 1996; 37: 712-7.

[16] Giordano A, Calcagni ML, Verrillo A, *et al.* Assessment of sympathetic innervation of the heart in diabetes mellitus using 123I-MIBG. Diabetes Nutr Metab 2000; 13: 350-5.

[17] Estorch M, Carrió I, Berná L, López-Pousa J, Torres G. Myocardial iodine-labeled metaiodobenzylguanidine 123 uptake relates to age. J Nucl Cardiol 1995; 2: 126-32.

[18] Sisson JC, Shapiro B, Meyers L, *et al.* Metaiodobenzylguanidine to map scintigraphically the adrenergic nervous system in man. J Nucl Med 1987; 28: 1625-36.

[19] Matsunari I, Schricke U, Bengel FM, *et al.* Extent of cardiac sympathetic neuronal damage is determined by the area of ischemia in patients with acute coronary syndromes. Circulation 2000; 101: 2579-85. [http://dx.doi.org/10.1161/01.CIR.101.22.2579]

[20] Makoto A, Hiroshi Y, Keiichi S, *et al.* Relationship between cardiac sympathetic function and baroreceptor sensitivity after acute myocardial infarction. Circ J 2002; 66: 247-52. [http://dx.doi.org/10.1253/circj.66.247]

[21] Henderson EB, Kahn JK, Corbett JR, *et al.* Abnormal I-123 metaiodobenzylguanidine myocardial washout and distribution may reflect myocardial adrenergic derangement in patients with congestive cardiomyopathy. Circulation 1988; 78: 1192-9. [http://dx.doi.org/10.1161/01.CIR.78.5.1192]

[22] Jacobson AF, Senior R, Cerqueira MD, *et al.* Myocardial iodine-123 meta-iodobenzylguanidine imaging and cardiac events in heart failure. Results of the prospective ADMIRE-HF (AdreView Myocardial Imaging for Risk Evaluation in Heart Failure) study. J Am Coll Cardiol 2010; 55: 2212-21. [http://dx.doi.org/10.1016/j.jacc.2010.01.014]

[23] Verberne HJ, Brewster LM, Somsen GA, van Eck-Smit BL. Prognostic value of myocardial 123I-metaiodobenzylguanidine (MIBG) parameters in patients with heart failure:a systematic review. Eur Heart J 2008; 29: 1147-59. [http://dx.doi.org/10.1093/eurheartj/ehn113]

[24] Kuwabara Y, Tamaki N, Nakata T, Yamashina S, Yamazaki J. Determination of the survival rate in patients with congestive heart failure stratified by 123I-MIBG imaging:a meta-analysis from the studies performed in Japan. Ann Nucl Med 2011; 25: 101-7. [http://dx.doi.org/10.1007/s12149-010-0452-0]

[25] Matsuo S, Nakajima K, Nakata T. Prognostic value of cardiac sympathetic nerve imaging using long-term follow-up data - ischemic vs. non-ischemic heart failure etiology. Circ J 2016; 80: 435-41. [http://dx.doi.org/10.1253/circj.CJ-15-0952]

[26] Verschure DO, Veltman CE, Manrique A, *et al.* For what endpoint does myocardial 123I-MIBG scintigraphy have the greatest prognostic value in patients with chronic heart failure? Results of a pooled individual patient data meta-analysis. Eur Heart J Cardiovasc Imaging 2014; 15: 996-1003. [http://dx.doi.org/10.1093/ehjci/jeu044]

[27] O'Neill BJ, Pflugfelder PW, Singh NR, *et al.* Frequency of angiographic detection and quantitative

assessment of coronary arterial disease one and three years after cardiac transplantation. Am J Cardiol 1989; 63: 1221-6.
[http://dx.doi.org/10.1016/0002-9149(89)90182-3]

[28] Schroeder JS, Hunt AS. Chest pain in heart-transplant recipients. N Engl J Med 1991; 324: 1805-7.
[http://dx.doi.org/10.1056/NEJM199106203242509]

[29] Kavanagh T, Yacoub MH, Mertens DJ, *et al.* Cardiorespiratory responses to exercise training after orthotopic cardiac transplantation. Circulation 1988; 77: 162-71.
[http://dx.doi.org/10.1161/01.CIR.77.1.162]

[30] Hosenpud JD, Morton MJ, Wilson RA, *et al.* Abnormal exercise hemodynamics in cardiac allograft recipients 1 year after cardiac transplantation. Circulation 1989; 80: 525-32.
[http://dx.doi.org/10.1161/01.CIR.80.3.525]

[31] Pflugfelder PW, Purves PD, McKenzie FN, Kostuk WJ. Cardiac dynamics during supine exercise in cyclosporine-treated orthotopic heart transplant recipients: assessment by radionuclide angiography. J Am Coll Cardiol 1987; 10: 336-41.
[http://dx.doi.org/10.1016/S0735-1097(87)80016-5]

[32] Estorch M, Campreciós M, Flotats A, *et al.* Sympathetic Reinnervation of Cardiac Allografts Evaluated by 123I-MIBG Imaging. J Nucl Med 1999; 40: 911-6.

[33] Scognamiglio R, Avogaro A, Casara D, *et al.* Myocardial dysfunction and adrenergic cardiac innervation in patients with insulin-dependent diabetes mellitus. J Am Coll Cardiol 1998; 31: 404-12.
[http://dx.doi.org/10.1016/S0735-1097(97)00516-0]

[34] Scott LA, Kench PL. Cardiac autonomic neuropathy in the diabetic patient:does ^{123}I-MIBG imaging have a role to play in early diagnosis? J Nucl Med Technol 2004; 32: 66-71.

[35] Nagamachi S, Jinnouchi S, Nakahara H, *et al.* 123I-MIBG myocardial scintigraphy in diabetic patients: relationship to autonomic neuropathy. Nucl Med Commun 1996; 17: 621-32.
[http://dx.doi.org/10.1097/00006231-199607000-00014]

[36] Zhao C, Shuke N, Yamamoto W, *et al.* Comparison of cardiac sympathetic nervous function with left ventricular function and perfusion in cardiomyopathies by ^{123}I-MIBG SPECT and ^{99m}Tc-tetrofosmin electrocardiographically gated SPECT. J Nucl Med 2001; 42: 1017-24.

[37] Solanki KK, Bomanji J, Moyes J, Mather SJ, Trainer PJ, Britton KE. A pharmacological guide to medicines which interfere with the biodistribution of radiolabelled meta-iodobenzylguanidine (MIBG). Nucl Med Commun 1992; 13: 513-21.
[http://dx.doi.org/10.1097/00006231-199207000-00006]

[38] Di Carli MF, Bianco-Batlles D, Landa ME, *et al.* Effects of autonomic neuropathy on coronary blood flow in patients with diabetes mellitus. Circulation 1999; 100: 813-9.
[http://dx.doi.org/10.1161/01.CIR.100.8.813]

[39] Zola B, Kahn JK, Juni JE, Vinik AI. Abnormal cardiac function in diabetic patients with autonomic neuropathy in the absence of ischemic disease. J Clin Endocrinol Metab 1986; 63: 208-14.
[http://dx.doi.org/10.1210/jcem-63-1-208]

[40] Stevens MJ, Raffel DM, Allman KC, *et al.* Cardiac sympathetic dysinnervation in diabetes: implications for enhanced cardiovascular risk. Circulation 1998; 98: 961-8.
[http://dx.doi.org/10.1161/01.CIR.98.10.961]

CHAPTER 12

Standardization of ^{123}I-*meta*-iodobenzylguanidine Heart-To-Mediastinum Ratio: Technical Aspects

Koichi Okuda[1,*], **Kenichi Nakajima**[2], **Chiemi Kitamura**[3] and **Yumiko Kirihara**[3]

[1] *Department of Physics, Kanazawa Medical University, 1-1 Daigaku, Uchinada, Kahoku, Ishikawa 920-0293, Japan*

[2] *Department of Nuclear Medicine, Kanazawa University Hospital, 13-1 Takara-machi, Kanazawa, Ishikawa 920-8641, Japan*

[3] *FUJIFILM RI Pharma Co., Ltd., 14-1, kyobashi 2-Chome, Chuo-Ku, Tokyo 104-0031, Japan*

Abstract: The heart-to-mediastinum ratio (HMR) in planar images has been used for the evaluation of cardiac ^{123}I-*meta*-iodobenzylguanidine (MIBG) uptake. However, the HMR values are influenced by both collimators and the cardiac and mediastinal regions of interests (ROI). Two technical developments in semi-automated ROI setting software and a calibration method for HMR values were described in this article.

Keywords: ^{123}I-MIBG, Heart-to-mediastinum ratio, Multicenter study, Planar imaging, Quantification, Region of interest, smartMIBG, smartMIBG-HF, Standardization, Washout rate.

INTRODUCTION

^{123}I-*meta*-iodobenzylguanidine (MIBG) has been used for over 25 years in Japan. Both ^{123}I-MIBG planar and single-photon emission computed tomography (SPECT) imaging are performed clinically, and these images are subsequently visually and quantitatively evaluated. The heart-to-mediastinum ratio (HMR) and washout rate (WR) are contemporary parameters for the evaluation of cardiac ^{123}I-MIBG uptake [1]. However, the HMR is affected by both the characteristics of the collimator and the delineation of the region of interest (ROI). Consequently, we have proposed technical solutions to standardize the quantification of HMR. In this chapter, we describe two technical developments: a software program for semi-automated ROI setting in ^{123}I-MIBG planar imaging [2] and a calibration

* **Corresponding author Koichi Okuda:** Department of Physics, Kanazawa Medical University, 1-1 Daigaku, Uchinada, Kahoku, Ishikawa 920-0293, Japan; Tel: 076-286-2211; Fax: 076-286-2620; E-mail: okuda@kanazawa-med.ac.jp

Shinro Matsuo (Ed.)

method for HMR values, which incorporates the characteristic differences of collimators [3 - 6]. These investigations are collaborative studies with Kanazawa University (Kanazawa, Japan), Kanazawa Medical University (Kahoku, Japan), and FUJIFILM RI Pharma Co., Ltd (Tokyo, Japan).

A Software Program for Semi-Automated ROI Setting

In 2011, we developed a software program for semi-automated ROI setting in ^{123}I-MIBG planar imaging (Fig. **1**). This program is called *smartMIBG* [2]. The *smartMIBG* can automatically delineate a mediastinal ROI when operators manually select a cardiac ROI on a planar image. For comparison with *smartMIBG*, operators manually select both cardiac and mediastinal ROIs in a conventional manner. Manual ROI setting for the cardiac and mediastinal regions induces a large variation of HMR values [7]. Thus, we focused on ROI definition using a software program to minimize such variations. The developed software has a higher reproducibility of ROI settings than manual operation and yields HMR values with high test-retest reliability. Consequently, we integrated *smartMIBG* with a risk estimation model for patients with chronic heart failure, called *smartMIBG-HF*. This program can successfully estimate cardiac mortality rates using the risk model [8, 9].

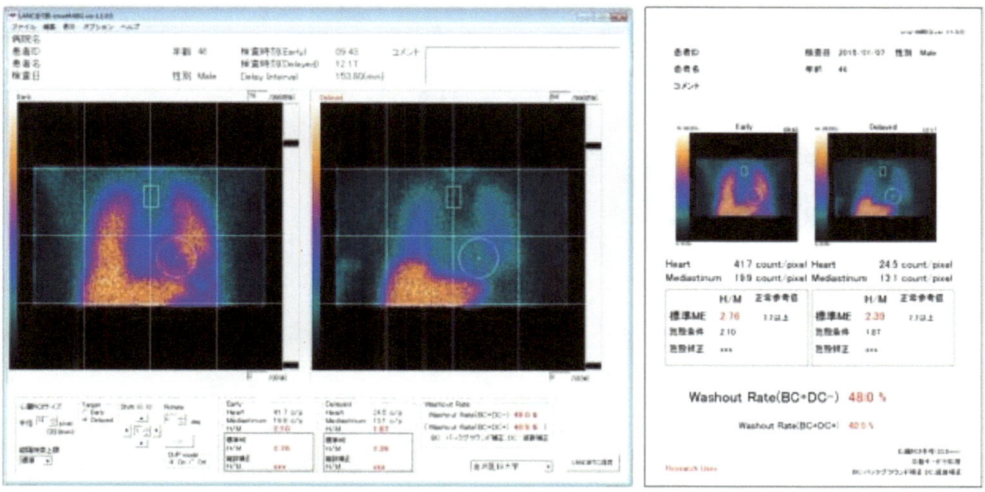

Fig. (1). A software program for semi-automated ROI setting in ^{123}I-MIBG planar imaging. (Left) Simultaneous calculation of early and delayed HMR values as well as WR. (Right) A report on the MIBG scan, HMR, and WR. *HMR*, heart to mediastinum ratio; and *WR*, washout rate.

HMR Calibration Methods for Characteristics of Gamma Cameras

The radioisotope, ^{123}I, has a couple of energy peaks, 159 keV (83%) and 529 keV (1.4%). Since photons with energy 529 keV are able to pass through the septa of a collimator, the image quality of ^{123}I-MIBG planar and SPECT scans is consequently degraded. These high-energy photons also influence the HMR values. Therefore, the use of medium-energy collimators is recommended in ^{123}I-MIBG imaging [10]. However, there are many kinds of collimators with different characteristics that can be used in nuclear medicine. Firstly, we sought to perform image acquisition using the ^{123}I-triple energy window (TEW) [5]. However, we could not standardize the acquisition condition using the TEW method. Therefore, we proposed a standardization method using a dedicated ^{123}I–MIBG phantom for the calibration of HMR values derived from various collimators. The phantom structure is flat and dedicated for planar imaging. It facilitates the calculation of calibration factors for combinations of gamma cameras and collimators. We performed a multicenter study to standardize HMR values in Japan and Europe based on the ^{123}I–MIBG phantoms. In the Japanese multicenter phantom study, we determined the relationship between the calibration factors and the collimators [6]. The average calibration factor ranged from 0.55 for a low-energy high-resolution (LEHR) collimator to 0.95 for a medium-energy low-penetration (MELP) collimator (Fig. **2**). Using this calibration method, cross-sectional multicenter studies were performed in Japan to distinguish between dementia patients with Lewy bodies from those with Alzheimer's disease [11, 12].

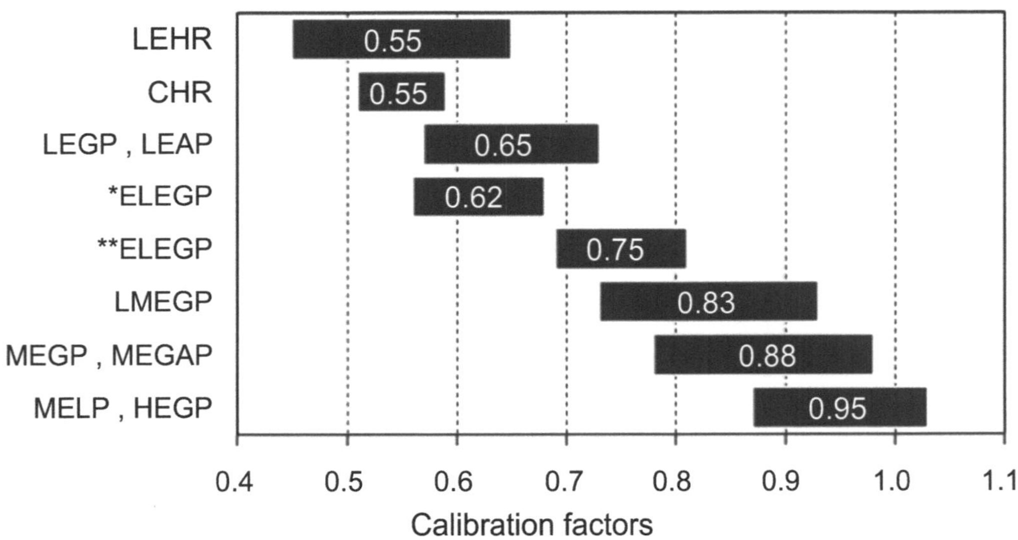

Fig. (2). Relationship between calibration factors and collimators in multicenter phantom studies. The values show the average of the calibration factors, and the bars represent the range of the mean ± 2*standard deviation. An *ELEGP collimator is used in a Millennium VG gamma camera system manufactured by GE. An **ELEGP collimator is also used in Infinia, Discovery, and Optima gamma camera systems by GE. *LEHR*, low-energy high-resolution; *CHR*, cardiac high-resolution; *LEGP*, low-energy general-purpose; *LEAP*, LE all-purpose; *ELEGP*, extended low-energy GP; *LMEGP*, low-medium-energy GP; *ME*, medium-energy; *MEGAP*, ME general-all-purpose; *MELP*, ME low-penetration; and *HEGP*, high-energy GP.

SUMMARY

We have proposed several technical solutions to standardize the quantification of HMR values. Our developed software programs and phantom are useful tools for minimizing the differences in HMR values acquired from different observers and hospitals.

CONSENT FOR PUBLICATION

Not applicable.

CONFLICT OF INTEREST

K.O. and K.N. have collaborative research work with FUJIFILM RI Pharma, Co. Ltd., Tokyo, Japan, supplier of I-123 MIBG in Japan. C.K and Y.K. are employed by FUJIFILM RI Pharma, Co. Ltd., Japan.

ACKNOWLEDGEMENTS

Declared none.

REFERENCES

[1] Merlet P, Valette H, Dubois-Randé JL, *et al.* Prognostic value of cardiac metaiodobenzylguanidine imaging in patients with heart failure. J Nucl Med 1992; 33(4): 471-7. [PMID: 1552326]

[2] Okuda K, Nakajima K, Hosoya T, *et al.* Semi-automated algorithm for calculating heart-t--mediastinum ratio in cardiac Iodine-123 MIBG imaging. J Nucl Cardiol 2011; 18(1): 82-9. [http://dx.doi.org/10.1007/s12350-010-9313-4] [PMID: 21104360]

[3] Nakajima K, Verschure DO, Okuda K, Verberne HJ. Standardization of ^{123}I-*meta*-iodobenzylguanidine myocardial sympathetic activity imaging: phantom calibration and clinical applications. Clin Transl Imaging 2017; 5(3): 255-63. [http://dx.doi.org/10.1007/s40336-017-0230-2] [PMID: 28596948]

[4] Nakajima K, Okuda K, Matsuo S, *et al.* Standardization of metaiodobenzylguanidine heart to mediastinum ratio using a calibration phantom: effects of correction on normal databases and a multicentre study. Eur J Nucl Med Mol Imaging 2012; 39(1): 113-9. [http://dx.doi.org/10.1007/s00259-011-1963-1] [PMID: 22009380]

[5] Nakajima K, Matsubara K, Ishikawa T, *et al.* Correction of iodine-123-labeled meta-iodobenzylguanidine uptake with multi-window methods for standardization of the heart-t--mediastinum ratio. J Nucl Cardiol 2007; 14(6): 843-51. [http://dx.doi.org/10.1016/j.nuclcard.2007.08.002] [PMID: 18022111]

[6] Nakajima K, Okuda K, Yoshimura M, *et al.* Multicenter cross-calibration of I-123 metaiodobenzylguanidine heart-to-mediastinum ratios to overcome camera-collimator variations. J Nucl Cardiol 2014; 21(5): 970-8. [http://dx.doi.org/10.1007/s12350-014-9916-2] [PMID: 24942608]

[7] Somsen GA, Verberne HJ, Fleury E, Righetti A. Normal values and within-subject variability of cardiac I-123 MIBG scintigraphy in healthy individuals: implications for clinical studies. J Nucl Cardiol 2004; 11(2): 126-33.

[http://dx.doi.org/10.1016/j.nuclcard.2003.10.010] [PMID: 15052243]

[8] Nakajima K, Nakata T, Yamada T, *et al.* A prediction model for 5-year cardiac mortality in patients with chronic heart failure using ^{123}I-metaiodobenzylguanidine imaging. Eur J Nucl Med Mol Imaging 2014; 41(9): 1673-82.
[http://dx.doi.org/10.1007/s00259-014-2759-x] [PMID: 24663289]

[9] Nakajima K, Nakata T, Doi T, *et al.* Validation of 2-year 123I-meta-iodobenzylguanidine-based cardiac mortality risk model in chronic heart failure. Eur Heart J Cardiovasc Imaging 2018; 19(7): 749-56.
[http://dx.doi.org/10.1093/ehjci/jey016] [PMID: 29415138]

[10] Henzlova MJ, Duvall WL, Einstein AJ, Travin MI, Verberne HJ. ASNC imaging guidelines for SPECT nuclear cardiology procedures: Stress, protocols, and tracers. J Nucl Cardiol 2016; 23(3): 606-39.
[http://dx.doi.org/10.1007/s12350-015-0387-x] [PMID: 26914678]

[11] Komatsu J, Samuraki M, Nakajima K, *et al.* (123)I-MIBG myocardial scintigraphy for the diagnosis of DLB: a multicentre 3-year follow-up study. J Neurol Neurosurg Psychiatry 2018.
[http://dx.doi.org/10.1136/jnnp-2017-317398]

[12] Yoshita M, Arai H, Arai H, *et al.* Diagnostic accuracy of 123I-meta-iodobenzylguanidine myocardial scintigraphy in dementia with Lewy bodies: a multicenter study. PLoS One 2015; 10(3): e0120540.
[http://dx.doi.org/10.1371/journal.pone.0120540] [PMID: 25793585]

CHAPTER 13

Image Diagnosis of Arteriosclerosis and Possibility of Early Intervention

Shinro Matsuo*

Department of Nuclear Medicine, Kanazawa University Hospital, Kanazawa, Ishikawa, Japan

Graduate School of Advanced Preventive Medical Sciences, Kanazawa, Japan

Abstract: Arteriosclerosis is a chronic disease and is related to infectious contributing factors. A hybrid SPECT/CT system may provide subclinical information of atherosclerosis noninvasively. The combined diagnosis of coronary artery calcification and myocardial perfusion imaging can be effectively used for the patients' monitoring and aggressive risk factor modification as well as optimal medical therapy. FDG PET/CT was employed to evaluate the inflammation of the vessels. This article aims at providing an updated overview about diagnosis of atherosclerosis by nuclear cardiology technique.

Keywords: Atherosclerosis, FDG, PET, SPECT/CT.

INTRODUCTION

Atherosclerosis is the number 1 cause of morbidity and mortality all over the world. Arteriosclerosis is a chronic disease affecting the entire arterial vessels, representing an inflammatory response in the vessels. The pathogenesis of atherosclerosis involves complex process leading to the formation of atherosclerotic plaque. The atherosclerosis gradually results in the restriction of the blood flow to one's organs and tissues, leading to severe health risks. The atherosclerosis is a specific form of arteriosclerosis caused by the buildup of fatty plaques, cholesterol, and some other substances on the artery walls.

The artery shows a three-layer structure consisting of the intima, the tunica media and the adventitia. The intima consists mainly of endothelial cells. Arteriosclerosis is the state or condition in which cholesterol (as oxidized LDL) are deposited inside the inner membrane, the wall of the artery becomes thicker,

* **Corresponding author Shinro Matsuo:** Department of Nuclear Medicine, Kanazawa University Hospital, 13-1 Takara-machi, Kanazawa 920-8641, Japan; Advanced Preventive Medical Sciences, Kanazawa University Graduate School, 13-1 Takara-machi, Kanazawa, Japan 920-8641; Tel: 81-76-265-2333; Fax: 81-76-234-4257; E-mail: smatsuo@med.kanazawa-u.ac.jp

and the blood vessel itself becomes harder. In atherosclerosis, the serum lipids etrate and deposit on the inner membrane, and the inner membrane is thickened. As a result, the vascular lumen becomes narrower than normal arteries.

Atherosclerosis is closely related to risk factors such as hypertension, hypercholesterolemia, diabetes and smoking. The vascular endothelial function is deteriorate affected by a cascade of pro-inflammatory responses.

A Hybrid SPECT/CT System

Calcification under 50 μm in size is generally considered microcalcification, which are a marker of cell death and inflammation and carry an increased risk of plaque rupture and indicates past-inflammation [1]. A computed tomography (CT) can be used to measure calcium scores to quantify the calcification of the coronary arteries [2 - 7]. A hybrid SPECT/CT system has been introduced recently to cardiology field of clinical medicine [7, 8]. The coronary artery calcification (CAC) is a marker of atherosclerosis, as shown in Table **1**. A CAC score has been shown to be related to the risk of future cardiovascular events since it can be used to estimate the total magnitude of atherosclerotic burden [9 - 11]. A hybrid SPECT/CT system may provide subclinical information of atherosclerosis non-invasively without any extra-cost. Recently emerging guidelines have recommended the use of CAC score for the risk-stratification of the patients with suspected coronary artery disease. Detection of coronary calcification using SPECT / CT is a quick non-invasive check and relatively easy to perform. Its only drawback is exposure to radiation.

Table 1. The calcium scale is a linear scale with 4 calcium score categories: The calcium score correlates directly with risk of events and likelihood of obstructive CAD.

0	no calcium
1-10	minimal
10–100	mild
100–400	moderate
400-1000	extensive
>1000	severely extensive

The electron-beam CT (EBCT) measurement of coronary artery calcification score established by the Agatston methods, quantitative evaluation of calcified plaque in coronary artery calcification area and the CT value (Hounsfield Unit; HU) are calculated. This value can be classified into stages according to the degree of calcification. As additional advantage, a recent advanced SPECT/CT system makes it possible to obtain myocardial perfusion imaging and coronary calcification information at the same time. Combined acquisition of SPECT and CT in a one-stop examination is more acceptable for the patients, since there is no extra-cost. Therefore, physicians can obtain perfusion and atherosclerotic information.

CAC in Patients with Normal Coronary Flow Reserve

Previous studies demonstrated that normal stress SPECT imaging is associated with low risk of cardiovascular risk. The patients with normal SPECT images are considered as having a risk of an annual event rate of 0.6-0.9% [12, 13]. Another previous clinical trial had shown a clear association between the extent of perfusion abnormalities and risk of coronary events. It was shown that the more perfusion defects are, the higher risk the patients have. However, the wide range of CAC scores in patients with normal MPI suggests that stress perfusion imaging is limited in its ability to delineate subclinical atherosclerosis. There is no evidence to compare the relative short and long-term risk for cardiac events among patients with both myocardial perfusion imaging and coronary calcium evaluation [14]. Another previous study showed that the cardiac event rate in elderly and diabetic patients with normal myocardial perfusion imaging was relatively higher than that in younger and non-diabetic patients. Subjects having normal myocardial perfusion study may differ in the stage of atherosclerosis and have a different atherosclerotic burden in the coronary artery. Then what about the patients with high CAC and normal myocardial perfusion imaging? Such patients with high CAC and normal SPECT might have low risk in the short-term but high risk in the long-term for cardiovascular events, since patients with high CAC have reportedly been regarded as high-risk patients [15]. According to the previous studies, patients with no ischemia on stress SPECT exhibit a stepwise increase in their risk of major cardiovascular events with increasing CAC scores. Therefore, this may indicate a warranty period, that is to say freedom of adverse events, might exist for normal stress myocardial perfusion imaging [16]. Even if the myocardial perfusion imaging is normal, the addition of the CAC score may improve the detection of coronary artery disease, particularly in severe multi-vessel coronary artery disease. The documentation of CAC as a hallmark or a clinical indicator of coronary atherosclerosis can be used to identify patients who require more intensive management of coronary risk factors.

Inflammation and Calcification

Inflammation is known to play an important role in the process of atherogenesis. Inflammatory markers such as high sensitive C-reactive protein (*hs*-CRP), tumor necrosis factor alpha (TNF-alpha), Interleukin-6 (IL-6) and so on, may aid in detecting subclinical atherosclerosis. However, the association between inflammatory markers and CAC is weak, since coronary disease attributes concomitantly to coronary risk factors. CRP is also non-specific and inflammation is an unrelated condition. The approach to use these biomarkers as part of a broader risk stratification is a subject of future investigation.

Evaluation of Atherosclerosis by SPECT/CT

CAC score data obtained by SPECT/CT can provide information on decision-making in the patient's management, showing the rate of absolute and relative progression of calcification. In the patients with high calcium scoring, the efficacy of statins may be reflected by the reduction of the progression of coronary atherosclerosis [17]. Coronary CT angiography may be used to diagnose the coronary artery disease. In patient with severe calcification, coronary CT angiography is useless because of the artifact of calcification. When SPECT/CT is applied to diagnose the suspected coronary artery disease in an early stage, such patients with high CAC do not have to undergo coronary CT angiography. Therefore, the evaluation of CAC by SPECT/CT is an interesting strategy for the diagnostic work-up of patients [18]. A recent clinical trial revealed that CAC testing in asymptomatic individuals can be cost-effective [19]. Since high CAC makes it difficult to evaluate coronary artery stenosis, SPECT/CT might be useful for the decision-making process with regard to performing CT angiography. Along with CAC evaluation presence or absence of ischemia could be evaluated by SPECT/CT.

The evaluation of CAC is reasonable approach for cardiovascular risk stratification in asymptomatic patients with intermediate cardiovascular event risk [20]. With the uncertainty in cardiovascular disease, we believe that the only way to determine the best strategy is to conduct SPECT/CT testing to identify coronary artery disease in selected patients for more or less intensive treatments.

Inflammation and FDG

The role of ^{18}F-FDG PET had been documented in monitoring the therapeutic outcome of various treatment for atherosclerotic disease [21, 22]. It is well known that human brain cells, myocardial cells and malignant tumors use glucose as an energy source, but inflammatory cells of the arteriosclerotic lesion also take up glucose well. FDG, which has a structure similar to glucose, is taken into cells in the same way as glucose, but it is suitable for imaging as it is not metabolized immediately.

FDG is an abbreviation for fluoro-deoxy-glucose. The metabolism stops early in the glycolysis, after a certain period of stay, it diffuses into the blood and is excreted from the kidney into the urine [21]. The recent PET exam can be performed simultaneously with a CT, which is called PET / CT. Although FDG is taken in the arteriosclerotic lesion, FDG can quantitatively evaluate the activity of inflammatory cells, especially macrophages, in plaque. Since it is known that the number of macrophages / smooth muscle cells is large in the lesion in which FDG accumulates, this suggests that the instability of plaque can be selectively depicted. In addition, it is known that FDG accumulates at a high level in hypoxic stimulated macrophages, and that FDG accumulates at the initial stage of foam cell formation. Furthermore, the possibility that FDG accumulates on M1 macrophage has been reported.

The quantitative evaluation of FDG accumulation using SUV (standardized uptake value) is possible. This SUV is also used to follow the course of diagnosis and treatment effect. FDG accumulation in arteriosclerotic lesions is used for the detection of inflammation in patients with hyperlipidemia, angina pectoris, diabetes mellitus and so on. When FDG-PET was administered to a patient with carotid arteriosclerosis, the FDG accumulation in the arterial wall was significantly high in symptomatic carotid artery stenosis patients, and it is suggested that it is related to the subsequent onset of cerebral infarction. Rudd *et al.* reported positive findings in the carotid plaque by ^{18}F -fluorodeoxyglucose (FDG) PET, positive findings in the carotid artery on the symptomatic side, and macrophage / smooth muscle cell infiltration histologically. Even in verification using an animal model of arteriosclerosis, infiltration of macrophages and FDG uptake is highly correlated, and the possibility that inflammation of arteriosclerosis can be evaluated by PET is considered. Besides this, accumulation in the artificial blood vessel and uptake into the aneurysm are shown to be associated with subsequent rupture of the aneurysm. FDG accumulation of coronary vessels will be taken as a clinical image. The accumulation of FDG has also been shown to correlate with the number of macrophages. These findings suggest that FDG can quantitatively evaluate macrophage activity, and it is possible to selectively visualize plaque instability. It is known that arteriosclerotic diseases are deeply involved in inflammatory diseases. The accumulated long-term inflammation is also associated with coronary calcification, and it is known that inflammation is involved in the breakdown of plaque [21, 23].

Intensive statin therapy has significantly improved the clinical outcomes of patients with ischemic heart disease [24, 25]. FDG PET/CT was employed to evaluate the inflammation of the vessels. Attempts have been made to prevent the onset of symptomatic disease by intervening therapeutically against such unstable plaque. Patients who had lesions in the carotid artery and had uptake of FDG received simvastatin and the uptake of FDG decreased. Arteriosclerosis progresses in patients with hyperlipidemia, but the accumulation of FDG is not changed by a diet alone, or it is partially strengthened, whereas FDG in the aorta after drug therapy with statin has almost disappeared [26, 27]. We believe that lesions with high activity of arteriosclerosis disappear, which will lead to the prevention of cerebral infarction afterwards.

In this way, physicians use statins to treat patients with hyperlipidemia, but this treatment will reduce not only the LDL cholesterol but also the systemic inflammatory markers. By imaging the arteriosclerotic lesion with FDG-PET, it is possible to anticipate the onset of the disease and receive appropriate treatment

Arteriosclerosis can be visualized by the latest imaging diagnostic techniques. There are various examination methods, it is becoming possible to diagnose arteriosclerosis appropriately and to grasp its condition. Diagnostic imaging of arteriosclerosis in this chapter would help you make a research as to early intervention. Among them, FDG-PET [28], a nuclear medicine diagnostic method, is a diagnostic method that can diagnose active inflammation. An effective preventive method is developed by accurately evaluating arteriosclerosis.

LIMITATION

Some degree of atherosclerosis is almost universally present in otherwise healthy adult persons. This does not mean all the subjects with atherosclerosis should be screened by FDG-PET. The subjects who should be screened need to be decided by further study. It might be dependent on the the cost/effect ratio.

CONSENT FOR PUBLICATION

Not applicable.

CONFLICT OF INTEREST

The author (editor) declares no conflict of interest, financial or otherwise.

ACKNOWLEDGEMENTS

Declared none.

REFERENCES

[1] Shaw LJ, Raggi P, Schisterman E, Berman DS, Callister TQ. Prognostic value of cardiac risk factors and coronary artery calcium screening for all-cause mortality. Radiology 2003; 228(3): 826-33. [http://dx.doi.org/10.1148/radiol.2283021006] [PMID: 12869688]

[2] Matsuo S, Nakae I, Matsumoto T, Horie M. Impact of endothelial dysfunction on left ventricular remodeling after successful primary coronary angioplasty for acute myocardial infarction- Analysis by quantitative ECG-gated SPECT. Ann Nucl Med 2006; 20(1): 57-62. [http://dx.doi.org/10.1007/BF02985592] [PMID: 16485576]

[3] Matsuo S, Nakajima K, Kinuya S. Clinical use of nuclear cardiology in the assessment of heart failure.

World J Cardiol 2010; 2(10): 344-56.
[http://dx.doi.org/10.4330/wjc.v2.i10.344] [PMID: 21160612]

[4] Matsuo S, Matsumoto T, Nakae I, *et al.* Prognostic value of ECG-gated thallium-201 single-photon emission tomography in patients with coronary artery disease. Ann Nucl Med 2004; 18(7): 617-22.
[http://dx.doi.org/10.1007/BF02984584] [PMID: 15586636]

[5] Rozanski A, Gransar H, Shaw LJ, *et al.* Impact of coronary artery calcium scanning on coronary risk factors and downstream testing the EISNER (Early Identification of Subclinical Atherosclerosis by Noninvasive Imaging Research) prospective randomized trial. J Am Coll Cardiol 2011; 57(15): 1622-32.
[http://dx.doi.org/10.1016/j.jacc.2011.01.019] [PMID: 21439754]

[6] Polonsky TS, McClelland RL, Jorgensen NW, *et al.* Coronary artery calcium score and risk classification for coronary heart disease prediction. JAMA 2010; 303(16): 1610-6.
[http://dx.doi.org/10.1001/jama.2010.461] [PMID: 20424251]

[7] Matsuo S, Nakajima K, Akhter N, *et al.* Clinical usefulness of novel cardiac MDCT/SPECT fusion image. Ann Nucl Med 2009; 23(6): 579-86.
[http://dx.doi.org/10.1007/s12149-009-0279-8] [PMID: 19572098]

[8] Matsuo S, Nakajima K, Okuda K, Kinuya S. The relationship between stress-induced myocardial ischemia and coronary artery atherosclerosis measured by hybrid SPECT/CT camera. Ann Nucl Med 2011; 25(9): 650-6.
[http://dx.doi.org/10.1007/s12149-011-0517-8] [PMID: 21779962]

[9] Berman DS, Rozanski A, Rana JS, Shaw LJ, Wong ND, Min JK. Screening for coronary artery disease in diabetic patients: a commentary. J Nucl Cardiol 2009; 16(6): 851-4.
[http://dx.doi.org/10.1007/s12350-009-9129-2] [PMID: 19690936]

[10] Berman DS, Wong ND, Gransar H, *et al.* Relationship between stress-induced myocardial ischemia and atherosclerosis measured by coronary calcium tomography. J Am Coll Cardiol 2004; 44(4): 923-30.
[http://dx.doi.org/10.1016/j.jacc.2004.06.042] [PMID: 15312881]

[11] Rozanski A, Gransar H, Wong ND, *et al.* Clinical outcomes after both coronary calcium scanning and exercise myocardial perfusion scintigraphy. J Am Coll Cardiol 2007; 49(12): 1352-61.
[http://dx.doi.org/10.1016/j.jacc.2006.12.035] [PMID: 17394969]

[12] Matsuo S, Nakajima K, Horie M, Nakae I, Nishimura T. Prognostic value of normal stress myocardial perfusion imaging in Japanese population. Circ J 2008; 72(4): 611-7.
[http://dx.doi.org/10.1253/circj.72.611] [PMID: 18362434]

[13] Matsuo S, Nakajima K, Yamasaki Y, Kashiwagi A, Nishimura T. Prognostic value of normal stress myocardial perfusion imaging and ventricular function in Japanese asymptomatic patients with type 2 diabetes--a study based on the J-ACCESS-2 database. Circ J 2010; 74(9): 1916-21.
[http://dx.doi.org/10.1253/circj.CJ-10-0098] [PMID: 20631452]

[14] Matsuo S, Matsumoto T, Takashima H, *et al.* The relationship between flow-mediated brachial artery vasodilation and coronary vasomotor responses to bradykinin: comparison with those to acetylcholine. J Cardiovasc Pharmacol 2004; 44(2): 164-70.
[http://dx.doi.org/10.1097/00005344-200408000-00004] [PMID: 15243296]

[15] Hachamovitch R, Hayes SW, Friedman JD, Cohen I, Berman DS. Comparison of the short-term survival benefit associated with revascularization compared with medical therapy in patients with no prior coronary artery disease undergoing stress myocardial perfusion single photon emission computed tomography. Circulation 2003; 107(23): 2900-7.
[http://dx.doi.org/10.1161/01.CIR.0000072790.23090.41] [PMID: 12771008]

[16] Schenker MP, Dorbala S, Hong EC, *et al.* Interrelation of coronary calcification, myocardial ischemia, and outcomes in patients with intermediate likelihood of coronary artery disease: a combined positron emission tomography/computed tomography study. Circulation 2008; 117(13): 1693-700.

[http://dx.doi.org/10.1161/CIRCULATIONAHA.107.717512] [PMID: 18362235]

[17] Achenbach S, Ropers D, Pohle K, *et al.* Influence of lipid-lowering therapy on the progression of coronary artery calcification: a prospective evaluation. Circulation 2002; 106(9): 1077-82. [http://dx.doi.org/10.1161/01.CIR.0000027567.49283.FF] [PMID: 12196332]

[18] Einstein AJ, Johnson LL, Bokhari S, *et al.* Agreement of visual estimation of coronary artery calcium from low-dose CT attenuation correction scans in hybrid PET/CT and SPECT/CT with standard Agatston score. J Am Coll Cardiol 2010; 56(23): 1914-21. [http://dx.doi.org/10.1016/j.jacc.2010.05.057] [PMID: 21109114]

[19] van Kempen BJ, Spronk S, Koller MT, *et al.* Comparative effectiveness and cost-effectiveness of computed tomography screening for coronary artery calcium in asymptomatic individuals. J Am Coll Cardiol 2011; 58(16): 1690-701. [http://dx.doi.org/10.1016/j.jacc.2011.05.056] [PMID: 21982314]

[20] Greenland P, Alpert JS, Beller GA, *et al.* 2010 ACCF/AHA guideline for assessment of cardiovascular risk in asymptomatic adults: executive summary: a report of the American College of Cardiology Foundation/American Heart Association Task Force on Practice Guidelines. Circulation 2010; 122(25): 2748-64. [http://dx.doi.org/10.1161/CIR.0b013e3182051bab] [PMID: 21098427]

[21] Matsuo S, Yoshinaga K. 18F-FDG PET viability assessment for the improvements of prognosis of the patients with left vwntricular dydfunction -Is this ready for the clinical practive? -. Ann Nucl Cardiol 2016; 2(1): 53-5. [http://dx.doi.org/10.17996/ANC.02.01.53]

[22] Matsuo S, Mochizuki T, Takeda S, *et al.* Cardiac time-of-flight PET for evaluating myocardial perfusion with 13N-ammonia: phantom studies for estimation of defect and heterogeneity. Ann Nucl Cardiol 2016; 2(1): 73-8. [http://dx.doi.org/10.17996/ANC.02.01.73]

[23] Tatsumi M, Cohade C, Nakamoto Y, Wahl RL. Fluorodeoxyglucose uptake in the aortic wall at PET/CT: possible finding for active atherosclerosis. Radiology 2003; 229(3): 831-7. [http://dx.doi.org/10.1148/radiol.2293021168] [PMID: 14593193]

[24] Tahara N, Kai H, Ishibashi M, *et al.* Simvastatin attenuates plaque inflammation: evaluation by fluorodeoxyglucose positron emission tomography. J Am Coll Cardiol 2006; 48(9): 1825-31. [http://dx.doi.org/10.1016/j.jacc.2006.03.069] [PMID: 17084257]

[25] Ogawa M, Magata Y, Kato T, *et al.* Application of 18F-FDG PET for monitoring the therapeutic effect of antiinflammatory drugs on stabilization of vulnerable atherosclerotic plaques. J Nucl Med 2006; 47(11): 1845-50. [PMID: 17079818]

[26] Nakahara T, Strauss HW. From inflammation to calcification in atherosclerosis. Eur J Nucl Med Mol Imaging 2017; 44(5): 858-60. [http://dx.doi.org/10.1007/s00259-016-3608-x] [PMID: 28062896]

[27] Derlin T, Wisotzki C, Richter U, *et al.* In vivo imaging of mineral deposition in carotid plaque using 18F-sodium fluoride PET/CT: correlation with atherogenic risk factors. J Nucl Med 2011; 52(3): 362-8. [http://dx.doi.org/10.2967/jnumed.110.081208] [PMID: 21321276]

[28] Yoshinaga K. Current Japanese ministry of health, labor, and welfare approval of cardiac positron emission tomography. Ann Nucl Cardiol 2015; 1: 106-7. [http://dx.doi.org/10.17996/ANC.01.01.106]

CHAPTER 14

Nuclear Cardiology for the Diagnosis of Takotsubo Syndrome

Shinro Matsuo*

Department of Nuclear Medicine, Kanazawa University Hospital, Kanazawa, Japan

Graduate School of Advanced Preventive Medical Sciences, Kanazawa, Japan

Abstract: Takotsubo syndrome is characterized by a transient reversible left ventricular dysfunction. Takotsubo syndrome has been associated with different neurological conditions. The heart-to-mediastinum ratio of MIBG was decreased and acute washout rate was increased in the acute phase of Takotsubo syndrome extended abnormal findings of ^{123}I-BMIPP. Such information by cardiac metabolism imaging can be used as an important tool for detecting myocardial injury and diagnosing disease. This article aims at providing an updated overview about diagnosis of Takotsubo syndrome by nuclear cardiology technique.

Keywords: BMIPP, FDG, Fusion imaging, MIBG, Takotsubo syndrome.

INTRODUCTION

Takotsubo syndrome is an acute clinical condition mimicking acute myocardial infarction. Initially described in 1991 by Sato *et al* in Japan [1], the typical angiographic appearance with apical ballooning and hyperconsractility of the basal segments of the left ventricle has given the name of Takotsubo cardiomyopathy. Takotsubo syndrome is more likely to occur in elderly women and is characterized by wide reversible constriction disorders centered on the apex of the left ventricle [1 - 3]. Clinical manifestation includes sudden onset of chest pain and shortness of breath. Takotsubo syndrome is characterized by a transient reversible left ventricular dysfunction [3 - 5]. Takotsubo syndrome has been associated with different neurological conditions. It has been reported that Takotsubo syndrome is triggered by the consequence of hemorrhagic and ischemic stroke, mainly involving insular cortex and the central autonomic network. Catecholamine release might be related to the apical wall motion abno-

* **Corresponding author Shinro Matsuo:** Department of Nuclear Medicine, Kanazawa University Hospital, 13-1 Takara-machi, Kanazawa 920-8641, Japan Advanced Preventive Medical Sciences, Kanazawa University Graduate School, 13-1 Takara-machi, Kanazawa, Japan 920-8641; Tel: 81-76-265-2333; Fax: 81-76-234-4257; E-mail: smatsuo@med.kanazawa-u.ac.jp

rmalities and cardiac sympathetic nerve dysfunction seems to play an important role. This article aims at providing an updated overview about diagnosis of Takotsubo syndrome by nuclear cardiology technique [6 - 9].

As a positron emission tomography (PET) examination to evaluate blood flow, we can use ^{13}N-ammonia as a radiopharmaceutical in our country to examine the state of blood flow in myocardium. For quantification, PET is developing technologies that enable the evaluation of myocardial blood flow with higher accuracy than SPECT [9, 10]. The report of patients with Takotsubo syndrome showed that a decrease in the coronary blood flow reserve (CFR) of the apex was observed by ^{13}N-ammonia study, and even though the left ventricular wall motion abnormality was normalized, the decrease in CFR of the apex occurred. Coronary vasodilatation is normalized within 3 to 5 months [9]. Coronary blood flow waveforms performed in the acute phase of the development of Takotsubo syndrome using the Doppler guide wire by coronary artery examination are almost normal patterns but the decline in coronary blood flow reserve is recognized in the left anterior descending branch, the left circumferential branch and the right coronary artery. In the chronic phase, coronary blood flow reserve was normalized as with PET.

It has also been observed that it takes time to recover the functional impairment of the microcirculation. Regarding the cause of microcirculatory disturbance, spasm of epicardial coronary artery is excluded, but the presence or absence of spasm of micro coronary vessels at the resistance blood vessel level cannot be denied from the image of coronary angiography. There are cases in which lactic acid production, which is an indicator of myocardial ischemia, increases in the coronary sinus, although coronary vasospasm is not observed in the acetylcholine spasm provocation test. The micro coronary circulation disorder including micro coronary vasospasm which is the pathology of cardiac syndrome X seems to be related to symptoms, ST elevation and abnormal findings nuclear imaging at the time of occurrence of Takotsubo syndrome.

In previous clinical reports, it is stated that Takotsubo syndrome often resembles acute coronary syndromes such as acute myocardial infarction and unstable angina. There is a report that about 1% of all patients who were diagnosed with acute myocardial infarction have been diagnosed as Takotsubo syndrome. It is difficult not only to obtain information on the extent of myocardial disorder in electrocardiogram diagnosis, but it is possible to obtain information on myocardial damage and myocardial viability by using myocardial perfusion imaging, for grasping the severity and prognosis.

Quantitative gated SPECT depicts the precise wall motion abnormalities [11]. Apical wall akinesis and dyssynchorny can be observed in Takotsubo syndrome [11].

Fatty Acid Metabolism Myocardial Scintigraphy (^{123}I-BMIPP)

^{123}I-beta-methy-iodophenyl pentadecanoic acid (BMIPP) shows the same pharmacokinetics as a fatty acid *in vivo*, and it is taken into cardiomyocytes and then is transferred into lipid pools and mitochondria [12]. As the methyl group exists in the β position as a side chain, it is less susceptible to β oxidation and remains a long time in myocardial cells. Myocardial ischemia is known to cause a decrease in fatty acid utilization in myocardium and shifts from fatty acid metabolism to glucose metabolism. ^{123}I-BMIPP imaging can detect a microcirculation abnormality at the cell level by evaluating myocardial fatty acid metabolic abnormality. Perfusion and metabolism are mismatched with less uptake of ^{123}I-BMIPP than thallium uptake, and this has been reported among myocardial infarction or angina patients, indicating ischemic myocardium. Recent studies have shown that perfusion and metabolic information may improve risk stratification of patients with coronary artery disease. It has been shown that the characteristics of metabolic abnormality patterns in patients with Takotsubo syndrome are different from those of acute myocardial infarction [13]. In the acute phase of patients with Takotsubo syndrome, ^{123}I-BMIPP showed a decrease in uptake at the apical part of myocardium and showed impaired fatty acid metabolism in non-infarcted myocardium [13, 14]. The metabolic blood flow mismatch region observed in the acute phase was finding similar to the stunning myocardium. Even in the subacute phase, the metabolic blood flow mismatch region is shown in Takotsubo syndrome. Metabolic blood flow mismatch is believed to represent an area at risk, reflecting transient ischemic injury or metabolically stunned myocardium. The metabolic abnormality region in the apex of the apex in Takotsubo syndrome is said to be small compared to the disorder of acute myocardial infarction in the anterior descending lining. The time course of myocardial perfusion and fatty acid metabolism in patients with left ventricular dysfunction in Takotsubo syndrome improves blood flow abnormality promptly and fatty acid metabolism gradually improves after the improvement of blood flow [13]. Semi-quantitative analysis of cardiac metabolic abnormalities can evaluate the extent of myocardial injury and diagnose the disease condition accurately. The metabolic abnormality of Takotsubo syndrome is a distinctly different region from the defect of myocardial perfusion imaging and is observed only in the apex of the left ventricle [13]. It is most important to differentiate it from the myocardial infarction of the anterior descending coronary artery, but in the electrocardiogram, ST depression of aVR is observed. In the case where ST elevation in V1 lead is not recognized, it can be distinguished with myocardial infarction by 90% or more, aVR. The presence of a positive T wave at the time point suggests Takotsubo syndrome [15]. Confirming a diagnosis becomes possible by clarifying the extent and severity of the injured myocardium by imaging in cases electrocardiogram suspected or cases which cannot be diagnosed by electrocardiogram. In Takotsubo syndrome, abnormality of metabolism detected by ^{123}I-BMIPP is more extensive than blood flow abnormality in many cases [13]. It is possible to diagnose events at onset as memory imaging [13, 16]. However, in the case of the obstruction of the distal part of the entire lower descending branch where the anterior descending branch is wrapped around the apical part (so-called wrapped LAD), it is difficult to distinguish between Takotsubo syndrome and myocardial infarction only by electrocardiogram. There is a possibility that the discrimination by the fusion image described later can be helpful. Extended abnormal findings of ^{123}I-BMIPP Such information by cardiac metabolism imaging can be used as an important tool for detecting myocardial injury and diagnosing disease.

^{18}F Fluorodeoxyglucose PET

^{18}F fluorodeoxyglucose (FDG) is an analogue of glucose allowing non-invasive evaluation of glucose metabolism. ^{18}F-FDG is usually transported into the cell through the glucose transporter protein at the cell membrane, depending on the concentration gradient of glucose from outside to the inside of the cell. Previous study showed that a unique pattern of transient myocardial glucose abnormalities can occur after severe emotional stress or physical stress in Takotsubo syndrome [17, 18].

Neurotransmitter Imaging for Cardiomyopathy and Takotsubo Syndrome

The cause of Takotsubo syndrome is suggested microcirculatory disorder, catecholamine myocardial disorder, localized myocarditis transient plaque rupture, coronary spasm and the like. Although it is also called Takotsubo cardiomyopathy, it is not suitable for calling cardiomyopathy, as it merges with various diseases, so it would be appropriate to call it as Takotsubo syndrome. Nuclear cardiology imaging obtains information that is close to the pathology of Takotsubo syndrome and is widely used in clinical practice to accumulate evidence [3 - 6]. In this article, including the latest findings of Takotsubo syndrome, we describe the characteristics of the disease condition and the practical use of the nuclear cardiology technique.

^{123}I-MIBG scintigraphy is a test often used for prognostic evaluation of heart failure because it can visualize cardiac sympathetic nerve [19]. The sympathetic nervous function can be accurately known by measuring the ratio of the mediastinum interval by the frontal image of the heart (planar image) and measuring the sympathetic disturbance in the whole heart. Akashi and colleagues evaluated by ^{123}I-MIBG observation that the heart-to-mediastinum ratio was decreased and acute washout rate was increased in the acute phase of Takotsubo syndrome as shown in Fig. (**1**) [20]. While the cardiac interval ratio evaluates cardiac sympathetic dysfunction abnormality of the whole heart, local evaluation can be made by using SPECT image. By SPECT, the site of sympathetic dysfunction abnormalities in Takotsubo syndrome can be accurately depicted [21]. Sympathetic dysfunction often occurs in the apex of the apex and the degree of disability is often more extensive than in the region of metabolic abnormality. ^{123}I - MIBG often causes prolonged extensive anomalies centered on the apex seen from the acute phase. Follow-up observation with ^{201}Tl, ^{123}I-BMIPP and ^{123}I-MIBG showed an accumulation of apical cord accumulation, prolonging the abnormality of ^{123}I-MIBG in the highest range. Recovery is said to recover in the order of ^{201}Tl, ^{123}I – BMIPP and ^{123}I - MIBG. The abnormality of ^{123}I-MIBG may fix irreversibly. Diagnosis by ^{123}I-MIBG imaging can be used supplementarily in subacute or chronic phase.

It has been reported that, in patients with pheochromocytoma, continued high plasma catecholamine concentrations cause reversible cardiomyopathy [22]. Symptoms of pheochromocytoma associated with catecholamine-induced cardiomyopathy are similar to symptoms in takotsubo syndrome. Also, myocardial histological changes in takotsubo cardiomyopathy are remarkably similar to those seen in cardiotoxicity of catecholamines in animals and humans [23]. In Takotsubo syndrome, it is known that it is at a high level of norepinephrine, but the aforementioned microvascular spasm and stunning are caused by a decrease in the incorporation of ^{123}I-MIBG in myocardium as a whole in pheochromocytoma [24, 25].

Left ventricular wall motion disorder that occurs in cases with subarachnoid hemorrhage often occurs in the apex of the apex and shows findings consistent with Takotsubo syndrome. In Takotsubo syndrome, a series of changes such as ischemia in the hypothalamus and local norepinephrine release, cardiac dysfunction and ECG abnormality occur in the onset of subarachnoid hemorrhage. In cerebral blood flow scintigraphy taken in patients with Takotsubo syndrome caused by stress, an increase in blood flow in the hippocampus, thalamus, basal ganglia, and brainstem is captured [26]. It is suggested a relationship between hippocampal hyperactivity and sympathetic excitement, which is an important observation in considering the pathogenesis of Takotsubo syndrome. It is triggered by the sympathetic nerve in the brain excited by the earthquake such as cerebral ischemia, earthquake and mental stress due to a train accident [1, 2]. In an experimental model of catecholamine-induced cardiomyopathy, in psychologically stressed rats, a decrease in inotropic response to norepinephrine associated with a decrease in myocardial β-adrenergic receptor has been reported. The blood catecholamine level in patients with takotsubo syndrome is high, and the concentration of norepinephrine is particularly high. It stimulates beta 2 adrenergic receptors that are abundant in the apex of the apex, resulting in stunning eventually resulting in contractile failure (catecholamines cardiomyopathy). The imaging of the sympathetic function by ^{123}I-MIBG can aid in diagnosis in accurately assessing such conditions of Takotsubo syndrome. It is known that there is a close relationship between dysfunction of the dopamine receptor transporter in the brain striatum in Lewy body disease and Parkinson's disease and cardiac sympathetic dysfunction abnormality. To understand the relationship between adrenaline secreted by anxiety and extreme tension, Heart - Brain Interaction including noradrenaline and the secretion of dopamine secreted at happiness, it is important to understand the pathology of Takotsubo syndrome and prevent recurrence.

Fusion Image of Takotsubo Syndrome

The left ventricular wall motion disorder of Takotsubo syndrome cannot be explained in the dominant region of the coronary artery. In the SPECT image, although it is possible to depict the degree and extent of the abnormality of the blood flow, experience is needed to understand the relation with the dominant part of the coronary artery. Data of SPECT and CT coronary angiography are transferred to a workstation, and these two tomographic images are aligned on the basis of the apex and interventricular groove on software [27]. Then, from the data of CT coronary angiography, the coronary artery tree is extracted by volume rendering. The information of the SPECT is displayed in the actual form of the heart, and the coronary artery is converted to 3D and displayed at the same time. As a result, the relationship between the traveling of coronary artery CT and abnormal blood flow in Takotsubo syndrome becomes obvious [27]. Coronary artery stenosis causes a flow decrease in the dominant region of the coronary artery. For example, in the case of a myocardial infarction in the anterior descending branch (# 6), a decrease in blood flow is recognized in the antero-septum region and apex of LV. In Takotsubo syndrome, a wide range of blood flow disorders, metabolic abnormalities, sympathetic dysfunction abnormalities are observed centered on the apical region, but it can be proved by fusion images that this abnormality is not related to coronary artery culprit lesion [27]. Attempts to simultaneously detect coronary arteriosclerosis using SPECT/CT multifunction machines have also been attempted to identify this [28].

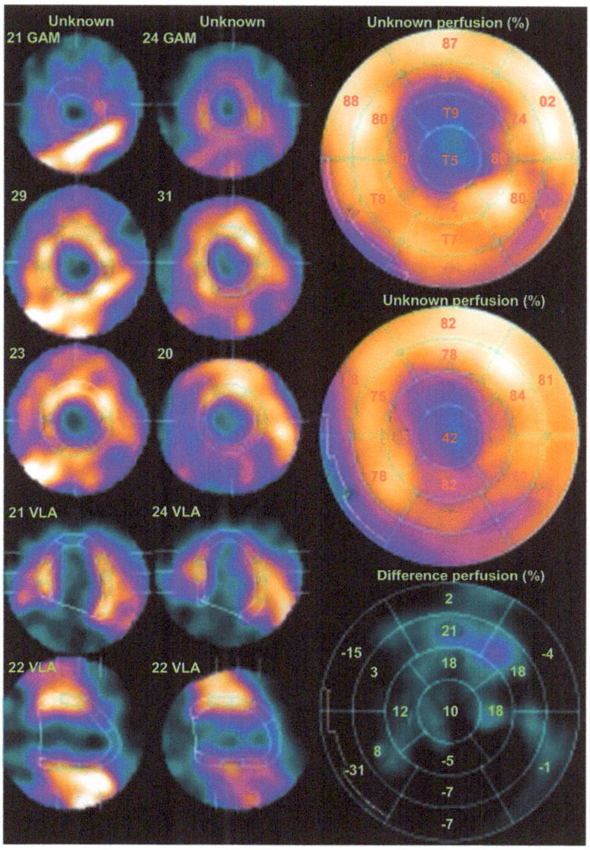

Fig. (1). ^{123}I-MIBG imaging of patient with takotsubo cardiomyopathy.

In a 66 - year - old woman with Takotsubo cardiomyopathy, a cardiac sympathetic nerve dysfunction was found in the center of the apex. The heart-to-mediastinum ratio of the delayed image was 1.9 (normal range 2.3 - 3.7), and it showed a decreased MIBG uptake.

Various Nuclear Medicine Tests used for Takotsubo Syndrome

By various nuclear medicine examinations, we can approach the condition of Takotsubo syndrome [29, 30]. By using ^{99m}Tc pyrophosphate scintigraphy, myocardial damage in the acute phase of Takotsubo syndrome can be observed. In addition, it has been reported that gallium accumulation did not occur in the apex of the apex, which is a lesion site in patients with acute osteoarthritic syndrome. Gallium scintigraphy is used as an aid in the diagnosis of myocarditis, but severe inflammation as seen in myocarditis is negative because there is no accumulation of gallium. Using heart pool scintigraphy, we can measure left ventricular function and right ventricular function. If pulmonary embolism is suspected in the acute ECG, it is recommended to perform pulmonary blood flow scintigraphy to diagnose pulmonary embolism. Kidney function is deeply related to the prognosis of patients with Takotsubo syndrome. It is known that the hospitalization period is long and the cardiovascular event rate is high in cases where the estimated glomerular filtration amount (eGFR) is poor. Nuclear medicine examination is a noninvasive examination and unlike a contrast medium, there is almost no adverse effect on kidney function, so it is an examination method suitable for management of patients with Takotsubo syndrome [30]. In the future, it is desirable to accumulate experience of many cases and to clarify further pathological conditions.

CONCLUSION

Takotsubo syndrome involves left ventricular apical metabolic and sympathetic abnormalities as well as perfusion, including apical wall motion abnormality. A nuclear cardiology approach for Takotsubo syndrome provides better understanding for the patient management.

CONSENT FOR PUBLICATION

Not applicable.

CONFLICT OF INTEREST

The author declares no conflict of interest, financial or otherwise.

ACKNOWLEDGEMENTS

Declared none.

REFERENCES

[1] Sato H, Tateishi H, Uchida T, *et al.* Takotsubo cardiomyopathy due to multivessel spasm.Clinical aspect of myocardial injury: from ischemia to heart failure. Tokyo: Kagakuhyouronsha 1990; pp. 56-64.

[2] Matsuo S, Tanaka T, Takahashi M, *et al.* A case of cardiac contusion by train accident. Shinzo 1993; 25: 1241-6.

[3] Tsuchihashi K, Ueshima K, Uchida T, *et al.* Transient left ventricular apical ballooning without coronary artery stenosis: a novel heart syndrome mimicking acute myocardial infarction. Angina Pectoris-Myocardial Infarction Investigations in Japan. J Am Coll Cardiol 2001; 38(1): 11-8. [http://dx.doi.org/10.1016/S0735-1097(01)01316-X] [PMID: 11451258]

[4] Prasad A, Lerman A, Rihal CS. Apical ballooning syndrome (Tako-Tsubo or stress cardiomyopathy): a mimic of acute myocardial infarction. Am Heart J 2008; 155(3): 408-17. [http://dx.doi.org/10.1016/j.ahj.2007.11.008] [PMID: 18294473]

[5] Kawai S, Kitabatake A, Tomoike H. Guidelines for diagnosis of takotsubo (ampulla) cardiomyopathy.

Circ J 2007; 71(6): 990-2.
[http://dx.doi.org/10.1253/circj.71.990] [PMID: 17527002]

[6] Inami T, Kataoka M, Shimura N, *et al.* Left ventricular dysfunction due to diffuse multiple vessel coronary artery spasm can be concealed in dilated cardiomyopathy. Eur J Heart Fail 2012; 14(10): 1130-8.
[http://dx.doi.org/10.1093/eurjhf/hfs103] [PMID: 22713288]

[7] Ito K, Sugihara H, Kawasaki T, *et al.* Assessment of ampulla (Takotsubo) cardiomyopathy with coronary angiography, two-dimensional echocardiography and 99mTc-tetrofosmin myocardial single photon emission computed tomography. Ann Nucl Med 2001; 15(4): 351-5.
[http://dx.doi.org/10.1007/BF02988242] [PMID: 11577760]

[8] Matsuo S, Nakae I, Tsutamoto T, Okamoto N, Horie M. A novel clinical indicator using Tc-99m sestamibi for evaluating cardiac mitochondrial function in patients with cardiomyopathies. J Nucl Cardiol 2007; 14(2): 215-20.
[http://dx.doi.org/10.1016/j.nuclcard.2006.10.022] [PMID: 17386384]

[9] Feola M, Chauvie S, Rosso GL, Biggi A, Ribichini F, Bobbio M. Reversible impairment of coronary flow reserve in takotsubo cardiomyopathy: a myocardial PET study. J Nucl Cardiol 2008; 15(6): 811-7.
[http://dx.doi.org/10.1007/BF03007363] [PMID: 18984457]

[10] Matsuo S, Mochizuki T, Takeda S, *et al.* Cardiac time-of-flight PET for evaluating myocardial perfusion with ^{13}N-ammonia: phantom studies for estimation of defect and heterogeneity. Ann Nucl Cariol 2016; 2: 73-8.
[http://dx.doi.org/10.17996/ANC.02.01.73]

[11] Matsuo S. Phase analysis using gated myocardial perfusion single-photon emission computed tomography imaging for evaluating cardiac dyssynchrony. Circ J 2012; 76(8): 1832-3.
[http://dx.doi.org/10.1253/circj.CJ-12-0636] [PMID: 22664418]

[12] Kawai Y, Tsukamoto E, Nozaki Y, Morita K, Sakurai M, Tamaki N. Significance of reduced uptake of iodinated fatty acid analogue for the evaluation of patients with acute chest pain. J Am Coll Cardiol 2001; 38(7): 1888-94.
[http://dx.doi.org/10.1016/S0735-1097(01)01634-5] [PMID: 11738290]

[13] Matsuo S, Nakajima K, Kinuya S, Yamagishi M. Diagnostic utility of ^{123}I-BMIPP imaging in patients with Takotsubo cardiomyopathy. J Cardiol 2014; 64(1): 49-56.
[http://dx.doi.org/10.1016/j.jjcc.2013.10.019] [PMID: 24331764]

[14] Matsuo S, Nakajima K, Yamashina S, *et al.* Characterization of Japanese standards for myocardial sympathetic and metabolic imaging in comparison with perfusion imaging. Ann Nucl Med 2009; 23(6): 517-22.
[http://dx.doi.org/10.1007/s12149-009-0269-x] [PMID: 19521747]

[15] Kosuge M, Ebina T, Hibi K, *et al.* Simple and accurate electrocardiographic criteria to differentiate takotsubo cardiomyopathy from anterior acute myocardial infarction. J Am Coll Cardiol 2010; 55(22): 2514-6.
[http://dx.doi.org/10.1016/j.jacc.2009.12.059] [PMID: 20510222]

[16] Matsuo S, Nakamura Y, Takahashi M, Mitsunami K, Kinoshita M. Myocardial metabolic abnormalities in hypertrophic cardiomyopathy assessed by iodine-123-labeled beta-methyl-branched fatty acid myocardial scintigraphy and its relation to exercise-induced ischemia. Jpn Circ J 1998; 62(3): 167-72.
[http://dx.doi.org/10.1253/jcj.62.167] [PMID: 9583441]

[17] Yoshida T, Hibino T, Kako N, *et al.* A pathophysiologic study of tako-tsubo cardiomyopathy with F-18 fluorodeoxyglucose positron emission tomography. Eur Heart J 2007; 28(21): 2598-604.
[http://dx.doi.org/10.1093/eurheartj/ehm401] [PMID: 17921529]

[18] Kobylecka M, Budnik M, Kochanowski J, *et al.* Takotsubo cardiomyopathy: FDG myocardial uptake

pattern in fasting patients. Comparison of PET/CT, SPECT, and ECHO results. J Nucl Cardiol 2017. [PMID: 28054182]

[19] Matsuo S, Nakajima K, Nakata T. Prognostic value of cardiac sympathetic nerve imaging using long-term follow-up data - ischemic *vs*. non-ischemic heart failure etiology. Circ J 2016; 80(2): 435-41. [http://dx.doi.org/10.1253/circj.CJ-15-0952] [PMID: 26638869]

[20] Akashi YJ, Nakazawa K, Sakakibara M, Miyake F, Musha H, Sasaka K. 123I-MIBG myocardial scintigraphy in patients with "takotsubo" cardiomyopathy. J Nucl Med 2004; 45(7): 1121-7. [PMID: 15235057]

[21] Matsuo S, Matsumoto T, Nakae I, *et al.* Noninvasive identification of myocarrial sympathetic and metabolic abnormalities in a patient with "Takotsubo"cardiomyopathy. Int Med J 2005; 12: 143-4.

[22] Suga K, Tsukamoto K, Nishigauchi K, *et al.* Iodine-123-MIBG imaging in pheochromocytoma with cardiomyopathy and pulmonary edema. J Nucl Med 1996; 37(8): 1361-4. [PMID: 8708774]

[23] Akashi YJ, Goldstein DS, Barbaro G, Ueyama T. Takotsubo cardiomyopathy: a new form of acute, reversible heart failure. Circulation 2008; 118(25): 2754-62. [http://dx.doi.org/10.1161/CIRCULATIONAHA.108.767012] [PMID: 19106400]

[24] Chen W, Dilsizian V. Cardiac sympathetic disturbance in Takotsubo cardiomyopathy: primary etiology or a compensatory response to heart failure? JACC Cardiovasc Imaging 2016; 9(8): 991-3. [http://dx.doi.org/10.1016/j.jcmg.2016.01.026] [PMID: 27344419]

[25] Christensen TE, Bang LE, Holmvang L, *et al.* (123)I-MIBG scintigraphy in the subacute state of Takotsubo cardiomyopathy. JACC Cardiovasc Imaging 2016; 9(8): 982-90. [http://dx.doi.org/10.1016/j.jcmg.2016.01.028] [PMID: 27344416]

[26] Suzuki H, Matsumoto Y, Kaneta T, *et al.* Evidence for brain activation in patients with takotsubo cardiomyopathy. Circ J 2014; 78(1): 256-8. [http://dx.doi.org/10.1253/circj.CJ-13-1276] [PMID: 24284957]

[27] Matsuo S, Nakajima K, Akhter N, *et al.* Clinical usefulness of novel cardiac MDCT/SPECT fusion image. Ann Nucl Med 2009; 23(6): 579-86. [http://dx.doi.org/10.1007/s12149-009-0279-8] [PMID: 19572098]

[28] Matsuo S, Nakajima K, Kinuya S. Coronary artery atherosclerosis measured by a hybrid SPECT/CT camera Atherosclerosis risk factors, prevention and treatment. NOVA publishers 2012; pp. 163-70.

[29] Matsuo S, Nakajima K, Akhter N, *et al.* Diagnostic and prognostic cardiac imaging in cardiomyopathies Cardiomyopathies: Causes, Effects and Treatment. NOVA publishers 2009; pp. 35-43.

[30] Vitale C, Rosano GM, Kaski JC. Role of coronary microvascular dysfunction in Takotsubo cardiomyopathy. Circ J 2016; 80(2): 299-305. [http://dx.doi.org/10.1253/circj.CJ-15-1364] [PMID: 26763468]

CHAPTER 15

Small Rodent Animal Positron Emission Tomography/Single Photon Emission Tomography

Hiroshi Wakabayashi*

Department of Nuclear Medicine, Kanazawa University Hospital, 13-1 Takara-machi, Kanazawa, Ishikawa 920-8641, Japan

Abstract: The recent development of noninvasive radionuclide and hybrid imaging systems may promote preclinical cardiovascular research. Molecular imaging advances beyond the traditional imaging paradigm of detecting morphological contrasts and aims to explore the physiological and pathological molecular processes at cellular and sub-cellular levels within intact living subjects. Molecular imaging typically uses targeted tracers that bind specific molecular targets with high affinity. Single-photon emission computed tomography (SPECT) and positron emission tomography (PET) provide distinct advantages over morphological imaging modalities regarding the detection of signals on a molecular level. Monitoring of small rodent animal models of cardiac diseases utilizing noninvasive imaging is a unique approach and is essential to further understand the dynamic processes of diseases. Here, we review the applications of SPECT and PET in small animal research.

Keywords: Molecular imaging, PET, SPECT, Small rodent.

INTRODUCTION

The recent development of noninvasive radionuclide and hybrid imaging systems may promote preclinical cardiovascular research. Molecular imaging advances beyond the traditional imaging paradigm of detecting morphological contrasts and aims to explore the physiological and pathological molecular processes at cellular and sub-cellular levels within intact living subjects. Molecular imaging typically uses targeted tracers that bind specific molecular targets with high affinity. The recent introduction of various novel tracers for radionuclide approaches allows the noninvasive characterization of multiple essential molecular targets, such as activation of the sympathetic nervous [1, 2] and the renin-angiotensin-aldosterone system [3], glucose metabolism [4], inflammatory [5], angiogenesis [6 - 8], and apoptosis [9 - 11].

* **Corresponding author Hiroshi Wakabayashi:** Department of Nuclear Medicine, Kanazawa University Hospital, 13-1 Takara-machi, Kanazawa, Ishikawa 920-8641, Japan; Tel: 81-76-265-2333; Fax: 81-76-234-4257; E-mail: wakabayashi@staff.kanazawa-u.ac.jp

Small rodent animal models of cardiac diseases help researchers study disease pathology or treatment efficacy before beginning clinical studies. Longitudinal monitoring utilizing noninvasive imaging is a unique approach and is essential to further understand the dynamic processes of diseases.

Positron emission tomography (PET) and single-photon emission computed tomography (SPECT) are the two primary forms of nuclear imaging currently employed by researchers. Both imaging systems are based on the fundamental principles of detecting gamma rays and building three-dimensional images. PET and SPECT provide distinct advantages over morphological imaging modalities regarding the detection of signals on a molecular level. Recent developments in multi-pinhole collimators and image reconstruction methodology have led to millimeter resolution in small rodent animal in SPECT [12], although PET provides superior temporal resolution. Conversely, neither method is suitable for morphological evaluation compared with computed tomography (CT) and magnetic resonance imaging (MRI). Constructions of hybrid scanners (such as PET/CT, PET/MRI, PET/SPECT/CT, and SPECT/CT) are preferred in a cardiac research field. Here, we review the applications of SPECT and PET in small animal research.

Radionuclides Used for SPECT and PET

To label carrier molecules, we used short half-lives radionuclides such as rubidium-82 (^{82}Rb, half-life (T½) 78 s), oxygen-15 (^{15}O, T½ 2.1 min), nitrogen-13 (^{13}N, T½ 10 min), carbon-11 (^{11}C, T½ 20 min), gallium-68 (^{68}Ga, T½ 68 min), or fluorine-18 (^{18}F, T½ 110 min) for PET and longer half-lives radionuclides such as technetium-99m (^{99m}Tc, T½ 6.01 h) and iodine-123 (^{123}I, T½ 13.27 h) for SPECT.

Myocardial Perfusion Image

Perfusion SPECT provides essential information for the accurate diagnosis of patients with coronary artery disease. Assessment of myocardial perfusion using SPECT has become an indispensable diagnostic tool for ischemic heart disease in clinical settings [13, 14]. Additionally, myocardial perfusion images are critical to understand the pathological process of cardiac diseases; therefore, molecular tracer images are obtained in addition to myocardial perfusion images. For SPECT imaging, ^{201}Thallium, ^{99m}Tc- methoxyisobutylisonitrile (MIBI), and ^{99m}Tc-tetrofosmin (TF) have been widely used. In addition, the use of PET tracers, such as ^{13}N ammonia (NH_3), ^{82}Rb, ^{15}O-water, ^{18}F-fluorobenzyl triphenyl phosphonium (FBnTP), and ^{18}F-Flurpiridaz, has also popularized. Novel tracers have demonstrated the stability of the perfusion defect size over time and the magnitude of the redistribution [15 - 17].

Normal myocardial perfusion distribution differs based on attenuation artifact, partial volume effect, cardiac or respiratory motion blurring effect, and methodological differences [18, 19]. Commercially available software packages have been used to accurately analyze cardiac nuclear imaging in small animal studies. A standard reference database may help in the accurate evaluation of the perfusion defect [20]. In mice with myocardial infarction (MI), reports have shown that the size of an MI quantified by commercial software was accurately correlated with the size of the MI confirmed by 2,3,5-Triphenyl tetrazolium chloride staining as well as the gold standard method autoradiography [21, 22]. In rats with MI, ^{99m}Tc-MIBI SPECT with measurements of the MI from commercially available software can help to objectively assess the extent and severity of ischemic injury [20]. The commercial software can support the assessment of perfusion defect size accurately in a clinical setting.

Cardiac Function

Imaging modalities enable the quantification of left ventricular function parameters (end-diastolic volume, end systolic volume, and ejection volume) and wall motion abnormalities using commercially available software. The use of a pinhole collimator in conjunction with gated SPECT enables the measurements of left ventricular function in rats [19]. The small animal PET also provides the cardiac function assessment, and the serial monitoring of LV function is critical to confirm the recovery or progression of disease in rat models. However, care should be taken as the function parameters may differ depending on each examination [23].

Glucose Metabolism

The most commonly used clinical PET tracer to assess myocardial glucose metabolism is ^{18}F-fluorodeoxyglucose (^{18}F-FDG). ^{18}F-FDG is a glucose analog that enters cardiomyocytes primarily *via* glucose transporters (GLUT) 1 and 4 and is subsequently trapped in the cell by a phosphorylation reaction catalyzed through hexokinase. Under normal resting conditions, most energy is derived from long-chain fatty acids in the myocardium. During exercise, the heart switches substrate preference from the fatty acid to glucose. In response to glucose loading and insulin administration, the energy source also rapidly changes to glucose. Insulin/glucose mixture injection 30 min before ^{18}F-FDG administration can maximize cardiac uptake in small rodent animals [4]. In another method, ^{18}F-FDG PET under hyperinsulinemic-euglycemic clamping conditions by high serum insulin concentrations allows the visualization of glucose consumption [24]. For the assessment of the inflammatory reaction within the myocardium, ^{18}F-FDG PET is useful to monitor inflammatory activity after acute MI and myocarditis. In addition, gated ^{18}F-FDG-PET enables the combined molecular and functional imaging of LV function in small rodent animals [25, 26].

Cardiac Sympathetic Nerve Imaging

The autonomic nervous system plays a critical role in most cardiovascular diseases. Attenuated sensitivity to neurotransmitters as well as enhanced sympathetic activity may lead to numerous heart pathologies. Evaluation of the sympathetic innervation of the heart can provide essential data on the etiology and progression of heart diseases.

When the heart fails and cardiac output falls, the sympathetic nervous system becomes overactivated to constrain the fall in mean arterial pressure. The chronic sympathetic overactivity results in cardiac remodeling [27] and mortality in patients with heart failure [27, 28]. Past studies suggest an essential role of cardiac sympathetic nervous tone and chronic catecholamine overexposure in cardiac hypertrophy, fibrosis, and right and left ventricular failure [29, 30]. Nuclear imaging of the sympathetic nervous system with radio-labeled catecholamine analogs provides measures of global as well as regional sympathetic activity. This technique has facilitated the study of the cardiac nervous system in both healthy and diseased hearts and has contributed significantly to an improved understanding of heart failure pathophysiology. ^{11}C-epinephrine (EPI), ^{11}C-hydroxyephedrine (HED), ^{11}C-phenylephrine (PHEN), and ^{123}I-metaiodobenzyl-guanidine (MIBG) have a high affinity to the presynaptic neuronal catecholamine transporter (uptake-1) [1, 2] and are available for direct analysis of myocardial sympathoadrenal activation by PET or SPECT imaging system. However, ^{123}I/^{131}I-MIBG may have a different uptake mechanism due to nonneural uptake-2 in rat hearts [31].

Angiogenesis Monitoring

Angiogenesis is an essential process in infarct healing and post-MI LV remodeling [8]. Therefore, noninvasive imaging of angiogenesis may improve risk stratification after MI. Angiogenesis imaging can also afford the evaluation of therapeutic interventions aimed at angiogenesis stimulation. αvβ3 integrin-avid agents, a family of cell surface receptors, have been used to visualize angiogenesis in postinfarct animal models. ^{18}F- and ^{68}Ga-labeled galacto-arginine-glycine-aspartate (RGD) has high affinity to αvβ3 integrin receptors, which are known to be overexpressed on the endothelial surface involved in neoangiogenesis in MI [32].

Apoptosis Imaging

Many investigations have examined the role of apoptotic cell death in ischemic disease and heart failure. Tissue hypoxia activates the suicide program of cardiac myocytes. Apoptosis and necrosis may independently contribute to myocyte cell death after MI [33]. Annexin-V (AV) has an affinity for binding to the externalized PS and is the most frequently studied tracer for apoptosis. For radiolabeling of this molecule, ^{18}F-, ^{68}Ga-, and ^{99m}Tc-labeled AV have been used to detect apoptosis [34]. Imaging of apoptosis can also detect the cardioprotective effects of a conditioned mesenchymal stem cell patch grafted in a rat model of acute MI [35] and would be useful in screening for drugs that have been shown to induce synergistic cardiac toxicity [36].

Artifact of SPECT and PET

Attenuation artifact, partial volume effect, cardiac or respiratory motion blurring effect, and methodological differences impact the results of a patient examination. A critical problem of both SPECT and PET imaging is the attenuation of emissions in tissue. Although tissue attenuation in cardiac PET images is much smaller in rodents than in humans, its influence on quantification should not be ignored when comparing results from rodents of different body sizes. The reduction in cardiac activity is also significantly higher in obese rats than in lean rats. Attenuation correction is indispensable for the accurate comparison of cardiac tracer activity [37].

Unlike human studies, preclinical studies utilize a variety of protocols that depend on the research group. For example, perfusion SPECT has been performed in a broad range of injection dose (from 37 MBq/rat up to 450 MBq/mouse) and time of starting acquisition (from 2 min to 60 min post-injection) [38]. Although the roles of noninvasive imaging modalities such as SPECT and PET are increasing, researchers must bear in mind their limitations to avoid pitfalls.

CONCLUSION

Small-animal SPECT and PET can provide *in vivo* measurements of physiology, metabolism, and molecular targets of heart diseases. Additionally, longitudinal monitoring of experimental models utilizing the noninvasive imaging is essential to understand the dynamic processes of heart diseases. Although some artifact might affect the results, these tools certainly offer the opportunity to investigate aspects of cardiovascular pathophysiological processes.

CONSENT FOR PUBLICATION

Not applicable.

CONFLICT OF INTEREST

The author (editor) declares no conflict of interest, financial or otherwise.

ACKNOWLEDGEMENTS

Declared none.

REFERENCES

[1] Higuchi T, Schwaiger M. Imaging cardiac neuronal function and dysfunction. Curr Cardiol Rep 2006; 8: 131-8.
[http://dx.doi.org/10.1007/s11886-006-0024-z]

[2] Higuchi T, Schwaiger M. Noninvasive imaging of heart failure: neuronal dysfunction and risk stratification. Heart Fail Clin 2006; 2: 193-204.
[http://dx.doi.org/10.1016/j.hfc.2006.02.003]

[3] Higuchi T, Fukushima K, Xia J, *et al.* Radionuclide imaging of angiotensin II type 1 receptor upregulation after myocardial ischemia-reperfusion injury. J Nucl Med 2010; 51: 1956-61.
[http://dx.doi.org/10.2967/jnumed.110.079855]

[4] Higuchi T, Nekolla SG, Jankaukas A, *et al.* Characterization of normal and infarcted rat myocardium using a combination of small-animal PET and clinical MRI. J Nucl Med 2007; 48: 288-94.

[5] Taki J, Wakabayashi H, Inaki A, *et al.* 14C-Methionine uptake as a potential marker of inflammatory processes after myocardial ischemia and reperfusion. J Nucl Med 2013; 54: 431-6.
[http://dx.doi.org/10.2967/jnumed.112.112060]

[6] Higuchi T, Bengel FM, Seidl S, *et al.* Assessment of alpha(v)beta(3) integrin expression after myocardial infarction by positron emission tomography. Cardiovasc Res 2008; 78: 395-403.
[http://dx.doi.org/10.1093/cvr/cvn033]

[7] Higuchi T, Wester HJ, Schwaiger M. Imaging of angiogenesis in cardiology. Eur J Nucl Med Mol Imaging 2007; 34: S9-S19.
[http://dx.doi.org/10.1007/s00259-007-0436-z]

[8] Sherif HM, Saraste A, Nekolla SG, *et al.* Molecular imaging of early alphavbeta3 integrin expression predicts long-term left-ventricle remodeling after myocardial infarction in rats. J Nucl Med 2012; 53: 318-23.
[http://dx.doi.org/10.2967/jnumed.111.091652]

[9] Taki J, Higuchi T, Kawashima A, *et al.* Effect of postconditioning on myocardial 99mTc-annexin-V uptake: comparison with ischemic preconditioning and caspase inhibitor treatment. J Nucl Med 2007; 48: 1301-7.
[http://dx.doi.org/10.2967/jnumed.106.037408]

[10] Taki J, Higuchi T, Kawashima A, *et al.* Detection of cardiomyocyte death in a rat model of ischemia and reperfusion using 99mTc-labeled annexin V. J Nucl Med 2004; 45: 1536-41.

[11] Taki J, Higuchi T, Kawashima A, *et al.* (99m)Tc-Annexin-V uptake in a rat model of variable ischemic severity and reperfusion time. Circ J 2007; 71: 1141-6.
[http://dx.doi.org/10.1253/circj.71.1141]

[12] Golestani R, Wu C, Tio RA, *et al.* Small-animal SPECT and SPECT/CT: application in cardiovascular

research. Eur J Nucl Med Mol Imaging 2010; 37: 1766-77.
[http://dx.doi.org/10.1007/s00259-009-1321-8]

[13] Hendel RC, Berman DS, Di Carli MF, *et al.* ACCF/ASNC/ACR/AHA/ASE/SCCT/SCMR/SNM 2009 Appropriate Use Criteria for Cardiac Radionuclide Imaging: A Report of the American College of Cardiology Foundation Appropriate Use Criteria Task Force, the American Society of Nuclear Cardiology, the American College of Radiology, the American Heart Association, the American Society of Echocardiography, the Society of Cardiovascular Computed Tomography, the Society for Cardiovascular Magnetic Resonance, and the Society of Nuclear Medicine. J Am Coll Cardiol 2009; 53: 2201-29.
[http://dx.doi.org/10.1016/j.jacc.2009.02.013]

[14] Hachamovitch R, Berman DS, Shaw LJ, *et al.* Incremental prognostic value of myocardial perfusion single photon emission computed tomography for the prediction of cardiac death: differential stratification for risk of cardiac death and myocardial infarction. Circulation 1998; 97: 535-43.
[http://dx.doi.org/10.1161/01.CIR.97.6.535]

[15] Higuchi T, Fukushima K, Rischpler C, *et al.* Stable delineation of the ischemic area by the PET perfusion tracer 18F-fluorobenzyl triphenyl phosphonium after transient coronary occlusion. J Nucl Med 2011; 52: 965-9.
[http://dx.doi.org/10.2967/jnumed.110.085993]

[16] Stegger L, Heijman E, Schafers KP, *et al.* Quantification of left ventricular volumes and ejection fraction in mice using PET, compared with MRI. J Nucl Med 2009; 50: 132-8.
[http://dx.doi.org/10.2967/jnumed.108.056051]

[17] Kim DY, Kim HS, Reder S, *et al.* Comparison of 18F-Labeled Fluoroalkylphosphonium Cations with 13N-NH3 for PET Myocardial Perfusion Imaging. J Nucl Med 2015; 56: 1581-6.
[http://dx.doi.org/10.2967/jnumed.115.156794]

[18] Wu MC, Gao DW, Sievers RE, *et al.* Pinhole single-photon emission computed tomography for myocardial perfusion imaging of mice. J Am Coll Cardiol 2003; 42: 576-82.
[http://dx.doi.org/10.1016/S0735-1097(03)00716-2]

[19] Vanhove C, Lahoutte T, Defrise M, *et al.* Reproducibility of left ventricular volume and ejection fraction measurements in rat using pinhole gated SPECT. Eur J Nucl Med Mol Imaging 2005; 32: 211-20.
[http://dx.doi.org/10.1007/s00259-004-1649-z]

[20] Wakabayashi H, Taki J, Inaki A, *et al.* Quantification of myocardial perfusion defect size in rats: comparison between quantitative perfusion SPECT and autoradiography. Mol Imaging Biol 2018.
[http://dx.doi.org/10.1007/s11307-018-1159-1]

[21] Constantinesco A, Choquet P, Monassier L, *et al.* Assessment of left ventricular perfusion, volumes, and motion in mice using pinhole gated SPECT. J Nucl Med 2005; 46: 1005-11.

[22] Roelants V, Delgaudine M, Walrand S, *et al.* Myocardial infarct size quantification in mice by SPECT using a novel algorithm independent of a normal perfusion database. EJNMMI Res 2012; 2: 64.
[http://dx.doi.org/10.1186/2191-219X-2-64]

[23] Szymanski MK, Kruizinga S, Tio RA, *et al.* Use of gated 13N-NH3 micro-PET to examine left ventricular function in rats. Nucl Med Biol 2012; 39: 724-9.
[http://dx.doi.org/10.1016/j.nucmedbio.2011.12.009]

[24] Lapa C, Arias-Loza P, Hayakawa N, *et al.* Whitening and impaired glucose utilization of brown adipose tissue in a rat model of type 2 diabetes mellitus. Sci Rep 2017; 7: 16795.
[http://dx.doi.org/10.1038/s41598-017-17148-w]

[25] Bousquenaud M, Maskali F, Poussier S, *et al.* Acipimox-enhanced (1)(8)F-fluorodeoxyglucose positron emission tomography for characterizing and predicting early remodeling in the rat infarct model. Int J Cardiovasc Imaging 2012; 28: 1407-15.
[http://dx.doi.org/10.1007/s10554-011-9983-2]

[26] Zhong M, Alonso CE, Taegtmeyer H, *et al.* Quantitative PET imaging detects early metabolic remodeling in a mouse model of pressure-overload left ventricular hypertrophy *in vivo*. J Nucl Med 2013; 54: 609-15.
[http://dx.doi.org/10.2967/jnumed.112.108092]

[27] Cohn JN. Sympathetic nervous system in heart failure. Circulation 2002; 106: 2417-8.
[http://dx.doi.org/10.1161/01.CIR.0000037105.14195.B6]

[28] Azevedo ER, Kubo T, Mak S, *et al.* Nonselective *versus* selective beta-adrenergic receptor blockade in congestive heart failure: differential effects on sympathetic activity. Circulation 2001; 104: 2194-9.
[http://dx.doi.org/10.1161/hc4301.098282]

[29] Davila DF, Bellabarba G, Hernandez L, *et al.* Plasma norepinephrine, myocardial damage and left ventricular systolic function in Chagas' heart disease. Int J Cardiol 1995; 52: 145-51.
[http://dx.doi.org/10.1016/0167-5273(95)02459-A]

[30] Grassi G. Role of the sympathetic nervous system in human hypertension. J Hypertens 1998; 16: 1979-87.
[http://dx.doi.org/10.1097/00004872-199816121-00019]

[31] Rischpler C, Fukushima K, Isoda T, *et al.* Discrepant uptake of the radiolabeled norepinephrine analogues hydroxyephedrine (HED) and metaiodobenzylguanidine (MIBG) in rat hearts. Eur J Nucl Med Mol Imaging 2013; 40: 1077-83.
[http://dx.doi.org/10.1007/s00259-013-2393-z]

[32] Laitinen I, Notni J, Pohle K, *et al.* Comparison of cyclic RGD peptides for alphavbeta3 integrin detection in a rat model of myocardial infarction. EJNMMI Res 2013; 3: 38.
[http://dx.doi.org/10.1186/2191-219X-3-38]

[33] Kajstura J, Cheng W, Reiss K, *et al.* Apoptotic and necrotic myocyte cell deaths are independent contributing variables of infarct size in rats. Lab Invest 1996; 74: 86-107.

[34] Todica A, Zacherl MJ, Wang H, *et al.* *In-vivo* monitoring of erythropoietin treatment after myocardial infarction in mice with [(68)Ga]Annexin A5 and [(18)F]FDG PET. J Nucl Cardiol 2014; 21: 1191-9.
[http://dx.doi.org/10.1007/s12350-014-9987-0]

[35] Godier-Furnemont AF, Tekabe Y, Kollaros M, *et al.* Noninvasive imaging of myocyte apoptosis following application of a stem cell-engineered delivery platform to acutely infarcted myocardium. J Nucl Med 2013; 54: 977-83.
[http://dx.doi.org/10.2967/jnumed.112.112979]

[36] Gabrielson KL, Mok GS, Nimmagadda S, *et al.* Detection of dose response in chronic doxorubicin-mediated cell death with cardiac technetium 99m annexin V single-photon emission computed tomography. Mol Imaging 2008; 7: 132-8.
[http://dx.doi.org/10.2310/7290.2008.00015]

[37] Hayakawa N, Yamane T, Arias-Loza AP, *et al.* Impact of tissue photon attenuation in small animal cardiac PET imaging. Int J Cardiol 2017; 227: 257-60.
[http://dx.doi.org/10.1016/j.ijcard.2016.11.119]

[38] Vrachimis A, Hermann S, Mathe D, *et al.* Systematic evaluation of 99mTc-tetrofosmin *versus* 99mTc-sestamibi to study murine myocardial perfusion in small animal SPECT/CT. EJNMMI Res 2012; 2: 21.
[http://dx.doi.org/10.1186/2191-219X-2-21]

SUBJECT INDEX

A

Abnormal BMIPP imaging 125
Abnormal BMIPP uptake 120, 125, 135, 136
Abnormalities 8, 237, 238, 239, 240
  cardiac sympathetic dysfunction 239, 240
  metabolic 8, 237, 239, 240
  myocardial glucose 238
Abnormalities of cardiac autonomic innervation 180
Absence of ischemia 45, 230
Accumulation, regional BMIPP 132
ACH provocation 154
Activation, myocardial sympathoadrenal 248
Activity, myocardial 41, 164
Acute chest pain 94, 97, 124, 125, 127, 128, 150, 208
Acute coronary syndrome 17, 62, 98, 113, 123, 125, 126, 166, 236
Acute myocardial infarction (AMI) 45, 46, 89, 90, 91, 114, 115, 116, 117, 118, 119, 120, 121, 122, 125, 136, 137, 150, 151, 157, 166, 203, 206, 207, 216, 235, 236, 237
Acute Myocardial Infarction Trial 188
Adding BMIPP imaging 126
Adenosine 1, 22, 72, 73, 74, 76, 78, 79, 88
Adenosine triphosphate 72, 73, 105
Adrenergic imaging 176, 177, 179, 182, 183, 187, 188, 192, 193, 194
  clinical use of 192, 194
Amount of residual ischemic myocardium 45
Anaerobic metabolic circuit 35
Angina, suspected 93, 94
Angiogenesis 245, 248
Antipsychotics 214
Apex, myocardial 207
Apoptosis 34, 245, 249
Area, myocardial salvage 89
Arrhythmias 36, 90, 181, 190, 216, 218
Arrhythmic events 182
  non-fatal 181, 182
Arteriosclerosis 227, 229, 231, 232
Artery 39, 89, 116, 123, 137, 231
  carotid 231
  culprit 123
  left anterior descending 39, 116, 137
  left main 89
Asian society of cardiovascular imaging (ASCI) 97
Assessing reversible ischemic dysfunction 35
Atherosclerosis 61, 62, 94, 227, 228, 229, 230, 232
  coronary 62, 229, 230
  subclinical information of 227, 228
  burden 61, 228, 229
Attenuation 1, 7, 69, 94, 95, 249
  correction (AC) 1, 7, 69, 249
  higher CT 94, 95
  internal 94, 95

B

Biomarkers, cardiac 98
Blood flow 5, 6, 9, 33, 58, 62, 67, 74, 96, 214, 217, 218, 227, 236, 237, 239, 240
  absolute myocardial 62, 74
  coronary 217, 218
  interpreting normal myocardial 5
  resting 33
Blood flow abnormalities 59, 237, 238
BMIPP 120, 114, 115, 126, 135, 157, 164
  delayed 126
  diffusion of 114, 115
  distribution of 157, 164
  exercise stress 114
  extent score of 120, 135
BMIPP and perfusion 150, 159, 160, 165
  agents 165
  defects 150, 159
  SPECT 160
BMIPP scan 112, 113, 117, 118, 122, 124, 126, 127, 128, 129, 134, 137, 151, 156
  second 151

single 113
BMIPP scintigraphy 105, 113, 118, 122, 123, 124, 126, 127, 131, 132, 133, 136
evaluated 124
BMIPP score 133, 152, 155, 156
total 152
BMIPP-sestamibi mismatch 119, 120, 131
evaluated 131
BMIPP severity scores 124, 133, 134
BMIPP Single-photon emission 155
BMIPP SPECT and tetrofosmin SPECT 121
BMIPP-tetrofosmin 121
BMIPP-tetrofosmin mismatch 116, 121
BMIPP-tetrofosmin SPECT 121
BMIPP/thallium dual-isotope SPECT 122
BMIPP-thallium mismatch 118, 119, 120, 122, 123, 130, 131, 132, 133
evaluated 119
large 120, 132
larger 131
BMIPP uptake 115, 123, 129, 130, 131, 133, 148, 157, 160, 161
concordant 130
discordant 123, 129, 130, 131, 133
myocardial 148, 157, 160
reduction of 115, 129
reductions in 157, 161
Brain natriuretic peptide (BNP) 23, 129, 136, 160, 177, 180, 181, 182, 188, 205, 209
Brown adipose tissue (BAT) 148

C

Cadmium zinc telluride (CZT) 7, 62, 165
Canadian cardiovascular society (CCS) 75
Cardiac autonomic innervation 180
Cardiac autonomic neuropathy, diabetic 218
Cardiac computer tomography (CCT) 87, 92, 93, 96, 97
Cardiac dysfunction 132, 133, 239
Cardiac magnetic resonance (CMR) 35, 36, 67, 87, 88, 89, 90, 91, 92, 97, 98
Cardiac magnetic resonance imaging 87
Cardiac output (CO) 177, 217, 248
Cardiac resynchronization therapy (CRT) 23, 47, 48, 135, 158, 160, 176, 177, 183, 184, 185, 186
Cardiac sympathetic activity 186, 203, 205, 206, 207, 208, 209, 213
impairments of 205
Cardiomyopathies 8, 91, 147, 163, 164, 185, 191, 193, 239
alcoholic 8
catecholamine-induced 239
mitochondrial 147, 163, 164
non-ischemic 91, 185, 191, 193
restrictive 8
Cardiovascular diseases 113, 124, 154, 213, 230, 248
Catecholamines 107, 238, 239
Cells 106, 230, 237
myocardial 230, 237
normal myocardial 106
Chronic coronary artery disease 128, 129, 130, 131, 132, 147, 166
Chronic kidney disease (CKD) 3, 4, 154
CMR imaging 90
CMR viability imaging 91
Compartment model, one-tissue 72
Concentrations, myocardial 148
Concordant defects 113
Congestive heart failure (CHF) 8, 135, 136, 183, 205, 206, 209, 216
Contractile proteins 34
Contractile reserve 38, 44, 117, 118, 129
myocardial 129
Conventional SPECT 6, 7
Coronary angiography 89, 116, 118, 125, 127, 128, 236
Coronary arteries 2, 43, 57, 58, 59, 60, 61, 62, 87, 88, 93, 94, 95, 97, 126, 128, 150, 157, 228, 229, 236, 240
epicardial 57, 58, 236
left anterior descending 60, 61
right 60, 97, 236
Coronary artery bypass grafting (CABG) 19, 29, 32, 46, 47, 99, 150, 151, 152
Coronary artery calcification (CAC) 62, 99, 227, 228, 229, 230

Coronary artery distribution 159
Coronary calcification 57, 61, 62, 228, 231
Coronary CT angiography 59, 97, 159, 230
Coronary flow reserve (CFR) 33, 34, 236
Coronary heart disease 93, 94
Coronary intervention 5, 18, 39, 57, 58, 59, 62, 63, 121, 150, 151
  percutaneous 5, 39, 121
Coronary occlusion 114, 116
Coronary revascularization therapy 21
Coronary revascularization treatment 18, 22
Coronary risk factors 62, 229, 230
Coronary stenosis 113, 124, 128, 152
  severe 113, 124, 128
  significant 124, 152
CT Angiography 57, 58, 59
CT attenuation correction 6, 7
CT coronary angiography 57, 59, 240
CT coronary angiography in patients 93
CT perfusion imaging 96
Cytosol, myocardial 111

D

Data 87, 126
  functional imaging 87
  stress thallium 126
Decreased BMIPP uptake 127, 150
Defect scores 120, 160
  high BMIPP 120
  higher BMIPP 160
Defibrillator, implantable cardioverter 176, 177, 188, 190
Denervation supersensitivity 179, 181
Detecting myocardial injury 235, 238
Diabetes mellitus (DM) 3, 153, 155, 215, 218, 231
Diffusion of nonmetabolized BMIPP 114, 149
Dilatation, ischemic 20, 62
Dilated cardiomyopathy 8, 9, 21, 110, 134, 135, 136, 147, 157, 188, 204
Dipyridamole 73, 76, 78, 88
Diseases 3, 4, 92, 94, 95, 136, 154, 227
  chronic 227
  chronic kidney 3, 4, 154
  myocardial 92, 136
  obstructive 94, 95
Disorder 236, 238, 239, 240
  left ventricular wall motion 239, 240
  myocardial 236, 238
DMIPP dimethyl iodophenyl pentadecanoic acid 108
Dobutamine echocardiography 119
Dobutamine stress 73
Dobutamine stress echocardiography (DSE) 31, 32, 35, 36, 38, 44, 46, 47, 121, 129, 130
Dynamic processes 245, 246, 249
Dysfunction 8, 33, 35, 62, 204, 205
  diastolic 204, 205
  mitochondrial 8
  post-stress 62
  reversible ischemic 33, 35

E

Echocardiography 48, 90, 98, 112, 119, 120, 121, 131, 135, 137, 163, 184
Ejection fraction (EF) 2, 30, 62, 69, 72, 120, 124, 129, 132, 176, 177, 187, 188
Electrocardiography 123, 128, 203, 206
ELEGP collimator 224
Endomyocardial biopsies 91
End-systolic volume (ESV) 16, 19, 20, 21, 47, 184, 186
Ergonovine 126, 127

F

Fatal arrhythmia 107, 181, 216
Fatty acid analogues, radiolabeled 107
Fatty Acid Metabolic Imaging 104
Fatty acid metabolism 105, 106, 114, 126, 133, 147, 148, 157, 237
  abnormalities of 133
  improved myocardial 135
Fatty acids 104, 105, 106, 107, 108, 109, 110, 111, 114, 147, 148, 237, 247
  branched-chain 108, 109
  evaluating myocardial 237
  free 9, 43, 105, 106, 148
  radiolabeled straight-chain 109

straight-chain 107, 108, 109
Fatty acid translocase (FAT) 106, 112
Fatty acid transporters 106
Fatty acid uptake 106, 130, 148
regulating myocardial 106
FDG accumulation 231
FDG PET-assisted management 32, 33, 46
FDG PET imaging 41
FFA metabolism 43
Fibrosis 8, 34, 90, 91, 92, 130, 157, 248
diffuse 91, 92
myocardial tissue 157
Flow reserve 2, 7, 35, 57, 58, 59, 62, 63, 128, 129, 236
coronary blood 2, 236
myocardial 7, 62, 63, 128, 129
reduced coronary 57, 58
reduced myocardial blood 59
regional myocardial 35
Food and drug administration (FDA) 16, 67, 68, 178
Fractional flow reserve (FFR) 59, 62, 77, 92, 95, 96, 97
Free fatty acids (FFA) 43, 105, 106, 148

G

Gadolinium 90
increased volume of distribution for 90
Gallium accumulation 241
Gated stress perfusion imaging 21
Glucose metabolism 38, 43, 133, 237, 238, 245, 247
myocardial 247
Glycogen 34

H

Heart diseases 59, 89, 114, 136,152, 153, 161
chronic ischemic 114, 152, 153
detecting chronic ischemic 153
developing ischemic 161
nonischemic 114, 136
non-ischemic 153
obstructive ischemic 89
suspected ischemic 59
Heart failure 8, 17, 29, 135, 136, 182, 183, 205, 209, 216
congestive 8, 135, 136, 183, 205, 209
ischemia-induced 17
ischemic 29, 182, 216
non-ischemic 216
Heart rate variability (HRV) 181
Heart transplantation 217
Hibernating myocardium 17, 18, 31, 33, 34, 35, 43, 46, 48, 104, 118, 129
chronic 35
High global CAD risk 98
Hybrid Imaging 57, 245
Hypertrophic cardiomyopathy 8, 132, 133, 134, 136, 147, 157, 164, 203, 204, 209
asymptomatic 134
Hypertrophy, myocardial 204

I

IHDA 17-iodoheptadecanoic acid 108
IHXA 16-iodohexadecanoic acid 108
Imaging 6, 31, 37, 41, 42, 57, 58, 105, 112, 129, 165, 235, 238, 245, 246, 248, 249
cardiac metabolism 235, 238
dual isotope 165
magnetic resonance 6, 31, 37, 112, 129, 246
myocardial fatty acid 105
noninvasive 245, 246, 248, 249
non-invasive 57, 58
rest-redistribution 41, 42
Imaging modalities 29, 35, 67, 98, 245, 246, 247
diagnostic 67
morphological 245, 246
Imaging paradigm, traditional 245
Imaging systems, hybrid 245
Imaging techniques, nuclear 121, 129, 134
Implantable cardioverter defibrillators (ICD) 176, 177, 179, 182, 184, 188, 189, 190, 191, 192, 193, 216
Infarction, cerebral 231, 232
Information, anatomical 57, 58, 63, 95, 159
Innervation, reduced myocardial 72
Intermediate global CAD risk 98
Intramyocardial hemorrhage 89

Iodine-123 meta-iodobenzylguanidine 192, 203, 204, 209
Iodine stabilization 104, 107, 110
IPPA iodophenyl pentadecanoic acid 108
Ischemic burden 18, 19, 21, 88
Ischemic cardiomyopathy group 157
Ischemic episodes, repetitive 33, 126
Ischemic heart disease 4, 57, 61, 96, 104, 105, 110, 112, 113, 115, 123, 128, 136, 147, 148, 149, 154, 163, 164, 166, 188, 193, 217, 218, 231, 246
Ischemic myocardium 4, 38, 44, 123, 126, 130, 237

J

Jeopardy, myocardial 29, 33, 48

L

LAD, proximal 94, 95
Late gadolinium enhancement (LGE) 88, 90, 91, 92, 157, 158
Late gadolinium enhancement imaging 44, 89
Left bundle branch block (LBBB) 48, 72
Left Ventricular assist device (LVAD) 176, 177, 183, 186, 187, 188
Left ventricular ejection fraction (LVEF) 3, 16, 17, 18, 20, 21, 23, 30, 35, 45, 47, 59, 133, 136, 153, 157, 160, 179, 180, 181, 182, 184, 185, 187, 188, 189, 190, 191, 192, 216
Left ventricular function 16, 37, 39, 114, 129, 131, 133, 134, 136, 247
Left ventricular mechanical dyssynchrony (LVMD) 15, 22, 23
Left ventricular outflow tract (LVOT) 204, 209
Lesions 57, 60, 122, 162, 163, 230, 231, 232
  arteriosclerotic 230, 231, 232
  culprit 57, 60, 122
  sarcoid 162, 163
Low attenuation plaque 94, 95
  central 94, 95
LVAD therapy 187, 188
LV dysfunction 29, 30, 31, 34, 35, 40, 42, 43, 46, 47, 48
  chronic ischemic 30, 31, 34, 40, 47
  ischemic 29, 35, 40, 48
  severe chronic ischemic 46
LVEF improvement 30, 46, 160
LV function, regional 30, 41, 42
LVOT obstruction 205
LV remodeling 29, 46, 47, 48
  prevention of 29, 46, 47, 48

M

Macrophages 148, 231
Magnetic resonance imaging (MRI) 6, 29, 31, 35, 36, 37, 44, 45, 48, 87, 88, 112, 129, 157, 246
Major adverse cardiac events (MACE) 61, 96, 160
Mechanical dyssynchrony 15, 22, 23, 48, 184, 186
  left ventricular 15, 22, 23
Mediastinal ROIs 223
Medium-energy low-penetration (MELP) 224
Metabolic imaging, clinical applications of fatty acid 104, 105
Mismatch BMIPP uptake 113, 119, 129, 131
Mismatched BMIPP 136
Mitochondrial Function Imaging 7
Myocardial ablation 209
Myocardial contractility 2
Myocardial CT perfusion image 93
Myocardial damage 8, 9, 91, 147, 148, 149, 150, 151, 154, 157, 161, 166, 205, 236, 241
Myocardial disarray 132
Myocardial energy requirements 105
Myocardial enhancement 44
Myocardial enzymes 122
Myocardial fibrosis 91, 130, 158
  diffuse 91
Myocardial function 8
Myocardial imaging 59, 87
Myocardial infarction 18, 38, 110, 114, 115, 121, 125, 128, 130, 131, 153
  chronic 131

large acute 121
non-acute 130
non-fatal 18
prior 38, 110, 114, 115, 125
stable 153
stable angina and old 128
Myocardial injury 17, 91, 127, 161, 237
direct 161
ischemia-related 17
Myocardial ischemia 1, 4, 17, 18, 20, 21, 58, 59, 72, 75, 77, 88, 96, 104, 123, 125, 126, 166, 216, 236, 237
acute 125
identified 123
prior 126
severe 20
Myocardial membrane 106
Myocardial metabolic changes 148
Myocardial metabolism 71, 107, 110, 111, 116, 130, 136, 147
evaluating 71
global 160
Myocardial oxygen consumption, regional 72
Myocardial perfusion 5, 6, 15, 17, 88, 93
correct 6
evaluating 88
gated 3
global 15
normal 5, 93
regional 17
Myocardial perfusion distribution 5
Myocardial perfusion Image 4, 246
Myocardial perfusion imaging defect score 59
Myocardial perfusion polar maps 17
Myocardial perfusion tracers 58
Myocardial perfusion-wall motion correlation 17
Myocardial presynaptic 83
Myocardial response function 74
Myocardial salvage 89, 117
Myocardial scarring 33
Myocardial stress imaging 88
Myocardial stunning 17, 208
post-ischemic 17
Myocardial sympathetic innervation imaging 192
Myocardial tissue imaging 87
Myocarditis 241, 248

N

Necrosis, non-ischemic myocardial 21
Neurotransmitter, false 178
Neurotransmitter imaging 205, 207, 208, 209
Nitroglycerin 43
Non-calcified occlusion 94, 95
Noninvasive myocardial perfusion imaging 84
Noninvasive quantification 84
Nonischemic cardiomyopathy 90, 104, 105, 110, 112, 113, 132
Non-ischemic cardiomyopathy treatment evaluation 188
Non-sudden cardiac death (NSCD) 182
Norepinephrine 177, 178, 213, 239, 240
Normal myocardial perfusion distribution 247
Normal scan-annual event 78, 79
Normal stress perfusion 79, 125
Nuclear cardiology imaging 152, 238
Nuclear cardiology technique 63, 227, 235, 236, 238
Nuclear imaging 36, 37, 38, 48, 104, 105, 129, 136, 236, 246, 248
Nuclear imaging method 213, 218
Nuclear medicine examination 1, 241, 242

O

Obstruction, microvascular 89, 157
Old Myocardial Infarction 128
Oxidation metabolites 111, 112

P

Parametric Mapping Imaging 87
Pentadecanoic acid, methyl 104, 105
Perfusion, regional 17, 18
Perfusion abnormalities 17, 57, 60, 115, 130, 154, 166, 229
definitive myocardial 21
myocardial 18, 19, 23
Perfusion data, myocardial 15, 19, 20

Perfusion defects 3, 6, 59, 75, 77, 133, 150, 159, 181, 229, 247
  myocardial 3, 6
  reversible 75, 77
Perfusion findings, myocardial 20
Perfusion images, static myocardial 70
Perfusion imaging 1, 45, 93, 113, 123, 126, 132, 134, 136, 165, 216
  produced myocardial 93
  rest thallium 136
Perfusion scan, myocardial 59
Perfusion SPECT, myocardial 59, 62
Perfusion SPECT imaging 117
Perfusion tracers 7, 18, 109, 113, 116, 149, 157, 179, 180
  potential myocardial 109
Perfusion tracer uptake 113, 165
PET MPI tracers, 18F-labeled 71
Pheochromocytoma 239
Plaque 94, 95, 228, 231
  calcified 94, 95, 228
  non-calcified 94, 95
Plaque rupture, localized myocarditis transient 238
Predicting revascularization benefit 31
Prognostic assessments 147, 153, 156, 164, 165
Prognostic information 8, 67, 90
Progression, coronary stenotic 118
Protocols, stress-redistribution-reinjection 38, 39, 41
Pulmonary embolism 93, 97, 242
Pulmonary thromboendarterectomy 163

R

Radiation, ionizing 88
Radiation dose 96, 161, 166
Radiation field 161, 162
Radiation injuries 147, 161
Radiation therapy 161, 162
Radioiodine, free 110
Radionuclide, noninvasive 245
Radionuclide imaging 112, 177, 178, 192
  perfusion/metabolic 112
Radiopharmaceuticals 70, 105, 107, 213, 236
Receptor, myocardial β-adrenergic 240
Regions 127, 237
  coronary vasospastic 127
  metabolic blood flow mismatch 237
Renin-angiotensin-aldosterone system (RAAS) 177, 183, 245
Reperfusion therapy 43, 44, 45, 89, 90, 114, 115, 116, 117
  refused 43, 44
Residual Ischemic Myocardium 45
Rest perfusion imaging 113, 126
Rest thallium SPECT 119, 120
Resuscitated cardiac arrest 181, 182
Retention 42, 109, 111, 112
  prolonged myocardial 111
Revascularization Medical treatment 31
Revascularization procedures 17, 88
  reduced 88

S

Sarcoidosis, cardiac 21, 147, 162
Scores, ischemic perfusion 21
Segments 30, 34, 38, 40, 41, 45, 73, 88, 89, 114, 116, 117, 119, 130, 207
  fixed defect 40
  hypokinetic 38
  impaired LV 207
  jeopardized 45
  myocardial 130
Sensitivity and specificity 35, 75, 77, 124, 127, 152, 154
Septum, ventricular 132
Serum CK-MB elevations 151
Sestamibi SPECT 75, 119, 123, 130
Severe stenosis, confirming focal 94, 95
Single-photon emission, myocardial 87
Size, initial damaged myocardium 89
Spasm-reinduced arteries 127
Stable angina 123, 127, 128, 129
Stenosis, left main 94, 95
Strategy, invasive 19
Stress, pharmacological 1, 2, 62, 70, 73, 74, 89
Stress imaging 16, 22
Stress perfusion imaging 124, 125, 126, 128, 134, 229

Stress perfusion SPECT 124, 127
Stress/rest MPI, gated 17, 18, 19, 20, 23
Stress-rest protocol 38, 39, 41
conventional 38, 41
Stunned myocardium 18, 107, 118, 119, 120, 137, 151, 237
identifying 120
Stunning myocardium 237
Subarachnoid hemorrhage 158, 239
Substrates, abnormal myocardial 189
Sudden cardiac death (SCD) 180, 181, 182, 188, 189, 192, 204, 205, 206, 209, 218
Summed difference score (SDS) 16, 21, 153
Summed rest score (SRS) 16, 21
Summed stress score (SSS) 3, 16, 18, 19, 20, 21, 22, 79
Sympathetic dysfunction, cardiac 216
Sympathetic dysfunction abnormalities 239, 240
Sympathetic innervation, myocardial 213, 218
Sympathetic nerve 179, 213, 214, 216, 217, 238, 239
cardiac 213, 216, 217, 238
Sympathetic nerve activity 214, 215
Sympathetic nerve dysfunction 216, 218
Sympathetic nerve heart, normal 213, 214
Sympathetic nervous system (SNS) 72, 190, 218, 248
Synaptic spaces 178
System 2, 61, 72, 218, 227, 228, 248
hybrid SPECT/CT 2, 61, 227, 228
sympathetic nervous 72, 218, 248

T

Takotsubo cardiomyopathy 21, 136, 137, 147, 158, 159, 235, 238, 239, 241
Takotsubo syndrome
acute phase of 235, 239, 241
conditions of 240, 241
pathology of 238, 240
Takotsubo syndrome and myocardial infarction 238
Tetrofosmin perfusion imaging 117
Tetrofosmin SPECT 43, 118, 121, 125
Tissue characterization 91, 92
myocardial 36, 91
Tissue compartment, irreversible 165
Tissue doppler echocardiography 48
Tissues, myocardial 116, 137
Total defect scores (TDS) 151, 215
Tracers
adrenergic 177, 178, 192
diffusible 67, 68
fatty acid 8, 104, 107, 109, 147
novel 245, 246
radiolabeled 213
retained 67, 68
Tracer uptake 17, 18, 116, 164
myocardial 178
preserved perfusion 17
reduced 17, 178
regional 18, 179
Traces, labeled myocardial perfusion 15
Transcatheter septal ablation 206
Transient ischemic dilatation (TID) 19, 20, 22, 62
Transluminal attenuation gradient (TAG) 97
appropriate revascularization 17
invasive revascularization 4
Tricyclic antidepressants 214
Triglyceride deposit cardiomyovasculopathy 147, 163
Triple energy window (TEW) 224
Triple rule out (TRO) 93, 97, 99
Troponin, increased 122

V

Vasospastic angina 126, 127, 149, 150, 153
Ventricular arrhythmias 72, 177, 179, 180, 189, 192, 193, 204
lethal 179, 189
Ventricular dysfunction 8, 124, 131, 136, 216, 217, 218, 235, 237
left 8, 124, 131, 136, 216, 217, 218, 237
reversible left 136, 235
Ventricular fibrillation 181, 182, 191
Ventricular myocardium 45, 113, 204
ischemic left 45
left 113

Ventricular remodeling, left 21, 46, 187
Ventricular tachycardia (VT) 181, 182, 206, 209
Ventriculography, left 120, 123, 127, 128, 136, 206, 207
Vessel diameter, outer 94, 95
Vessels, stenotic 61, 128
Viability 32, 33, 39
  identifying 32, 33
  underestimation of 32, 39
Viability assessment 18, 29, 30, 31, 38, 41, 42, 43, 44, 47, 48, 91, 152
Viable myocardium 2, 17, 30, 31, 32, 33, 35, 38, 40, 41, 42, 43, 44, 45, 46, 47, 48, 104, 113, 118, 119, 121, 129, 130, 131, 149, 150, 165
  extent of 32, 46
  identifying 43
  ischemic 45

W

Wall thickness, myocardial 58
Washout rate, myocardial 8
WR acceleration 216, 218

www.ingramcontent.com/pod-product-compliance
Lightning Source LLC
LaVergne TN
LVHW070948210926
848482LV00002B/142